Disease, Health Care and Government in Late Imperial Russia

T0227534

This book addresses fundamental issues about the last decades of Tsarist Russia, contributing significantly to current debates about how far and how successfully modernisation was being implemented by the Tsarist regime. It focuses on successive outbreaks of cholera in the city of Saratov on the Volga, in particular contrasting the outbreak of 1892 – widely regarded at the time as a national fiasco and a transformative episode for the Russian Empire – with the cholera epidemics of 1904–1910 when – despite completely new scientific discoveries and administrative arrangements – Russia suffered another national outbreak of the disease.

The book sets these outbreaks fully in their social, economic, political and cultural context, and explains why a medical and social disaster – which had long since been overcome in other parts of Europe – continued much later in Russia. It explores autocratic government, urban renewal, public health and disaster management, including the management of widespread public hysteria and social unrest. The book further analyses the assimilation of Western medical knowledge and the resulting institutional and epistemological changes. Overall, it demonstrates that Russia's medical history was inseparably linked to the nature of the tsarist regime itself in its confrontation with modernity.

Charlotte E. Henze completed her doctorate at the University of Cambridge, UK, and is currently teaching History and Russian in Zurich, Switzerland.

BASEES/Routledge Series on Russian and East European Studies

Series editor:

Richard Sakwa, Department of Politics and International Relations, University of Kent

Editorial Committee:

Julian Cooper, Centre for Russian and East European Studies, University of Birmingham
Terry Cox, Department of Central and East European Studies, University of Glasgow
Rosalind Marsh, Department of European Studies and Modern Languages, University of Bath
David Moon, Department of History, University of Durham
Hilary Pilkington, Department of Sociology, University of Warwick
Graham Timmins, Department of Politics, University of Stirling
Stephen White, Department of Politics, University of Glasgow

Founding Editorial Committee Member:

George Blazyca, Centre for Contemporary European Studies, University of Paisley

This series is published on behalf of BASEES (the British Association for Slavonic and East European Studies). The series comprises original, high-quality, research-level work by both new and established scholars on all aspects of Russian, Soviet, post-Soviet and East European Studies in humanities and social science subjects.

Disease, Health Care and Government in Late Imperial Russia

Life and death on the Volga,
1823–1914

Charlotte E. Henze

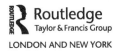
Routledge
Taylor & Francis Group

LONDON AND NEW YORK

First published 2011
by Routledge
2 Park Square, Milton Park, Abingdon, Oxfordshire OX14 4RN

Simultaneously published in the USA and Canada
by Routledge
711 Third Avenue, New York, NY 10017

First issued in paperback 2015

Routledge is an imprint of the Taylor & Francis Group, an informa business

Typeset in Times New Roman by RefineCatch Limited, Bungay, Suffolk

British Library Cataloguing in Publication Data
A catalogue record for this book is available from the British Library

Library of Congress Cataloging in Publication Data

Henze, Charlotte E.
    Disease, health care, and government in late Imperial Russia: life and
    death on the Volga, 1823–1914/Charlotte E. Henze.
        p. cm.

    Includes bibliographical references and index.

    1. Cholera—Russia (Federation)—Saratov—Epidemiology—History—19th century. 2. Cholera—Russia (Federation)—Saratov—Epidemiology—History—20th century. 3. Urban health—Russia (Federation)—Saratov—History—19th century. 4. Urban health—Russia (Federation)—Saratov—History—20th century. 5. Medical care—Russia (Federation)—Saratov—History—19th century. 6. Medical care—Russia (Federation)—Saratov—History—20th century. 7. Medical policy—Russia (Federation)—Saratov—History—19th century. 8. Medical policy—Russia (Federation)—Saratov—History—20th century. 9. Saratov (Russia)—Social conditions—19th century. 10. Saratov (Russia)—Social conditions—20th century. I. Title.

    RA644.C3H47 2011
    614.5'14094746—dc22

                                                                        2010027438

ISBN 13: 978-1-138-96777-9 (pbk)
ISBN 13: 978-0-415-54794-9 (hbk)

Contents

Figures and tables

Figures

Acknowledgements

In its original form this book was my PhD dissertation in the Department of History, University of Cambridge. It has subsequently been reworked into its present form as a monograph. Along the journey to the completion of the work, many people have graciously supported me. It is a great pleasure to express my gratitude here to those whose scholarship, generosity and friendship have made this book possible.

First, I would like to thank Dr Hubertus F. Jahn for supervising my dissertation at Clare College, Cambridge, and for giving me assistance and advice whenever needed. My sincerest gratitude goes to Professor Richard J. Evans, who most generously offered time, knowledge and academic expertise. His contributions to the history of cholera cannot be underestimated and his insightful work is closely interwoven with the story presented here. I also wish to express my deepest thanks to Professor Frank Snowden, whose fascinating lectures on the history of medicine I enjoyed while an exchange student at Yale University in 2000. Dr Kim Taylor deserves special thanks for selflessly sharing her research and knowledge with me in countless discussions on cholera. Her careful assessment and insights placed my understanding of the history of medicine on firmer ground and have greatly enriched my work. I am also indebted to Dr David Moon, whose scholarship and advice through long research summers in Helsinki and St Petersburg have proven invaluable, and to Professor Simon Dixon, who has provided important critique and suggestions for turning the dissertation into a book. Special mention is due to the anonymous referees of RoutledgeCurzon, whose careful reading and comments have helped to make this a better book. All errors of fact and omissions of knowledge remain of course my own responsibility.

I owe a great debt to the staff at the Slavonic Library of the University of Helsinki, the Cambridge University Library, the Library of the Academy of Sciences in St Petersburg, the Library of the Institute of Experimental Medicine in St Petersburg, the Russian State Historical Archive in St Petersburg, the Russian National Library, the University Library in Saratov, the Regional Library in Saratov, and the State Archive of *Saratov oblast'*. It is a particular pleasure to thank Irina Lukka for her constant support in the Slavonic Library of the University of Helsinki and, especially, for directing my attention to the lower Volga cities. In St Petersburg, Marina Pavlovna was a wonderful host and offered her invaluable knowledge and practical support beyond the call of duty in the Library of the Academy of Sciences. And finally, a special thank you goes to the Slavonic Library family for wonderful research festivals: Natalia Bashmakoff, Seymour Becker, David Moon, David Schimmelpenninck van der Oye, Richard Stites, the jazz version of historians, and finally, Alla Zeide.

Research for this book was supported by the University of Cambridge, and the Cambridge European Trust. A CITO scholarship facilitated research in Helsinki. During my PhD I received a substantial scholarship from the Geoffrey Elton Fund, which made it possible to finish my degree. I would like to extend my greatest thanks here to Lewis Elton, brother of Geoffrey Elton, for his friendship – and for a spectacular tour through London.

The completion of this manuscript took place in Zurich, Switzerland, which boasts an excellent educational system that allows teachers the opportunity to teach and pursue research. I would like to express my sincerest gratitude to Professor Alfred Baumgartner, Professor Christoph Meister, and Professor Hans-Peter Horlacher at the Kantonsschule Hohe Promenade, Zurich, for their continuing encouragement. Most especially I am grateful for their generous offer of leave to complete the research needed to finish this manuscript. I am deeply grateful to my colleague, Rahel Gastberger, and to our students with whom I enjoyed a journey by ship along the cholera's highway from Astrakhan' to Moscow. Special thanks also go to my colleagues Dr Franziska Baur, PD Markus Ehrengruber and Donat Maron for sharing their formidable insights into Russian culture, past and present, with me.

There are family and friends not yet mentioned who have remained by my side throughout. Alice Chapman and Kristin Semmens have shared the various writing stages of the dissertation with me at Cambridge and patiently tolerated my interest in bacteria. A special thank you to Sabine, Klaus and Judith von Heusinger, Alan Julseth, Marilen Rieder, Wilfried, Sigrid, Wolf-Dietrich and Cathrin Steppuhn, and Masha Zaborovskaia for their constant friendship, support and assistance. Rahel Gastberger and Elisabeth Goslicka have been an inexhaustible source of advice and humour while witnessing the final writing of the manuscript. Finally, I owe much to Brigitte Maass-Henze for being such a courageous sister, musician and strong scientist.

Conventions and abbreviations

BHM	*Bulletin for the History of Medicine*
Brokgauz-Efron	*Entsiklopedicheskii slovar' Brokgauz i Efrona*
GASO	*Gosudarstvennyi Arkhiv Saratovskoi Oblasti*
ISGD	*Izvestiia Saratovskoi Gorodskoi Dumy*
JfGO	*Jahrbücher für Geschichte Osteuropas*
MVD	*Ministerstvo vnutrennikh del*
ORVP	Obshchestvo russkikh vrachei v pamiat' N.I. Pirogova
PSZ	*Polnoe sobranie zakonov Rossiiskoi imperii, 2nd series*
RS	*Russkaia starina*
RGIA	*Rossiisskii Gosudarstvennyi Istoricheskii Arkhiv, St Petersburg*
SSO	*Saratovskii Sanitarnyi Obzor*
SZN	*Saratovskaia Zemskaia Nedelia*
VOGSPM	*Vestnik obshchestvennoi gigieny, sudebnoi i prakticheskoi meditsiny*
Zhurnal ORVP	*Zhurnal obshchestva Russkikh vrachei v pamiat' N.I. Pirogova*

Glossary

Duma	Duma (city council)
Desiatina	desiatina, equivalent to 1.09 hectares
Fel'dsher	feldsher (paramedic, medical assistant)
Glasnyi	deputy
Guberniia	province
Meshchanin	townsman
Oblast'	region
Pud	equivalent to 16.38kg
Sanitarnyi vrach	sanitary physician (physician-hygienist or medical inspector who was responsible for the collection of medical statistics and the supervision and control of public places such as marketplaces, schools, etc.)
Uezd	district within a province
Ukaz	decree, edict
Uprava	governing board on the provincial and municipal levels
Versta	equivalent to 1.06km
Zemstvo	zemstvo (elective councils in Russia on the provincial and district levels, 1864–1917)
Zemskoe sobranie	zemstvo assembly
Zemskaia uprava	zemstvo governing board

Note on Transliteration and Dates

All dates in this work are given according to the Julian calendar in use in Russia until 1918. It was 12 days behind the Gregorian calendar in the nineteenth century and 13 days behind in the twentieth century.

With a few exceptions, the Library of Congress system of transliteration has been followed. I have anglicised some names and archaic nineteenth century spellings have been modified to conform with modern Russian orthography.

Introduction

Epidemic diseases confound the modern world. AIDS and SARS were merely the most recent examples of the disastrous effects of humanity's encounters with dangerous micro-organisms. The impact of epidemics can be so disruptive that they have been thought to serve as impetus for political coups, revolutions and even the rise and fall of civilisations themselves.[1] To historians of modern Europe, the role of epidemics and their impact on society have therefore long held a particular fascination. Epidemic diseases such as smallpox, fever (typhus and typhoid) and tuberculosis have garnered their fair share of historiographical attention.[2] Most prominently, historical research has focused on epidemics of plague, the most deadly killer in late medieval Europe, and Asiatic cholera.[3] This disease from the Ganges River spread to Europe via Afghanistan and Russia as a result of the massive expansion of European, especially British, trade as Britain embarked on the process of industrialisation and empire-building. Cholera stood at the gates of Europe for the first time in 1823, when it reached the Russian city of Astrakhan'. This flare-up was brief and limited, however, and passed almost unnoticed.[4] Only in 1829 did cholera reappear in the Caspian region and henceforth become a threat to European Russia and the continent. Travelling along rivers and railways, the epidemic swept Europe in five successive waves (pandemics), capitalising upon overcrowded housing conditions, poor sanitation and water supply, which characterised the teeming cities in the throes of rapid urbanisation.[5] Cholera is indeed the classic epidemic disease of Europe's age of industrialisation and urbanisation.[6]

For historians on Russia the subject of cholera is bound to be particularly rewarding. Against the background of the European history of the disease, Russia's cholera experience stands out. The first nation to be afflicted by the disease on the continent was also the last to overcome it. As late as 1892, when the epidemic had gradually abated in western European countries, the tsarist empire was hit by the most devastating cholera onslaught of the nineteenth century. And, while the sixth pandemic (1899–1923) spared the industrial world almost entirely, cholera continued to present a permanent threat to Russia well into the twentieth century. The last major epidemic, in fact, attacked the country as late as 1925. Only the Soviet regime managed to eradicate the disease once and for all.

This book, by focusing on Saratov's cholera history in the period 1823–1914, will serve, in the first instance, as a case study through which opposing historiographical positions can be tested. Historical scholarship has utilised the epidemic as means to elucidate the workings and functioning of modern statecraft and society. In a seminal article, Asa Briggs most clearly outlined the historical dimensions and social significance of the 'disease of society':

> Whenever it threatened European countries, it quickened social apprehensions. Wherever it appeared, it tested the efficiency and resilience of local administrative structures. It exposed relentlessly political, social and moral shortcomings. It prompted rumours, suspicions, and at times violent social conflicts. It inspired not only sermons but novels and works of art. For all these reasons a study of the history of cholera in the nineteenth century is something far more than an exercise in medical epidemiology, fascinating in themselves though such exercises are; it is an important and neglected chapter in social history.[7]

In conformity with Briggs's position, Louis Chevalier, the second chief pioneer in the field, has put forward the claim that '*le choléra est un fait majeure de l'histoire générale de ces années, au même titre que les tourmentes politiques, les crises économiques ou les conflits sociaux.*'[8] For this reason, both Briggs and Chevalier called upon historical scholars to study cholera and its impact on European societies comparatively against an international background.

Their appeal has yielded a fruitful response. Over the last 50 years, historians have generated an extensive international literature on the history of Asiatic cholera and its impact on Western societies. Most studies have vindicated the insights of Briggs and Chevalier, revealing that the occurrence of a cholera crisis enables historians to explore the social fabric of a given community. In one of the earliest responses to Chevalier and Briggs, an examination of cholera's first visitation to Russia, Roderick E. McGrew confirmed their view, noting that 'cholera scored the European social consciousness, exacerbated contemporary tensions, intensified the impact of current social problems, and as it did so, revealed fundamental characteristics of European life and outlook'.[9] Building on these early studies, cholera's capability to illuminate the texture of modern European society has provided a guiding thread for many cholera studies to date.

Yet Briggs's and Chevalier's claims have also provoked criticism and dissent. Charles Rosenberg, who studied the cholera in the United States, concluded that the epidemic had no long-lasting impact on society.[10] Margaret Pelling regarded the attention directed to cholera by historians as 'more than optional'. She pointed out that in sheer terms of numbers cholera was much less significant as a cause of debility and death than other epidemic diseases such as the fevers, smallpox, measles and, most notably, tuberculosis.[11] It was mainly because of the extreme reaction by contemporaries to a novel and intractable disease, she argued, that historians came to elevate cholera into the role of a 'reform catalyst'.

The pivot of this study is Russia's cholera outbreak of 1892. For both historians of Russia and of cholera, Russia's medical tragedy in that year is a significant event. Traditionally, cholera historiography has predominantly examined Europe's first experiences with the disease in the 1830s and 1840s, mainly because it was assumed that these posed the greatest challenge to the afflicted societies. Once the terror caused by the unknown killer wore off and mortality figures lessened, both contemporaries' and historians' attention to the epidemic diminished as well. Two major monographs have redressed the imbalance by fundamentally questioning this evaluation. The cases of Hamburg in 1892 and Naples in 1884 demonstrate that the strain and pressure exerted by a severe cholera outbreak at a time when the disease was largely understood and therefore successfully controlled in most parts of western Europe was tremendous.[12] Russia's cholera outbreak in 1892 stands out because the cholera ravaged an entire nation on the European continent at an exceptionally late date. Accordingly, cholera's immediate impact on society was explosive. In large parts of the empire, the disease unleashed mass flight, attacks on doctors, and tumultuous riots which, while reminiscent of the dramatic first cholera experience across Europe, were now generally considered as anachronistic. It is hardly surprising, therefore, that the emergency of 1892 stirred up the whole country. The epidemic generated a great outpouring of articles and reports in medical journals and the mass newspaper press. Compelled to examine the causes of the ordeal, government officials, doctors and journalists produced an abundance of source material on all aspects related to the disease such as housing, diet and sanitary conditions. Moreover, their descriptions and analyses of the cholera's course amply document social tensions, the relations between governmental officials and the people they governed, and popular attitudes towards medical experts. Russia's cholera outbreak of 1892 undoubtedly confirms Asa Briggs's and Louis Chevalier's insight that Asiatic cholera provides a fruitful means of exploring life and living conditions in a given society.

Yet much more is at stake. It is of crucial interest for the debate between Briggs and Pelling that historians of Russia have credited the cholera of 1892 with having been a major transformative event for the empire. In conjunction with the devastating famine of the preceding year, the cholera is generally regarded as a landmark that defined the beginning of Russia's revolutionary era yielding consequences which shaped the whole period to the end of the tsarist regime. The twin disasters, historians have pointed out, amply demonstrated the incompetence of the autocratic state and thus discredited the old regime in the eyes of the educated public.[13] It mobilised public activity and debate to an unprecedented degree and set into motion a process of increasing alienation and conflict between the government and the population. Coinciding with the fundamental disruption of the socio-economic order during the 1890s and 1900s, the profound change in the country's political climate instigated by the dual crisis of the early 1890s eventually corroded the very foundations of the autocratic state. In addition, famine and cholera also inaugurated significant reforms in the field of public welfare and public health in order to prevent the recurrence of such disasters.[14] And finally, it has been shown that the epidemic played a crucial role in the coming of age of Russia's medical profession. The catastrophe gave the country's physicians an active role in public policies for the first time; it enhanced their status as scientific experts and thus granted them a new level of professional autonomy and corporate consciousness.[15]

Considering that the epidemic is commonly assessed as an event of historical significance, the striking neglect of it as subject for historical analysis is surprising. Partly, this needs to be explained by the fact that the medical history of late imperial Russia suffered general neglect after 1917 and therefore did not achieve independent stature inside or outside the Russian Empire or the Soviet Union.[16] Socialised medicine, however, has received considerable attention from Western scholars.[17] Western scholars have also uncovered epidemics and diseases as a topic for Russian history. Thus, John T. Alexander has written a pioneering social history of Russia's experience with bubonic plague during the reign of Catherine the Great. With regard to cholera, only Roderick McGrew has studied Russia's first outbreak in any detail.[18] The fifth and sixth cholera epidemics have been considered from only two points of view: in one article Nancy Frieden has analysed the epidemic's impact on medical professionalisation and in another article John Hutchinson has investigated the process by which the bacteriological revolution arrived in Russia.[19] Until now, there has been no study making the cholera of 1892 its focus of analysis as, for instance, Richard Robbins has done with the famine of 1891.[20] Because we lack a comprehensive study of the social, political and medical impact of Russia's fifth cholera outbreak, its historical significance, in fact, has as yet to be examined. At the same time, there has been no compelling explanation of the political, social, economic and cultural circumstances that accounted for the continuing existence of a medical and social disaster in Russia that other European countries had overcome long before. For the disastrous outbreak in 1892 did not remain a single episode. After a brief reappearance in the Caspian region in 1904, cholera came back to Russia in 1907 and this time infected the whole empire for several years, culminating in a severe outbreak as late as 1910. The analysis of cholera's return in the early twentieth century highlights the lessons provided by the epidemic in 1892 and thus further illuminates its social, political and medical impact.

Cholera historiography has thus far focused its attention on the urban centres most affected by the disease. However, in late-nineteenth and early-twentieth-century Russia, cholera was a disease of the countryside even more than it was of teeming cities.[21] The epidemic ravaged a huge territory of enormous ethnic, social and cultural diversity, all of which significantly affected the course of the outbreak. Despite its presence empire-wide, cholera remained a local disease. This book takes account of the variety of Russia's cholera experience by singling out the city of Saratov as a case study. The choice was an obvious one. Located on the Volga River, one of the great epidemiological highways for the *vibrio cholerae* to Europe, the city ranked as one of the places in Russia most severely hit since cholera's first visitation to the continent in 1830. Towards the end of the nineteenth century, Saratov was particularly vulnerable to the disease. In the midst of rapid economic transition, the city suffered all the high-risk symptoms of a favourable breeding ground for the cholera bacillus: mass poverty, malnutrition and susceptibility to illness brought about by staggering numbers of peasant migrants. An urban environment marred by sanitary neglect and a frightening quality of medical health provision compounded the problem. Notoriously unhealthy,

Saratov was empire-wide infamous for its high incidence of diseases and deaths caused by poverty, malnutrition and squalor. Poor harvests, famines and epidemics were regular occurrences in the period under consideration. When cholera approached the city in the summer of 1892, it found perfect conditions to produce a medical calamity. In addition, the city also became the centre of some of the most violent cholera riots witnessed in the empire in that year. Epitomising the worst aspects of the cholera in 1892, Saratov provides an ideal prism through which to understand the onslaught. Moreover, the city's experience with cholera in 1892 paralleled the course of the disease in the big urban centres at the lower Volga. Throughout the period under consideration, the cholera history of the Volga capital typified the regional experience with the disease.

This analysis of Saratov's fight against cholera offers insight into some of the key questions concerning state and society in late imperial Russia. First, the book sheds light on the nature of local government in the autocratic state. The quality and scope of local governmental activity has been a constant theme for historians who have extensively investigated local initiative in the fields of education, public health and poor relief, the major areas of responsibility assigned to the newly elected self-governing institutions (zemstvo) by the Great Reforms in 1864.[22] These studies have rectified too simplistic juxtapositions of local liberal-minded reformers fighting against an oppressive autocratic regime. They offer instead a more complex picture, which delineates the strengths and weaknesses of both sides: the space for autonomy as well as the constraints imposed on local government in late imperial Russia. Delegating anti-epidemic combat to the local level, in particular, proved to be a very contentious issue for the autocratic state. Reform legislation at first only transferred the management and financing for community welfare to local authorities, while keeping the highest authority over all matters of public health, including epidemic control, in the hands of the central government. Only in 1879 did recurrent cholera outbreaks force the government to vest the zemstvo and, later, the municipal duma with broad regulatory powers during epidemics. The fight against epidemics soon became an important field for negotiating local autonomy and central authority. And conversely, the mitigation of this conflict was crucial for any long-term containment of cholera. To the autocratic state, epidemics therefore represented not only a medical but also a political challenge. These larger political, institutional and medical developments have been most lucidly analysed by Nancy Frieden and John Hutchinson.[23] Yet to date, there is no study which examines the fight against cholera in late imperial Russia at a local level.[24] The study of cholera epidemics in late-nineteenth and early-twentieth-century Saratov allows one to discuss the political and administrative conflicts brought about by anti-epidemic combat as seen from a specific local perspective. This book will examine how local governing authorities assumed the responsibility for public health and how they translated their legal rights into practical policy. More importantly, it will analyse how the highly complex interaction of local and national authorities worked in practice during times of epidemic crisis. The focus on a particular locality also reveals the mechanisms by which local officials and medical authorities and the population coped with an overwhelming problem such as cholera. We see, as well, how diseases and epidemics were experienced by ordinary people.

Second, by focusing the investigation of cholera on the city of Saratov, this study becomes a part of Russia's urban history, a field of research which has been assessed by one scholar as 'sufficiently underexplored to be considered a "black spot" in our understanding of Imperial Russia'.[25] With an 86.6% rural population in 1897, studies of the pre-revolutionary Russian Empire have focused on the countryside. What is more, Russia's cities were not only looked on as insignificant in size but also as devoid of *civitas*. As 'service cities' (Michael Hittle), it was widely assumed, they did not enjoy the degree of local autonomy and independence that characterised their western European counterparts and thus failed to develop an urban citizenry which could take on an innovative and powerful role in the process of nation-building.[26]

Following the Great Reforms, however, Russia's urban centres became entangled in the empire's economic, political, administrative and social transformation. Under the impact of rapid industrial and economic development, of trade and migration, the country underwent what William Blackwell termed its 'first urban transformation'.[27] Western scholars have turned their attention to this process since the late 1960s and early 1970s. The empire's cities have been looked at from a wide array of themes covering economic and demographic growth, migration, ethnic diversity, the urban environment, poverty, urban life, consumer culture, cultural patronage, sexual identity, voluntary associations and many more.[28] However, only a few histories examine an individual city. Moreover, with rare exceptions (such as Odessa, Kiev, Kazan') existing local studies mostly focus on St Petersburg or Moscow.[29] Vital peripheral centres of Russia's urban development still need to be explored.

Due to its political, economic and social significance, Saratov is one of the provinces that has enjoyed the most attention from historians of late imperial and revolutionary Russia. Historians have, however, tended to focus on Saratov's political history and examined the province's and the city's significance as a centre of political radicalism.[30] As yet we know little about the socio-cultural history of late imperial Saratov. Epidemics, diseases, dirt, health and sex provide organising categories with which to discuss urban space, and with which to integrate the wider social and cultural history. For my study I take Briggs's assessment as my starting point. My premise is that the investigation of cholera in Saratov provides a means to analyse the profound social, economic and cultural changes and the strains brought about by rapid urban growth; it will look at glaring problems such as overcrowding, sanitation and the urban poor and will examine the efforts of the institutions of self-government to cope with the challenges caused by huge increases in population.

These first two themes are closely linked to a third major point. The history of modern Russia has for a long time been analysed and interpreted as distinct from that of 'the West'.[31] Since the Cold War Russia's process of political, social and economic development in the late nineteenth and early twentieth centuries has been widely regarded as belated and incomplete if compared with western Europe.

The country experienced a revolution because it deviated from the Western model of development. This idea of Russia's unfinished modernisation and its 'backwardness' has continued to appear in many scholarly works.[32] More recent works, however, have emphasised a common comparative model of European modernity of which Russia was a component part.[33] The study of cholera in Saratov between 1892 and 1910 provides a prism through which numerous aspects of Russia's variant of modernity can be viewed from a comparative perspective. Cholera, the 'ally of sanitary reforms' (Asa Briggs), is widely regarded as a catalyst of social modernisation. Russia's epidemic of 1892 brought about a widespread recognition of the country's need for extensive reforms. In Saratov, the epidemic highlighted the economic misery and in particular the social issues of poverty and destitution which had caused the outbreak. In the wake of the cholera, national and local government officials, medical experts and urban planners addressed the problems of sanitation, housing, poverty and social unrest. Extensive sanitary and medical reforms became the key for social modernisation and control. New concepts of hygiene and preventive medicine were to combat peasant backwardness and irrationality and to transform peasant superstition into rational and modernised behavioural norms. In St Petersburg, at the same time, the epidemic of 1892 inaugurated an era of unprecedented innovation and success in the field of modern laboratory medicine. In its drive to be modern and scientific Russia paralleled the larger movement of medical modernisation taking place across the globe at the time.[34] As elsewhere, modern medical science was also a sphere for interaction and conflicts between rulers and ruled, between the governmental authorities and the medical profession, between the doctors and the population. As the return of the epidemic to Saratov in 1904 showed, eradicating cholera involved more than updating the medical infrastructure. The fundamental problems of poverty and social antagonisms had to be addressed.

Methodology

Cholera appeals to social historians largely because of its potential for disclosing the workings of state and society on both the local and the central levels. The subject criss-crosses a multitude of governmental bodies, scientific institutions, official commissions, voluntary organisations and other social organisations. As a result, the history of cholera in Saratov relies upon an abundance of disparate sources. What is more, Russia's cholera epidemic of 1892 represents the country's best documented cholera visitation of the nineteenth century. Unlike most western European states, where the first and most shocking cholera experience in 1830–31 is often better recorded than subsequent encounters with the disease, Russia's epidemic of 1892 produced an outpouring of source material which surpassed the wealth of records of the first pandemic. Since the outbreak has been the subject of relatively little scholarly investigation, it was critical to begin the research process by sifting through a large quantity of printed primary material. Contemporary medical journals hold an abundance of valuable reports and analyses of the medical and administrative sides of the disease and have been

extensively used for this study. They were supplemented by the multitude of contributions in various volumes (*trudy, sborniki, protokoly, doklady, otchety*) of
medical societies, professional congresses and official scientific commissions on
both the national and local levels.

The medical and sanitary histories of late imperial Saratov, meanwhile, pose
some unique problems. Of particular importance for an investigation of the history
of urban sanitation and public health is the quantity and quality of statistical material which constitutes another important source basis for the present study. Until
the end of the nineteenth century, Russian cities – with the exception of the
capitals – very rarely came to be considered as objects of statistical and especially
medical-statistical research. It was only after the municipal reforms in 1871 and
1892, which transferred the responsibility of public health to the urban municipalities, that genuine urban medical statistics began to develop.[35] Because urban
statistics were still in their infancy, it is almost impossible to obtain sufficient and
accurate demographic data for Saratov until well into the twentieth century. The
first very rudimentary attempt by the municipality to collect information systematically on the city's mortality rates was made in 1893, one year after the devastating cholera epidemic. Medical statistical work developed slowly and for the first
time became institutionalised in the city in the form of a medical-statistical office
(*mediko-statisticheskii stol*) in 1904. In light of the constant shortage of material
and experienced personnel resources, the available statistics are far from satisfactory. Yet giving due allowance to the incompleteness and unreliability of the
material, central and local, official and unofficial statistical institutions did still
leave behind a broad array of sources, which contain a wealth of information
about many aspects of economic, social and cultural life in late-nineteenth-century
Saratov. Alongside the first elementary diagrams and tables depicting the city's
morbidity, mortality and birth rates, local physicians conducted research into
Saratov's most vulnerable places with regard to health. They investigated night
shelters, almshouses, bath-houses, hospitals and hiring markets; they analysed
water, food, salaries and prices; they examined the significance of seasonal work
from the standpoint of infectious diseases by describing the life of the migrants,
their living conditions and their work at the banks. Many of their articles were
published in the nationally renowned *Saratov Sanitary Review* (*Saratovskii
Sanitarnyi Obzor*), a supplement of the zemstvo edited *Saratov Zemstvo Weekly*
(*Saratovskaia Zemskaia Nedelia*), as well as in major national medical journals.
Providing the most valuable material on the causes, especially the social causes,
of diseases in the city, these works convey a detailed picture of the economic and
social conditions prevailing in Saratov on the eve of the cholera outbreak in 1892
and long thereafter. They thus form another basic source for the present study.
The medical investigations are complemented by material such as tourist guides,
reports and protokols from the city council, and newspaper articles to name just a
few. Finally, the most detailed and perceptive source for an analysis of the
cholera's course in Saratov in 1892 is the city's local press. From mid-June until
the end of July, cholera constituted the major topic in Saratov's newspapers. The
journalists of the *Saratov Herald* (*Saratovskii Vestnik*) and the *Saratov Leaflet*

(*Saratovskii Listok*) wrote on every aspect, past and present, of the epidemic and freely reported about the populace's riots and resistance. Their extensive coverage provides the backbone for the analysis of the city's experience with the disease.

The book is divided into five chapters. Chapter 1 surveys Russia's cholera history prior to 1892. The chapter delineates Russia's traditional epicentres and reviews early medical debates and governmental strategies to combat the disease; it further analyses the changes in Russia's anti-cholera defence after mid-century; and it discusses how the strong influence of Max von Pettenkofers's new medical discoveries challenged the autocratic state at the very core of its beliefs. The chapter explores the factors that explain why Russia's cholera experience diverged from western Europe after mid-century and thus provides the background for the analysis of Russia's fifth and sixth cholera pandemics.

Chapter 2 introduces Saratov city by analysing the factors that made Saratov so susceptible to diseases and specifically to epidemic cholera at the end of the nineteenth century. It scrutinises the circumstances that help to explain why Saratov was hit by one of the most devastating cholera onslaughts of the century as late as 1892. The chapter looks into the problems resulting from rapid economic and social development after the Great Reforms; it discusses the city's pattern of diseases and the existing medical infrastructure to control Saratov's health. In so doing, it establishes the basic local and medical context for this study.

Chapter 3 is the pivot of this book and analyses Saratov's cholera experience of 1892. The chapter begins by investigating the role of the national government in the epidemic. It examines the desperate efforts made by central authorities to prevent the cholera from crossing the Persian–Russian border by means of militarily enforced quarantine; and it describes the arrival of the *vibrio cholerae* at the Caspian Sea, in particular in Baku and Astrakhan', the two major centres from which the cholera spread across European Russia. The chapter then explores the epidemic as experienced in Saratov city, analysing anti-epidemic policies as conducted by local municipal and provincial authorities. It also discusses local medical strategies to contain the disease; and finally it uncovers popular responses to the cholera in the form of rioting, attacks on doctors and poisoning hysteria and examines the political, social and medical reasons for such public resistance.

Chapter 4 focuses on the cholera's impact on Saratov. The epidemic of 1892 provided an impetus for reform both from above and from below. The chapter examines the means by which the municipality, the educated elite and the medical profession addressed the causes of the disaster. It looks at the most important, cholera-related projects of urban renewal undertaken in Saratov by local and state authorities in the 1890s and 1910s; it further looks at the development of philanthropic work as a crucial means to confront the problem of the urban poor and it discusses the reasons for the limited success of these reform endeavours. The chapter further examines the rise of the medical profession and of medical knowledge as influential factors in the city's public life. Examining the social, political and medical impact of the epidemic in 1892 for the next two decades, the chapter also discusses the preconditions for the return of cholera in 1904.

Chapter 5 examines the return of the cholera to Saratov in 1904–1910. The significance of this cholera outbreak differed crucially from that in 1892. Within a decade, the bacteriological revolution had explained the causality of the disease and state policies to contain the *vibrio* had fundamentally changed. In addition, the relations between the medical profession, the population and the state had been altered. Mortality figures lessened and the social impact of the epidemic was far removed from the tumultuous events in 1892. And yet, cholera once again became a catalyst for social and political tensions. The chapter analyses the new medical and administrative basis for the country's cholera combat in the age of bacteriology; it examines the social and political challenge posed by the disease to Saratov's local governing authorities in a time of revolutionary upheaval and scrutinises the factors that hindered the successful eradication of the disease.

The conclusion returns to the debate instigated by Asa Briggs and Margaret Pelling and asks what the prevalence of cholera in Saratov during the period from 1892 until 1910 can tell us about the political, social and cultural transformation of the autocratic state in a time of its rapid urbanisation and modernisation.

1 Cholera in Russia

In the century ending in 1914, six epidemics of Asiatic cholera rampaged through the tsarist empire. With 44 cholera years since 1823 claiming more than 2 million human lives, Russia was the most frequently and most violently stricken country in Europe.[1] Using Astrakhan' as its entrance gate to Europe the *vibrio cholerae* infected Russia as the first country on the continent. During the second (1826–1837) and third (1841–1859) pandemics the empire was the immediate source for cholera in the rest of Europe and of North America. In Europe's history of the disease Russia's cholera experience played a pre-eminent role.

This chapter surveys and analyses Russia's cholera experience prior to 1892. In tsarist Russia, the cholera's first onslaught was by no means the worst. Violent epidemic outbreaks ravaged the empire during the Crimean War and between 1865 and 1871–72. And, while Russia's cholera history during the first three pandemics was quite similar to that of western Europe, its cholera path diverged from the rest of Europe after the middle of the century. Cholera continued to pose a medical challenge to the tsarist empire which, moreover, increasingly grew into a political threat as the century went on. These later cholera epidemics have been of little interest to scholars to date.[2] Although it is not and cannot be within the purview of this chapter to analyse each pandemic in detail, it is necessary to review earlier outbreaks and to compare them with political precautions and social responses evoked in Russia and elsewhere in order to understand why Asiatic cholera could create a major national medical, political and social calamity in the tsarist empire as late as 1892.

The chapter is divided into two parts. The first part surveys the course of the first three cholera pandemics in Russia. It traces the *vibrio*'s classic routes through Russia since 1823 and delineates the empire's major traditional epicentres; it further discusses Russia's earliest medical theories and initial governmental strategies to combat the cholera. The second part of the chapter examines Russia's cholera history after mid-century. As elsewhere in Europe, new medical discoveries, advanced by the Bavarian hygienist Max von Pettenkofer, affected the government's policing of epidemics. However, in Europe's only autocratic state the triumph of Pettenkofer's localist approach to epidemic diseases challenged the foundations of the state itself. Establishing the background for an analysis of the cholera outbreak in 1892, it is an essential purpose of this chapter to illustrate the conditions that explain why tsarist Russia, alone of all European states, was highly susceptible to epidemic cholera empire-wide until well into the twentieth century.

Empire of germs: cholera in Russia, 1823–1848

In 1823 cholera stood at the gates of Europe for the first time. The disease had left its endemic home, the Ganges-Brahmaputra Delta in West Bengal, in 1817; having reached Bangkok in 1820 and China in 1822, it had swept large parts of south-east Asia by 1824. During these same years, the cholera also travelled to the north following traders to the Punjab and across the whole of Persia to the Caspian Sea. In August 1823, the first cholera cases occurred in Baku and, one month later, the bacterium arrived in Astrakhan'. It was here that the European history of epidemic cholera began.[3]

Russia's response was swift. As soon as the cholera was reported from Tiflis in July, the Medical Council of the Ministry of Internal Affairs for the first time devised a set of recommendations and regulations to control the disease. With little medical understanding and experience with the cholera, the Medical Council suggested cutting any communication with other infected places; it emphasised the need to isolate the sick and provided basic standard means of treating the disease. These early instructions were published and disseminated among local doctors in the south.[4] In addition to providing information, the Medical Council's chairman General-Staff Doctor Reman also set up a Central Cholera Council charged with the task of collecting information on the unknown disease and issuing administrative measures for the fight against it.[5]

Though demonstrating an acute awareness of the threat, state action lagged behind events. Information about a mysterious, deadly disease which was moving across an unwieldy territory reaching from India to Africa and Asia was vague and slow to spread, and St Petersburg's initial efforts were bound to be too late. Medical experts dispatched from the capital to help with the cholera arrived in Astrakhan' on 4 November. After a tedious journey down the river they were informed that the disease had receded on 4 October, three days before they had left St Petersburg.[6] Meanwhile, in view of the unknown disease, Astrakhan' had launched an active campaign of self-defence. Policemen reported every suspected case of cholera to officials; the administration took responsibility for medical treatment and its costs and set up lazarettos in every borough of the city; it also advised people of individual measures of prevention such as eating a healthy diet and avoiding unripe fruits.[7]

The outbreak was too weak to test the efficacy of these measures. An unusually cold winter effectively stopped the spread of the disease before it could reach epidemic proportions.[8] All in all, the cholera's first visitation to Astrakhan' caused an estimated 392 cholera cases and 205 deaths.[9] Once the disease had disappeared, governmental efforts to combat the threat subsided as well. The Central Cholera Council was disbanded in 1824, and only revived in 1830 when it became the central medical-administrative body in the government's first large-scale anti-cholera campaign. Otherwise, Russia's first cholera encounter in Astrakhan' remained an isolated outbreak with no political, social or medical impact. For the next six years, official and public thinking ignored the possibility of a major epidemic attack.

But disaster was imminent. In 1829 cholera unexpectedly flared up in the city of Orenburg in the southern Ural. Since the region was well known for its good health and generally considered immune to diseases, cholera's appearance left medical experts at odds about both the epidemic's arrival and its predisposing causes.[10] It soon turned out that the disease had arrived by camel. As the most important military post of the Orenburg line, a military defence line to promote Russia's expansion towards Central Asia, Orenburg also hosted a large spring fair for trade with the Central Asian khanates. Caravans from Bukhara carried the disease across the Russian–Persian border and in August 1829 established Orenburg as the germ's second classic entry to Russia.

Unsettling rumours about a terrifying disease in Bukhara and Khiva were rife as early as June when trade with the approaching kirgis and other nomadic tribes was just about to be opened. Well aware of the latent threat, the Central Medical Council set up a special commission to investigate the rumoured epidemic. The commission, headed by Lieutenant-General Veselitskii, found two diseases, named Ova and Tagun, which were unknown both in their meaning and in their medical qualities. Infectious diseases, according to the caravan leaders, existed neither in the caravans nor at any of the places through which they passed. Moreover, since vast deserts separated the afflicted regions from the Russian border, the commission soothingly concluded that there was no medical threat to Russia. On 21 July, the caravans were permitted entry to Orenburg. Five weeks later, on 26 August, the first acknowledged cholera case was recorded.[11]

For the first time, the disease spread, infecting the entire Orenburg region. This was in marked contrast to Astrakhan's initial cholera outbreak. On 7 November cholera was reported from as far as Bugulma, a city 200 miles east of Kazan'. It then advanced further to Buguruslan (5 December), Menselinsk (2 January 1830), and Belebeevsk (6 January). By February 1830, when the epidemic subsided, Orenburg province had reported a total of 3,500 cholera cases, 865 of which had proved fatal.[12]

Such spread notwithstanding, cholera's reappearance on Russian soil was hardly noticed beyond the medical community. Alexander von Humboldt, who was just returning from his expedition to Siberia, became aware only in the capital that he had in fact passed through a region afflicted by cholera. Across the Orenburg area people remained calm. Everyday life was constrained by the establishment of a *cordon sanitaire* and other basic precautionary measures, yet cholera was not viewed as threatening and the situation seemed controllable. Not only was the outbreak numerically limited in its impact, but, more importantly, people still lacked any experience with the disease. Cholera had not yet created its fearful image and memories, the chief basis for the psychological resonance evoked by the epidemic in subsequent outbreaks. In Orenburg in 1829, it therefore still did not unleash hysteria, social panic or the tumultuous popular reactions which were to characterise the first pandemic all over Europe.[13]

In far-away St Petersburg, Orenburg's outbreak passed unnoticed as well. Unlike the plague, the cholera was still not considered a national problem and governmental circles took no measures to prevent the epidemic's spread. Such passivity could not only be ascribed to ignorance. In 1829–30, Russia's rulers were preoccupied with political issues of the highest magnitude. The outbreak of the July Revolution in Paris in 1830 ultimately questioned the legitimacy of the Holy Alliance, Europe's new order as established at the congress of Vienna in 1815. Nicholas I, firmly determined to halt Europe's revolutionary development by military means, ordered the general mobilisation of the Russian army. By the autumn of 1830, however, the cholera's move across European Russia had rendered the deployment of military troops to Prussia impossible.[14]

For all the while that the cholera was slowly subsiding in Orenburg, the germ continued to move across Persia and successfully entered Russia via the western border. In July 1830, Baku, Elizavetpol and Tiflis suffered violent attacks from the disease. With local authorities and the populace being unprepared, the epidemic relentlessly killed thousands of people.[15] Widespread panic, mass flight and the demoralisation of the public for the first time presaged a haunting spectacle for times to come. From the Caucasus, the germ travelled further along the western coast of the Caspian Sea and reached Astrakhan' on 4 July. Three weeks later, the disease was reported again from the Orenburg region, where it had attacked Gurev, a small settlement at the shore of the Caspian Sea.[16] Thus, by the end of the month, cholera had infected the entire western coastline of the Caspian Sea.

Events in Russia's south-east culminated in Astrakhan'. While the central government was slow to act, local authorities had indeed followed the epidemic with concern since its appearance in Orenburg. Already in November 1829, the governor of Astrakhan' considered it necessary to issue secret instructions about the establishment of quarantine measures in the case of a cholera outbreak. The following spring, he further instructed local district authorities to report the occurrence of cholera immediately to neighbouring districts and provinces. In many places, precautionary quarantine measures had been taken well before the epidemic arrived.[17] Yet despite such preparation, the epidemic's assault was devastating. The first scattered cases, which occurred in Astrakhan' province on 4 July, could still successfully be isolated in a quarantine station on the Caspian Sea. On 20 July, however, four people were stricken by cholera in the city of Astrakhan'. That day, the epidemic began in earnest. Within 10 days cholera developed into a full-scale catastrophe. By 15 August 1830, 3,633 people out of the city's 30,770 residents were reported to have fallen ill. After three weeks, more than 2,500 people had died.[18]

Confronted with such a killer, Astrakhan' was defenceless. Medical horror turned into social anarchy. This mysterious plague from the Ganges struck old and young, rich and poor, ordinary people and local officials with terrifying rapidity. While the disease relentlessly tortured its victims to death with violent spasms of vomiting and diarrhoea, there was no medical explanation and no defence against it.[19] Terrified and helpless, thousands of people took flight. Refugees from Astrakhan', at times more than 4,000 a day, spread the disease across the province and beyond.[20] For the first time in its history, cholera journeyed up the Volga, violently attacking Tsaritsyn on 4 August and Saratov on 8 August.[21] With unexpected fury and rapidity, a full-scale cholera epidemic erupted all over the lower Volga region. Local governments collapsed everywhere and the population on the river's lower reaches was gripped by fear and panic. A first-hand report from the German physician in Tsaritsyn described the atmosphere of anarchy and chaos:

> Lacking any help, consolation or reassurance, nobody showed the strength and determination to establish some sort of order or to gain trust; some of the city's residents took flight; all obedience ceased; nobody commanded since nobody wanted to obey; corpses lay unburied in the houses or were thrown in the graveyard as nobody was willing to dig the graves or to bury the dead.[22]

All the while that the disease ravaged the country's south, medical and governmental authorities learned their first lessons. Effective control of the epidemic depended on medical understanding of the disease. Here opinions were divided. During the outbreak in Astrakhan' in 1823, the Medical Council of the Ministry of Internal Affairs expressed a strongly contagionist view.[23] Cholera was transmitted through touching infected clothing or goods. The Medical Council further established that the disease occurred in hot, damp and cloudy weather, whereas it subsided in cold temperatures. Based on such a medical position, the Medical Council stressed the value of quarantine and sequestration to combat the epidemic.[24] Reman's early description of treatment and prophylaxis additionally suggested treating the patients with large doses of calomel and opium.[25] The cholera outbreak at Orenburg, however, thoroughly questioned the Medical Council's early medical assumptions.[26] In order to be able to explain the cause and transmission of the disease during wintertime, Russia's doctors proposed a more complex theory. Combining contagion with personal predisposition and local environmental conditions, it laid the foundations for the three basic cholera models which continued to be debated throughout the nineteenth century:

> a person who had contracted a tendency to the disease in a place where it prevails, arrives in an uninfected place, there takes ill, and communicates a diseased condition to the atmosphere of his new residence. Here the disease increases and spreads, seizing all whose constitutions are by nature predisposed to receive it.[27]

In the midst of wild speculations as to whether the cholera was an attack on the nervous system, a disease of the digestive tract, or a malady of the blood, medical practitioners resorted to an experimental armamentarium of preventive and therapeutic techniques. On the basis of various foreign, particularly British, sources doctors advised people to protect themselves from infection by leading a well-balanced way of life which involved, above all, a healthy diet, avoiding debauchery and excessive drinking.[28] To ease the cramps and stimulate circulation cholera patients were given hot baths and wrapped in warm sheets and blankets saturated with Spanish pepper or aromatic liquids such as Eau de Cologne.[29] In addition, doctors favoured large doses of purgatives, most prominently calomel and chloride mixed with salt, quinine, bismuth and opium, to detoxify the patient's body. Yet the most widely used of all treatments was blood-letting and depletion. Although generally discounted after the first pandemic as ineffective, depletion remained the most persistent remedy against cholera in Russia until the end of the nineteenth century.[30]

By contrast, state authorities were guided by non-medical considerations. In fact, governmental policy harshly contradicted the Medical Council's recommendations. On 8 July and 12 August, two major decrees on cholera relaxed quarantine rules and placed full responsibility for all measures regarding the epidemic, in particular quarantine, on the central government.[31] St Petersburg's chief coordinators of the anti-cholera campaign, Minister of Internal Affairs Count Zakrevskii and Finance Minister Count Kankrin, decidedly opposed expensive quarantine measures, pointing out that they threatened economic trade and social stability.[32]

On 12 September, however, the government radically changed its policies. Overrun by an unknown killer, Russia initiated Europe's great experiment in eradicating cholera with anti-plague defences. *Cordons sanitaires* were drawn around major infected areas. Quarantine and sequestration measures typically involved the isolation of the sick and the inspection and observation of travellers from suspect places; any articles and clothes were to be washed with a chlorine-lime solution, and papers and documents were to be fumigated.[33] Since medical personnel was lacking, the military and the police were employed to supervise the sanitary regime.

This policy was a complete failure. As the epidemic advanced through European Russia, military coercion actually aggravated the crisis. Terrified by a deadly disease and threatened by military force, the population responded with outbursts of collective phobia and fury directed at physicians and officials.[34] Historians of cholera widely agree that Russia presents Europe's most extreme case of terror and violence, unleashed by brutal and inhumane quarantine policies to combat the continent's first encounter with cholera. Nechkina concluded in strong terms that Russian anti-cholera policies in 1831 were conducted in an atmosphere of martial law leading to massive suffering and social unrest which paralysed the whole Volga region between Astrakhan' and Nizhnii Novgorod.[35]

Yet one needs to be careful in evaluating Russian policies as being the exception in Europe. During the first pandemic resorting to militarily enforced *cordons sanitaires* was a universal response. As Richard Evans pointed out, public order collapsed across eastern and central Europe in 1831.[36] In France's case, Louis Chevalier showed that the disease played a significant role in the political riots of April and June 1832 in Paris, even if it did not directly cause them.[37] And in Britain, popular resentment was directed towards the medical profession and resulted in attacks on hospitals across the country.[38] Likewise, the Habsburg Empire and Prussia experienced violent public disturbances.[39] In Europe's first encounter with cholera Russia's dramatic popular responses were by no means unique.

For a variety of reasons Russian quarantine policy was by no means as stringent and unified as Nechkina's otherwise pioneering analysis suggests. Although the Medical Council had opted for rigorous isolation and control measures since 1823, it had not defined what actually constituted effective quarantine procedures.[40] In fact, until mid-September very little was done to enforce quarantine regulations in general. Furthermore, the population could not as yet recognise the cholera and paid little attention to those regulations that were in existence.[41] In Russia's southern epicentre people took flight long before any state policies were employed. Moreover, quarantine measures varied highly from place to place, even when the epidemic was already sweeping through the country. McGrew, for instance, described Prince Golitsyn's moderate and circumspect handling of the cholera in Moscow in 1830. Russia's old capital, which experienced the culmination of the 1830 epidemic, escaped civil conflict, social anarchy and rebellion.[42] By necessity, quarantine policies throughout the epidemic were contested, inconsistent and hastily improvised. As McGrew's analysis convincingly demonstrated, the central government had, in practice, no control over medical and social events.[43]

Relentlessly moving forward, cholera established two major bacterial highways and defined the empire's most vulnerable epicentres. Starting from Astrakhan', the germ established the immense waterway of the Volga as its classic epidemiological route into the heart of European Russia and beyond it towards western Europe. Volga cities and provinces suffered the worst ravages in 1830. Within two and a half months cholera attacked, in order, Saratov, Kazan' and Nizhnii Novgorod. The epidemic reached Moscow province in September 1830 and from here travelled further to the Baltic provinces and western Europe. As in many subsequent outbreaks, the disease became less deadly as the germ moved from south to north. Mortality was highest in Astrakhan' (90%), followed by Saratov (70%), Kazan' (60%), and Moscow (50%).[44]

The Caucasus, Russia's second major epicentre, was also heavily devastated in 1830. From Baku, cholera spread to Elizavetpol', which recorded 4,557 cases and 1,655 deaths, and then violently attacked Tiflis, Erivan and Kars. At the same time, the germ advanced from Baku in a northerly direction. According to the authoritative estimates by Grigorii I. Arkhangel'skii, the intensity of the 1830 outbreak reached its pinnacle in Astrakhan's neighbouring province of Stavropol'.[45]

Finally, while moving from south to north, cholera also attacked the country along a second standard route. From Orenburg in the east the epidemic travelled westward to the river Don, then passed through Voronezh, Tambov, Kursk and manifested itself in the country's south-west. Russia's third national high-risk region was thus identified as the region of the Don Cossacks and Bessarabia, the provinces of Kherson, Ekaterinoslav, Poltava, Khar'kov, Chernigov, Voronezh, Vitebsk and Tambov. Although these provinces did not suffer as horribly as the provinces along the Volga River in 1830, the pattern was reversed in 1831. As in many later cholera visitations, the south-western provinces were most severely struck when the *vibrio* rolled back.

In fact, the renewed outbreak hit Russia even more severely. In the winter of 1830, cholera had already seriously infected the provinces of Podolia, Volhynia,

Kiev and Bessarabia. From Chernigov province, where the disease flared up in January 1831, the germ spread south and eastwards, affecting all the surrounding provinces.[46] Exploding with fury, the epidemic was much more deadly than its predecessor. In Bessarabia, cholera reached its maximum intensity of 20.3 per thousand, killing more than 10,000 people. These figures were followed by Chernigov (12.1), Poltava (13.1), Ekaterinoslav (10.1) Khar'kov (9.3), Tauride (10.2) and the Don Cossack Region (10.3).[47] Yet in other centres as well the epidemic had survived the winter. It appeared in Tambov in January, in Vologda in February, and in Moscow in March. In addition, Orenburg province, Arkhangel' and particularly the capital St Petersburg itself were severely struck. From Moscow, the germ eventually advanced city by city down the Volga River and again returned to Astrakhan' on 1 July 1831. With an estimated 466,000 victims, the second cholera year proved six times more deadly than its predecessor.[48] What is more, the disease caused massive social uprisings and violent revolts across the empire which even exceeded the disturbances of the preceding year.[49]

The historiography of cholera has predominantly discussed Russia's and Europe's first encounter with the disease. Not least the sheer number of deaths left in the epidemic's wake across the whole continent caused scholars to investigate the social, political and medical impact of cholera in the 1830s.[50] While the status of the epidemic as a means to explore the functioning of a given society has never gone unchallenged, the two major monographs by Richard Evans on Hamburg and Frank Snowden on Naples clearly call into question an understanding of the epidemic's significance on the basis of its demographic impact.[51] A comparative view of the six waves that afflicted the Russian empire in the nineteenth and twentieth centuries confirms their view. In fact, one of the most striking aspects about the Russian cholera in the 1830s is its very limited long-term political and social significance. As McGrew has laid out, the epidemic arrived at a crucial point in Russia's cultural development and indeed supported important developments in the field of medicine. Russia's experience with quarantine in particular raised violent professional debates amongst Russian and European medical experts about the nature and transmission of cholera. Yet despite its major ravages and the social and political violence brought about by the epidemic, cholera did not effect any political or administrative reform efforts.[52] Indeed, there is no evidence that the disastrous cholera experience of 1830–31 was of any state interest once the immediate impact of the epidemic faded. All the while the disease blanketed western Europe in 1832 and caused minor outbreaks in several Russian provinces until 1838, tsarist state authorities do not seem to have discussed the possibilities of preventing a future epidemic outbreak of cholera.[53] When cholera struck with renewed vigour in 1847, and with even higher force and virulence in 1848, Russia found itself ill-prepared. As McGrew stated:

> the epidemic's final tragedy was that this opportunity, like so many before and after, passed without the lessons being learned, and the victims of both disease and riots died to no purpose. (. . .) The Russian autocracy showed its

greatest strength as it defended itself, its greatest purpose as it destroyed its enemies, its greatest weakness as it prepared for the future.[54]

In the tsarist empire, administrative problems, drug and personnel shortages, the hatred of officialdom and of doctors, poisoning phobia and violent rioting would be normal occurrences until the beginning of the twentieth century.

Cholera finally subsided in Russia during the winter of 1831–32. While the disease most ferociously ravaged western Europe and north America, the tsarist empire was largely spared from further outbreaks in subsequent years. Only in 1838, when the disease came back from western Europe, did scattered cases of cholera occur in Volynsk, Grodno, Belostok, Vil'na and Minsk. After this time, this particular epidemic disappeared from Europe and Russia altogether.

A third pandemic, which lasted from 1841 to 1859, had reached Europe by 1844. Russia was once again invaded via the Persian–Russian border, claiming its first victims in the Caucasus on 16 October 1846.[55] Three days later, the disease was reported in Baku. The autumnal outbreak was not severe, yet cholera persisted until the following spring when it developed into a full-scale epidemic. What was more, the disease now spread from the Caucasus into European Russia. By mid-July 1847 cholera had been reported in Ekaterinoslav province and in the Don Cossack region. When the disease eventually arrived in the city of Astrakhan' on 4 July Russia was clearly in danger. Journeying along its familiar routes, the *vibrio* infected all of European Russia within four months. Although much milder than in 1831, the outbreak was twice as ferocious as in 1830, claiming an estimated 190,846 cholera cases and 77,719 deaths.[56]

Worse was to follow. Having established epidemic foci across the whole of European Russia, cholera survived the winter in the provinces of Chernigov, Poltava, Orel, Moscow, Kazan', Simbirsk and Orenburg, where it flared up in early 1848. At the same time as using its classic epidemiological highways, the disease extended radially from a multitude of already infected areas to adjacent provinces and regions. Taking Kazan' as a major starting point in Russia's northeast, the epidemic advanced both up and down the Volga; meanwhile the *vibrio* also spread from Moscow province, the second main centre in the very heart of Russia, into all neighbouring provinces. With such itineraries, the epidemic was even less predictable than in 1831. By May 1848, cholera was active from Arkhangel' in the north to Astrakhan' in the south. For the first time, the epidemic also crossed the Urals into Siberia, reaching Tobolsk on 1 July.[57]

Cholera's most terrifying attack of the century could hardly have appeared at a more inopportune moment for the Russian state authorities. Just as the first sporadic cholera cases were being reported from the country's south, France declared itself a republic on 25 February 1848. With the tide of revolutionary upheavals sweeping from Paris to Berlin and Vienna, the tsarist government faced the spectre of political revolution entering Poland as well as the Baltic and the western provinces. In the spring of 1848, when the cholera broke out with full force after ship traffic had opened on the Volga, the government's attention was absorbed with calling up the military and moving large numbers of troops into the western provinces. Compounding the political crisis, Russia suffered an empire-wide famine with catastrophic consequences for the country's economy.[58]

Given such context, the onslaught was explosive. In absolute numbers of sickness and death, the year 1848 was the most virulent and fatal of all cholera years that afflicted Russia in its epidemic history. With a total of 1,742,439 cholera cases, the epidemic slew 690,150 people over the course of the year.[59] The worst effects of the cholera outbreak were once again felt in the Don Cossack region, which recorded a total of 46,611 cases and 23,186 deaths (a mortality rate of 32.9 per thousand). The second hardest hit area was Russia's south-east, in particular the provinces of Voronezh (86,326 cases and 42,481 deaths) and Khar'kov (84,395 cases and 30,345 deaths). Finally, Podolia, Kiev and Chernigov continued to be the special high-risk regions in the south-west.[60]

With no medical explanation of the still mysterious disease, the tsarist state authorities this time abandoned their strategy of combating cholera with anti-plague defences. Following the first pandemic, the Russian government drew the same conclusions as most other European governments. *Cordons sanitaires*, it was widely concluded, could not halt the spread of cholera. Instead, soldiers and policemen evoked terror and panic among the population and thus contributed as much to the spread of the disease as to the collapse of public order.[61] In common with Britain, France and the German states, after 1831 the tsarist government indeed retreated from its strongly interventionist stance. For decades, quarantine policy to combat cholera was no concern of the Russian state. In 1841, Russia's first comprehensive quarantine legislation regulated in detail the establishment and implementation of quarantine measures both within the country and at the borders.[62] Yet the document only regulated prophylactic measures to eradicate plague. It mentioned neither cholera nor any other infectious diseases. During the third pandemic, quarantine precautions continued to be put into effect on a local level, especially at the country's traditional quarantine ports.[63] But the state did not attempt to halt the epidemic via means of such rigorous and stringent quarantine policies as implemented in 1830.[64]

Cholera remained endemic in Russia until 1859. All in all, the third pandemic was not only longer than the second but also proved to be more intensive and extensive. In particular, two severe outbreaks flared up during the turmoil of the Crimean War in 1853 and 1855. Once again, cholera claimed an estimated 100,083 deaths in 1853 and 131,327 lives in 1855.[65] It was only in 1859 that the epidemic finally subsided.

Cholera and medicine: 1850–1873

Up to this point, cholera history had evolved in Russia in much the same way as it had in western Europe. Cholera's violent course during the earliest two pandemics, the medical debates surrounding the disease, official policies of dealing with it as well as popular responses, all paralleled similar developments in Britain, France and the German states. By mid-century, however, Russia's cholera experience began to diverge from the western European pattern. New scientific explanations, most influentially advanced by the British physician John Snow and the Bavarian hygienist Max von Pettenkofer, inaugurated a sea-change in the medical understanding of the disease.[66] In addition, cholera now posed an even more existential threat to industrialising Europe. With large-scale movements of goods and people accompanying Europe's rapidly expanding mercantile and industrial enterprise, an outbreak of cholera at any principal European seaport severely endangered the whole continent. Apart from the medical danger, the costly closing of borders would damage the vital economic interests of Europe's industrialising nations. Finding new strategies to contain major epidemic diseases, in particular cholera, without harming trade and industry became a matter of great international concern.

It was cholera's second attack on Europe that sparked the debate. In 1851, government officials and medical authorities of 12 European states discussed the establishment of an internationally devised system of sanitary surveillance for the first time at a conference in Paris. The debate, interrupted by the Crimean War, continued at a series of international sanitary conferences which steadily accommodated scientific advances until the etiology of cholera was understood at the beginning of the twentieth century.[67] At all seven conferences the tsarist government was represented by delegations of the country's highest medical experts and governmental officials.

With negotiations ongoing, the cholera's fourth pandemic (1863–1875) demonstrated Europe's heightened vulnerability. For the first time, the *vibrio* deviated from its classic bacteriological highway and entered Europe via a different route. Starting from Mecca in May 1863, about 15,000 pilgrims carried the disease on the faster steamships of the day across the Red Sea to Suez. Killing more than 60,000 people within three months in Egypt, cholera journeyed further towards the Mediterranean Sea and severely afflicted Spain, Italy and France. Meanwhile, the *vibrio* also travelled from Constantinople across the Black Sea and reached Odessa on 27 July 1865. Although all of European Russia was infected the disease caused only sporadic outbreaks, none of which were comparable in their intensity to the attacks in 1830 and 1848.[68] Nonetheless, Russia, too, had become much more susceptible to epidemic assaults. In 1853, contemporaries in Moscow noted the arrival of the disease by train for the first time.[69] The country's growing railway network facilitated the epidemic's spread throughout the third and fourth pandemics. Spreading across Russia's immense territory, cholera lingered on until 1873, with two severe outbreaks in 1871 and 1872.[70] After 1873, all of Europe was free from the disease for the moment, including Russia.

In such an altered context Russia fundamentally reviewed its anti-epidemic defences. A new law, codified in 1866 in the context of Alexander II's liberal reforms, radically changed existing policies.[71] For the first time, quarantine legislation, hitherto confined to combat bubonic plague, was extended to yellow fever, smallpox and cholera. More importantly, in common with the authorities elsewhere in Europe, the Russian state greatly relaxed its approach to quarantine. In sharp contrast to the detailed instructions from 1841, the revised set of regulations was, in fact, strikingly lax and permissive.

To begin with, the Imperial authorities resorted to old strategies. In the case of an epidemic outbreak, Russia's new scheme of defence sought to save the empire from infection largely by sealing off the country's borders to Asia and Europe. Such a strategy of isolation, in fact, revived the arsenal of precautionary measures which had successfully eradicated plague from western Europe during the seventeenth and eighteenth centuries. Pioneered under Catherine the Great, the Russian government had gradually established a network of checkpoints and quarantine stations to prevent the importation of the deadly killer at the country's main points of entry. In Astrakhan', Odessa, Taganrog and Vasil'kov (near Kiev), Russia's principal quarantine institutions closely followed foreign experiences and anti-plague practices. Additional facilities were built to secure the Transcaucasian border. And finally, St Petersburg and Reval were equipped with special island quarantines.[72]

Yet in accord with international consensus the Russian state officially withdrew from the attempt to eradicate cholera by coercive means. Although the instructions still justified quarantine, isolation and disinfection, they were far milder than those that had governed plague in 1841. Under the new law, an incoming ship was interned for quarantine only if it reported any cases of infection. The quarantine period itself was cut down from 14 to 7 days. Instructions, moreover, were kept to an absolute minimum. In fact, the new document described almost no techniques for the implementation of disinfection measures. And as to land borders, it was simply stated that quarantine authorities should apply the same precautionary measures as those put into effect at ports. Since controls at the border were further relaxed, any epidemic could, in fact, easily enter the country.

Once the epidemic was in the country, governmental authorities abandoned any strategies of coercive prophylaxis. In 1841, state legislation had pursued vigorous policies in terms unimaginable elsewhere in Europe. Army and police encircled any places of infection; all communication between afflicted localities and neighbouring communities was severely forbidden; every house within a sanitary cordon was subjected to daily inspection and medical examination. While infected houses were isolated and disinfected, person-to-person contact was cut off through the closure of any public places such as schools, small businesses and churches. In addition to stipulating the total isolation of the population, the law also addressed the practical problems of maintaining the quarantine. It described in detail the build-up of quarantine stations, their equipment with medicine and doctors as well as methods and means of fumigation, sequestration, cleansing and disinfection; it regulated the provision of isolated communities with food and water; and it defined resolute fines or even imposed the death penalty on anybody breaking the quarantine.[73]

By contemporary standards, Russia's revised scheme of epidemic combat was impeccable. Moulded under the pressure of powerful interests of trade, the new policy of *laissez-faire* was, moreover, backed by latest scientific developments. Since 1831 the international medical community exhaustively debated the reasons for the failure of sanitary cordons and their disastrous effects on the course of the disease all over Europe. While the ubiquitous breakdown of quarantine defences had persuaded the majority of doctors that cholera was not a contagious disease, there was actually no explanation for the causes and mechanisms of the epidemic's spread. By 1860, however, the controversy between the adherents of contagionism, miasmatism and the moralist-psychologist stance entered a new phase. Max von Pettenkofer advanced a medical-scientific theory which seemed to verify the anti-contagionist view in a plausible way. Being the most vehement advocate of the localist school, Pettenkofer became the undisputed authority on epidemic prevention in Germany and France until the early 1880s.

Pettenkofer's 'ground-water' model accepted the existence of a germ or fungus as the causative agent of cholera, yet he concluded that this was carried neither by drinking water nor in infected clothes or goods. Rather, the decisive factor for the spread of the disease was the condition of the soil. Depending on its moisture content the soil could 'germinate' cholera provided it had been infected with a cholera germ. The process of germination created a miasma in which the disease was transmitted through the polluted air.[74] It followed from Pettenkofer's theory that any measures of quarantine, isolation or disinfection were useless against cholera. Massive state intervention, as propagated by the contagionists, was unsuccessful and ultimately pointless.

However, the view that the air was poisoned called for a large-scale clean-up of the environment. State regulation, according to Pettenkofer, had to concentrate on extensive sanitary reforms as long-term measures of prophylaxis. The only effective prevention against epidemic diseases, in particular cholera, were wide-ranging improvements in water supply and sewage disposal to reduce the possibility of creating an unhealthy miasma through the contamination of the soil.

In Russia, Pettenkofer's work won wide support. Foreign medical knowledge and experience with cholera had circulated through the empire since the epidemic's very first visitation on Russian soil. As early as 1822, doctors around the Caspian Sea read each other extracts from the work by Doctor Jameson, an English observer of the cholera in India.[75] Ten years later, Dr M.F.D. Markus's pioneering study of the cholera's sociology in Moscow and the correlation of the disease with the local ecology was firmly rooted in classic European medical thought.[76] Throughout the second pandemic Russian studies on cholera persistently stressed factors such as the condition of the soil, the quality of food and water, and the living and working environment as favourable to the epidemic's spread.[77] By mid-century, Russia's most eminent medical scientists unanimously advocated epidemic control through environmental change and sanitary reform. Figures such as Nicholas I. Pirogov (1810–1881), Evgraf A. Osipov (1841–1904), and Ivan I. Molleson (1842–1920) marshalled the need for public health reform in the strongest possible terms.[78] Yet Russia's most influential advocate of preventive medicine was the Swiss-born physician Friedrich F. Erismann (1841–1915). In his scientific capacities and all-round abilities as active promoter of public health reform the empire's leading hygienist was entirely equal to his own teacher, the illustrious Max von Pettenkofer himself.[79]

Above all, powerful political factors directed Russian medical thought. Historical scholarship has intensely disputed the hegemony of miasmatism as enmeshed in the socio-political struggles of a given community in the industrial age.[80] In the showcase of Germany Evans unravelled how Pettenkofer's theory, deeply entwined with the issue of quarantine, directly appealed to the specific economic interests and the political ideology of a society in an era of economic liberalism and free trade.[81] By contrast, in contemporary Naples anti-contagionism served as a vehicle for conservative and authoritarian purposes. Moreover, Neapolitan doctors, as Snowden argued, skilfully extrapolated Pettenkofer's doctrines in order to enhance their own professional standing and to gain a more influential position in local politics.[82]

Yet nowhere in Europe was the political leverage carried by cholera theories heavier than in the tsarist empire. Russia's controversy over contagionism, in fact, provides a fascinating model of the European contest. As for the Nicholaevan era, McGrew denied any reference to political or ideological purposes within the contagion debate.[83] However, the Crimean War (1853–56) profoundly changed the country's political and social life. Russia suffered more losses from disease than from battle.[84] Recurrent epidemics, particularly of plague and cholera, demonstrated that the central institutions failed miserably in Russia's 'undergoverned provinces'.[85] In all areas, the war heralded a turbulent process of renewal and innovation which ought to have overcome the country's decrepit administrative, social and economic structures and to reintegrate it with the European powers as a modern state. The problems that confronted the nation were familiar: reallocating responsibilities and functions in an autocratic state posed the greatest dilemma. Creating modern state structures without having the necessary financial, administrative and personal resources posed yet another set of problems. Medical reorganisation, following the tradition of Catherine the Great, became intrinsically linked to one of the most important and most challenging reform projects: the creation of local centres of authority as manifested in the institutions of the provincial zemstvo and their urban equivalent, the municipal duma.[86] According to the new constitutional practice, the responsibility for public health and its expenses was delegated to local authorities.

Medical doctrine forcefully buttressed the political programme. Pettenkofer's localist approach to diseases directly affected the state's policing of epidemics. As he insisted, the decisive factors in the cause of disease were the individual characteristics of the local environment. More than anything else, defeating diseases required profound knowledge about the particulars of topography and geography, flora and fauna, temperatures and rainfall. Since only local residents could gain such knowledge of the local ecology, full authority over public welfare was best delegated to them. It was solely local officials who were equipped to decide upon the specific remedies needed and to carry them out. Pettenkofer's philosophy provided a scientific rationale for decentralising the provision of medical care.[87]

In autocratic Russia, alone of all European states, localism went to the very core of the state's beliefs. The combination of medical theory and political programme proved explosive. At a landmark moment in the country's constitutional history, public health and medicine were set up in a field of manoeuvering the conflict over local autonomous interests within an autocratic state. Given such context, the devolution of the responsibility of public health to local authorities meant a lack of public health provision. As the case of Saratov will demonstrate, the state's centralised political and administrative structure hampered a substantial renewal of the urban infrastructure based on local initiative until far into the twentieth century. Lacking the most effective defence against the *vibrio cholerae*, the achievements of the sanitary reform movement, the Russian Empire remained highly vulnerable when cholera struck.

Against this background, Russia's revised quarantine legislation was oblivious to the country's needs. In fact, detailed and reasonably elaborate quarantine instructions would have been essential to offer the only possible effective protection to the nation. Whereas the new ordinances most weakly defined measures for the empire's ocean borders, they lazily suggested applying the same measures to Russia's wide and differentiated land borders with both Asia and the rest of Europe. Once the epidemic was in the country, the instructions did not provide for any medical surveillance at all. Only in 1892, when the epidemic was already moving faster than any governmental regulations could halt it, did the state issue a law on the sanitary observation of river transportation.[88] Important practical questions for implementing sanitary surveillance, such as the build-up of medical barracks and their provision with medical supplies and personnel, which had been regulated in rigorous detail in 1841, were now simply left to the goodwill of local authorities. It was precisely by ignoring the practical problems at a local level, as the analysis of Saratov's cholera epidemic in 1892 will show, that the tsarist government had not learned the most important lesson from all previous encounters with cholera. At the same time, the revised rules allowed free application of quarantine procedures. Whilst legislation, in theory, broke with Russia's tradition of strong state intervention, there was little change in the arrangements made for coping with the cholera during the outbreaks of 1871 and 1872. And when plague broke out in 1878 at Vetlianka, a small village at the Volga River in Astrakhan' province, the tsarist government demonstrated its willingness to enforce the most brutal quarantine measures if faced with a national health threat.[89] Lacking in rigidity, the quarantine regulations opened the way for local administrators to ignore contemporary medical opinion and, as it turned out, invited coercion. Such combination proved fatal in Russia's fifth encounter with cholera.

Yet the consequences of miasmatist theory reached far beyond 1892. Localism inevitably affected the complex relationships between the tsarist government and the medical profession. Entangled in the struggle between central power and local interests, the vast majority of doctors outside St Petersburg would reject modern laboratory medicine even as late as 1905. As we shall see, Pettenkofer's theory was much more congenial to them to validate their position and to use their medical knowledge to exercise power. Only by appreciating the complexity of the indissoluble connections between medical science and political interests is it possible to understand why Russia experienced the most devastating cholera outbreak of the century in 1892. And for these reasons, it was only in 1925 that Russia became free from cholera.

Conclusion

On the European continent, the Russian Empire was the country most frequently and most violently attacked by cholera over the course of the nineteenth century. Although Russian state policies, medical discussions and social responses paralleled developments in western Europe during the epidemic's early history, Russia's cholera experience began to diverge from the rest of the continent after 1850. The new quarantine legislation, revised under the pressure of powerful international economic interests, could not effectively protect a country which did not embark on sanitary reform before the end of the nineteenth century. At the same time, Pettenkofer's influential medical discoveries, which delegated anti-epidemic combat to the local level, challenged Europe's only autocratic state at the core of its political beliefs. The entanglement of medical theories and political programme was the major reason why Russia was just as unprepared for cholera's fifth visitation as it was for the epidemic's first.

2   Saratov on the eve of the epidemic

Saratov was a cholera-stricken place. The city was located at the dividing point between the two main tracts along which diseases travelled from one end of Russia to the other: the Volga from south to north and the Orenburg–Tambov route from east to west. In times of cholera Saratov was therefore particularly volatile. In 1830, the disease killed nearly 2,200 people out of 35,000 inhabitants within one month.[1] The second onslaught in 1848 again cost several thousand victims.[2] The third and fourth pandemics were less virulent, yet even in 1872 the city counted 2,468 cases and 1,422 deaths.[3] Such mortality figures placed Saratov in a row with Russia's traditional urban cholera centres: Astrakhan', Baku, Ekaterinoslav, Kiev, Kursk, Moscow, Orenburg, Podol'sk, Poltava, Tambov, St Petersburg, Voronezh and Chernigov.

To the central government in St Petersburg, Saratov was not only of geographical and medical significance, but also of social and political significance during cholera epidemics. The city was infamous throughout the empire for the violent social unrest which had been provoked by the epidemic in 1830 and which had threatened to paralyse local as well as national administrative authorities. Starting with the first pandemic, central officials consequently regarded Saratov as a key centre from which to coordinate Russia's defence against cholera. The establishment of the first national cholera commission in the city in 1830 secured Saratov's place in the medical history of Russia.[4]

It comes as no surprise that by the end of the nineteenth century cholera, held a prominent place in Saratov's collective memory. The city's first tourist guide, published in 1881, regarded the epidemics of 1830 and 1848 as a matter of course in Saratov's historical development.[5] Likewise, to the local historical society the recurrent occurrence of cholera presented a milestone in the city's history comparable to other major regional events such as the Pugachev revolt, the peasant emancipation and the plague at Vetlianka in 1878–79.[6]

Yet the most devastating cholera onslaught of the century hit Saratov and the empire as late as 1892 – at a time when in western European countries cholera epidemics abated as a result of dramatic sanitary improvements. From its outset in May until 1 December 1892, cholera claimed 555,010 cases in the empire, 267,880 of which proved fatal. European Russia counted 331,077 cases and 151,626 deaths.[7] In absolute numbers of sickness and death the 1892 epidemic was only exceeded by the outbreaks in 1831 (466,457 cases and 197,069 deaths) and 1848 (1,742,439 cases and 690,150 deaths).[8] With a mortality rate of 45.8 per thousand, however, the epidemic in 1892 was much more virulent than in any other preceding year.[9] Saratov, again, ranked among the most severely stricken places. Between 15 June and 31 August the city officially recorded 4,211 cholera cases and 2,210 (52.4%) deaths.[10]

Locally and nationally, such devastation was most alarming. Until mid-century, cholera had no medical explanation. Almost everywhere in Europe, the epidemic took a heavy toll of human life and caused massive social suffering by triggering off fear and violence. By 1892, however, cholera's epidemiology was established. Since John Snow's and Pettenkofer's findings in the 1850s and 1860s, the connection between the spread of the epidemic and conditions of sanitation and hygiene had been drawn. In western European countries, improvements in public health, sewage control, housing conditions and water supply, though not directly brought about by cholera epidemics, had indisputably led to a general decline of epidemic visitations. Finally, the discovery of the *vibrio cholerae* by Robert Koch in 1883 revealed the causal agent of the disease and provided the scientific explanation for the link between its dissemination and polluted water.[11] By contrast, in Saratov and the tsarist empire in general the earlier cholera outbreaks had not effected any improvement in sanitation and public health at all.

This chapter considers the factors that made Saratov such a favourable breeding ground for the bacillus as late as 1892. It introduces the city by surveying the economic and social changes following the Great Reforms; it looks at the problems resulting from urban expansion, rapid population growth and increased mobility; it investigates Saratov's medical topography and its pattern of diseases; finally, it discusses the available medical resources and facilities as well as the key administrative institutions controlling Saratov's health on the eve of the cholera outbreak in 1892. Establishing the local setting and the medical context, the chapter provides the basis for the discussion of the main topic of this study.

City on the Volga

In the shape of an amphitheatre, Saratov extended west of the River Volga. The heart of the city was located on the stage adjacent to the river. Stretching for seven versts along the Volga (from which it was separated by a sandbank), the town sloped upwards into a chain of hills by which it was enclosed to the north-west (*Sokolov* hills) and to the south-west (*Lysy* hills).

When founded in 1590 on the eastern side of the river, Saratov had originally begun as a military outpost to secure Russia's still unsettled south-eastern borderland. The fortress was refounded in 1674, four years after its invasion by Stenka Razin, and relocated at the right western bank of the river. Its new and safer location between hills and ravines placed Saratov in a position to gain economic importance, and it was founded as a town with a marketplace in its centre, offices for state representatives as well as a cathedral.[12]

Two important state-directed initiatives fostered Saratov's economic growth during the eighteenth century: the opening of salt mine operations at Lake Elton in the 1740s, 136 miles south-east of Saratov, and the settlement of the city and its hinterland by German, French and Swiss colonists as well as by religious sectarians and peasants under Catherine the Great. It was they who started to use the region's fertile soil for the growing of grain and who, already by the beginning of the nineteenth century, had vitally linked Saratov's future to the rich black earth lands in the northern part of the province.[13]

The Pugachev rebellion eventually marked the crucial turning point in Saratov's administrative history.[14] In order to establish control over Russia's unruly south-eastern area Catherine the Great bestowed upon Saratov the status of general governorship (*namestnichestvo*) and thus created a new regional administrative centre midway on the Volga between Kazan' and Astrakhan'. By the early nineteenth century, the former fortress was firmly incorporated into the administrative framework of the empire, holding out the promise of further development into a commercial pivot of the entire middle and lower Volga.

Saratov's development into a commercial centre of the entire middle and lower Volga region in the course of the nineteenth century was based on two main pillars: the Volga and the northern black earth districts of the province.[15] The appearance of the first steamboat on the river in the 1820s heralded a revolution in river transportation which fundamentally changed the economic life of the whole region. Astrakhan', Saratov, Samara, Simbirsk, Kazan' and eventually Tsaritsyn became booming centres of trade and commerce during the nineteenth century. Located on an increasingly efficient, cheap, fast and safe trading route from Central Asia through the Caspian up to the Baltic Sea, Saratov was passed by exported products from the south – fish from Astrakhan', salt from Lake Elton, oil from Baku – which were on their way to Rybinsk, Moscow and St Petersburg. Wood, in turn, went downstream towards Astrakhan'. Other cargo moving along the river included linseed-oil, cotton and cast iron.

Yet the most important product for the city's prosperity was grain. From 1870 Saratov was connected to its north-western districts (Serdolsk, Atkarsk, Saratov) through the construction of the Saratov–Tambov railway. At the same time, the first major rail link with Moscow in 1871 (Riazan'–Urals railway) provided access to the rich iron supplies of the Urals.[16] The connection to the central regions, the Baltic and Black Sea ports, and to the Caucasus and central Asia significantly activated the cultivation of grain in the former distant south-east area and offered the possibility for the production to reach the domestic as well as the foreign market. The favourable transportation network delineated the leading sectors of Saratov's booming economy at the end of the century: the province came to be a major producer of grain in the whole empire, and its capital emerged as an entrepôt for the processing and trans-shipment of grain from its huge agricultural hinterland.

It is difficult to gain an idea of the scale of Saratov's trading activities as reliable numbers are difficult to come by. Following the Bulletin of Finances, Industry, and Commerce (*Vestnik finansov, promyshlennosti i torgovli*), the city provided

17 million pud of bread at a total value of 11 million rubles in 1878. According to official data from the city duma, Saratov shipped 7 million pud of grain in 1880 while receiving 4 millon pud for further transportation via railway. In addition, there arrived 1,772,000 pud of fish, 3 million pud of salt, 16,775,000 pud of wood, and 3,625,000 pud of fruits, iron and paraffin. In total, the port processed 20 millon pud of grain, 3 million pud of fish and 4 million pud of salt. In 1897 it imported more than 56 million pud of freight to the value of 11 million rubles; 7.8 million pud to the value of 6.6 million rubles were shipped from the city.[17]

Although the role of industry in Saratov intensified, especially during the last decade of the nineteenth century, the city remained predominantly a commercial and administrative centre even as late as at the beginning of the twentieth century. To be sure, the biggest factories of the province (mills and distilleries) were concentrated first and foremost in the two cities of Saratov and Tsaritsyn. Most important was the processing of raw materials, above all food products such as grain, oil and tobacco, for trans-shipment on the river. Concerning milling, in particular, Saratov was second in importance only to Nizhnii Novgorod among the cities on the Volga. At the beginning of the 1890s the six mechanical mills in the city processed 8 million pud of flour.[18] The city also concentrated the whole tobacco production of the province, its second distinguishing industrial enterprise, as well as creameries.

Yet industrial development in Saratov needs to be understood in relative terms. In the 1890s Saratov was not a factory town. There were very few large-scale enterprises, and they occupied only 2,362 workers in total. An urban labouring population thus remained, even by the 1890s, relatively small. The largest factories in Saratov city at that time (mainly flour mills and tobacco firms) did not have more than 100 to 150 workers on their payroll.[19] The remaining enterprises, bell factories, saw-mills, printing houses and others, employed fewer than 100, and mostly fewer than 50 workers.

The situation gradually changed with the shift from agricultural commodities to the processing of raw material, especially metal. In the 1890s metal processing industry in Saratov was only in its incipience and included the Otto Bering factory (founded in 1888), four iron foundries built in 1891 and most notably the Volga steel works (*Volzhskii Staleliteinyi zavod*), which was built in 1898 in *Uvek*, the southern periphery of the city. In 1901, eventually, the city's largest employer was the Riazan'–Urals railway workshop, which employed 3,190 workers.

But even at the beginning of the twentieth century large-scale industrial enterprises in Saratov did not exist. Urbanisation along the Volga, as opposed to the Ural, was based on commercial and not industrial activity. Typical for Saratov, besides trade and commerce, were small privately owned mini-enterprises. Thus, in 1891, 2,362 workers were paralleled by 8,420 artisans, a number which rose to 20,903 in 1904.[20] They were working in tiny workshops as shoemakers, joiners, blacksmiths, bricklayers or in other crafts.[21]

As a new town which had developed more or less in accordance with prescribed plans, Saratov created the impression of being one of Russia's "well-built" cities.[22] The municipal plan most graphically illustrates the impact of planning and systematic regulation. Enclosed within a ring formed by the Great Garden Street (*Bol'shaia Sadovaia Ulitsa*), the whole city mainly consisted of regularly laid out quarters confined by straight and wide streets leading into two main directions – from the *Sokolov* hills to the Volga and from the *Lysy* hills to the Volga. Less regular streets and quarters were to be found in Saratov's north-eastern corner right at the river. This was Saratov's oldest part, the so-called old city (*staryi gorod*), which had been built before the first urban plan had been developed in 1812. From here, the city had extended over the nineteenth century.[23]

Commercial and industrial growth altered the physical appearance of the city almost beyond recognition. Gradually, the city centre shifted from its location right at the banks to what came to be the first administrative district, bound by the *Aleksandrovskaia, Konstantinovskaia, Astrakhanskaia* and *Moskovskaia* streets. At the end of the nineteenth century, this was Saratov's better-off district and a centre of commerce and trade. It contained the most fashionable shops of the city, a number of Saratov's best restaurants and luxurious hotels as well as public buildings such as the theatre and the redaction of the local newspaper.

Adjoining to the north-east was the second district confined by the *Nikol'skaia, Kamyshinskaia, Aleksandrovskaia,* and *Tartarskaia* streets. The distinguishing features of this relatively small area were the public buildings of the merchant society and the nobility. Finally, the third, and still central, district encompassed the territory of the *staryi gorod* in the north-eastern corner of the city as well as part of the area between the first and second districts and the river banks. It contained the old cathedral and main administrative buildings such as the court, the treasury and the provincial government.

Whereas the first, second and third districts concentrated Saratov's commercial activity, its administrative, financial and cultural life, the new factories were built on the city's margins, in particular in the south-eastern periphery. The newly arriving workers settled in the marginal fourth, fifth, sixth and seventh districts, which already emerged outside the city's confinement. In addition, three small suburbs developed at the end of the nineteenth century: the *Soldatskaia* settlement (*sloboda*) in the east, the *Monastyrskaia* settlement in the north, and the *Agafonovskii* and *Mikhailovskii* settlements in the north-east on one of the slopes of the *Lysy* hills.

Two ravines cut the city into three geographical parts thereby constituting three socially, economically and culturally distinct units with divergent medical histories. The bigger ravine, which was actually a whole system of ravines named *Glebuchev* after Saratov's governor (*voevoda*) Glebov in 1674, took its beginning at the bottom of the *Sokolov* hills in the north-west and ran through the whole city down to the Volga in the north-east. Criss-crossing one-fifth of the urban territory it provided a natural border between the city centre and Saratov's salubrious northern boroughs, known among the population as *gory* (hills). To the south, the centre was naturally confined by the *Beloglinskii* ravine, which crossed the city from the *Lysy* hills in the south-west to the Volga in the south-east and thus separated a third vicinity from the centre. It was these ravines which presented the most critical factor in the health of the city. A major sanitary problem, they put Saratov's population at a high risk of catching infectious diseases and epidemics.

Sites of infection

In 1885 N.V. Ekk read a paper to the Society of Russian Physicians (*obshchestvo russkikh vrachei*) in St Petersburg 'on the extraordinary mortality in Russia and the need for "sanitation"'.[24] The talk, which asserted that Russia's indisputably high mortality rates were caused by the lack of preventive measures against diseases, resulted in the establishment of a special commission in 1886 endowed with the task to investigate measures for improving the state of the nation's health. Although the famous *Botkin Commission*, named after its renowned head, the internist and court physician Sergei Botkin, soon ceased its activity, it spawned public concern about the empire's sombre medical conditions, especially in view of the renewed cholera menace facing Europe as of 1881.[25] From now on, at the latest, Russia's high mortality rates were officially recognised as a major cause of state concern.[26] Ekk's talk marked the beginning of Russia's programme of national sanitation (*ozdorovlenie*).[27]

The middle and lower Volga, as national and local reports agreed, was a particularly unhealthy place to live even when compared to most other parts of Russia.[28] In Saratov, death loomed large. Mortality figures for the years 1894–1906 establish the insalubrity of the city. Annual mortality rates ran up to rates of 36.8 to 45.5 per thousand during the years from 1893 to 1904. Examining the period from 1891 to 1903, P.N. Sokolov, sanitary physician in Saratov from 1894–1904, estimated an average annual mortality of 40.7 per thousand.[29] These figures did not only fall far behind international standards.[30] They also surpassed the average mortality rate of European Russia (36.7 per thousand), where some cities could favourably compare with western European capitals.[31] Reval's mortality rate, for instance, was 25.6 per thousand, Tver' stood at 23.5, and Kaluga at 23.2 per thousand. Even lower death rates were to be found in Khar'kov (19.7 per thousand) and Vitebsk (18.5).[32] Yet a rate of 40 per thousand, or even higher, was representative for cities on the middle and lower Volga, a region where life expectancy at birth generally was lower as in most other parts of European Russia. In Saratov, according to a local physician, it stood at 55 years in 1903.[33]

Outlining the reasons for these disastrous figures requires extreme caution. Given the scarcity of statistical material, the uncertainties of diagnosis and thus the vagueness of the classification of diseases, an estimation of the role of specific diseases in the overall mortality can only be an estimate at best. Almost 50% of Saratov's high mortality rate was attributed to the city's monstrous infant mortality, which accounted on average for 33% of the annual mortality of the city's population as a whole. At the beginning of the twentieth century, Saratov's annual infant mortality stood approximately at 41.4 per hundred live births.[34] The most common causes of infant death were all sorts of gastro-intestinal disorders, which on average carried away about 2,000 children annually.[35] Other childhood infections, notably measles, scarlet fever, diphtheria and smallpox, added another 200–300 deaths.[36]

Infant mortality was highest during the summer months, reaching its peak from mid-May until August. Adults of all age groups, by contrast, were severely and regularly affected by typhus and typhoid. Although the death rate from both diseases was relatively low, these maladies were endemic in late imperial Saratov and never ceased during the entire period under consideration.[37] Caused by inadequate sanitation, they frequently accompanied cholera epidemics. Just before the cholera outbreak in the summer of 1892, a severe typhus epidemic had absorbed the medical, financial and administrative resources of Saratov province.

These patterns of diseases were highly indicative of severe sanitary neglect, filth and unhygienic living conditions. In fact, according to a poignant article, published in *The Week* (*Nedelia*) in 1891, the pulse of Saratov's social life was to be found in the city's sanitary society. The article lamented, however, that 'unfortunately, the reason for the city's social life is Saratov's weakest spot, its unbelievable sanitary conditions.' It continued: 'Along the city flows an entire ocean of water yet within the city one will not find a glass of pure water. [. . .] In the Volga capital the cemeteries, for example, are built on the slopes of hills and the products of decay, together with urban sewage, flow down to the ground of a ravine into the river just at the opening of the reception pipe of the waterpipe.'[38] In fact, dirt and excrement, the unavoidable by-products of urban growth, presented the prime challenges facing Saratov one year before the cholera outbreak. As the article in *Nedelia* pointed out, the city's two major uncontrolled factors were sewage and water.[39]

Like most other Russian cities at the end of the nineteenth century, Saratov possessed no sewage system.[40] Sewage collection was contracted out to private entrepreneurs, who were paid to empty the urban cesspits of kitchen and domestic waste and to collect dead animals from the streets; these people also carted off the garbage to the municipal dump, where they dug the ditches to be filled with garbage. After 14 or 15 days the ditches were covered with sand.[41]

Constant demands in the newspapers for some regulation of the sewage problem reveal that the procedure was hardly organised at all, insufficiently controlled and almost not existent. The municipal dump was located beyond the city at the eastern side of the *Lysy* hills. The way to it was so badly constructed that it was impassable during spring and autumn. It was much too small, had long been overfilled, and as a result the whole place had turned into a cesspit swamp by 1888.[42] Worst of all, sewage percolated through the soil into a little ravine and travelled back into the city. Medical officials were not alone in pointing to the permanent threat the dump posed to the health of Saratov's inhabitants. Officers from the military camp complained that the dump severely contaminated the water in the wells used by the soldiers. Furthermore, it created a dreadful smell for the soldiers.[43]

Sewage collection was totally insufficient because the service confined itself to the buildings belonging to the municipality. The cleanliness of the tenement courtyards was left to private initiative and funds.[44] As a result, courtyards and streets functioned as cesspits as well as public urinals. A report to the municipal uprava in 1899 estimated that less than one-tenth of the urban waste was removed from the city.[45] The remainder stayed partly within the city limits, severely polluting streets, marketplaces and other important public spaces. Some was dispelled into the ravines and from here ran down into the Volga. During the winter lots of garbage and refuse were simply dumped into the Volga under the cover of snow.[46]

Complaints about the sanitary habits of Saratov's population filled the local newspapers. Sanitary facilities were bad throughout the city, yet nothing demonstrated the dismal state of waste removal practices better than the ravines. The *Glebuchev* ravine (respectively the *gory*), in particular, was infamous for its dramatic state of sanitation.[47] When Nikolai Chizhov, author of the canalisation project for Saratov, visited the city in 1901, he had to admit: 'Without doubt, those present and every inhabitant of Saratov in general acknowledge the sanitary horror of the Glebuchev ravine. I have heard about it for a long time, but what I have seen exceeds all my former imagination.'[48]

The ravines presented the most perilous breeding ground for infectious diseases in the whole city, in large part as a result of their housing without any consideration of building and sanitary regulations. In fact, the urban plan from 1812 had prohibited settlement there.[49] Yet as explosive population growth swamped available amenities and Saratov had no space for expansion, the ravines presented the only way out. At the end of the nineteenth century, they housed the large majority of Saratov's urban poor, especially the new arrivals who came to the city in search for work. In the words of a municipal medical report, these people lived "worse than animals". They were squeezed into little wooden hovels, which spread over the combs as well as the bottom of the ravine. Apartments were commonly used as multi-family dwellings. Most of them lacked windows and suffered from permanent dampness, especially if located at the bottom of the ravines. Courts and lanes were in the worst state imaginable, and the streets were so narrow and crooked that this area of the city was largely inaccessible.[50]

Yet most alarming in terms of cholera, both ravines had steadily developed into Saratov's universal sewer. Not only the ravine population, but also the residents of the adjacent central parts of the city used them as a fast and cheap way to get rid of their excrement. When Grigorii Khlopin, professor of hygiene and consultative member of the Medical Council of the Ministry of Internal Affairs, visited Saratov in 1908, he drew a grim picture of the *Glebuchev* ravine: earth-closets, stables, and cow-sheds scattered amongst the other buildings were cleared by simply heaping all the dung onto the slopes; watersheds of dirty water came from public wash houses and various trades; in addition, some of Saratov's entrepreneurs deliberately carried refuse to the ravine in order to fill it up and thus extend the plot of land on which they had built their business. Saturated with sewage, the soil of the ravines spawned an unbearable stench. Puddles, mud and moisture were omnipresent. Amidst the stench and debris, people moved freely in pursuit of domestic work. Children used the slopes as playgrounds and animals quickly conveyed dirt and disease-causing agents from the ravine to the adjacent courts and other parts of the city.[51]

To make matters worse, the ravines were hazardously linked with Saratov's second microbial circuit, the river banks.[52] There, much of the garbage accumulated, which was directly discharged into the Volga through the ravines and a few drain pipes. A powerful factor in Saratov's trade and commercial activity, the banks also collected all the waste from those industrial factories, in particular mills and saw-mills, which were located on the river, and during navigation time, the refuse from the ships and barges as well.

Notoriously unhealthy, life on the banks deeply impacted the health of the whole city. The large majority of sailors, peddlers, clerks, and workers at the mills, numbering an estimated 4,000 people daily, lived in the *Glebuchev* ravine or on the banks themselves.[53] They spent the whole day at the Volga using the river water for domestic and economic purposes. People caught fish, which was later sold at the marketplace; fruit vendors washed their vegetables and fruits; laundresses washed the linens of the whole city. Bathing in the Volga was also a popular recreation. Not surprisingly, when it came to diseases and epidemics, the bacterial exchange between the banks and the ravines was rapid and intensive. Both areas faced the highest morbidity and mortality rates in Saratov, and it was here that most people would fall victim in the summer of 1892.

The sanitary havoc created by the lack of proper sewage disposal was only exacerbated by Saratov's inadequate water supply system.[54] Several sources provided drinking water to the population. The residents of the city centre could gain water from a water-supply system based on water pipes which had been built

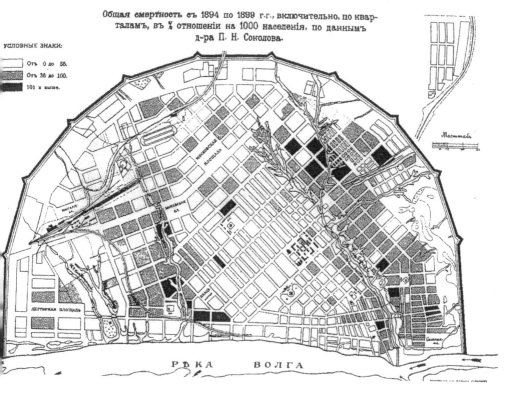

Figure 1 Saratov's mortality, 1894–1899, N.I. Matveev, *Gorod Saratov v sanitarnom otnoshenii* (Saratov, 1906).

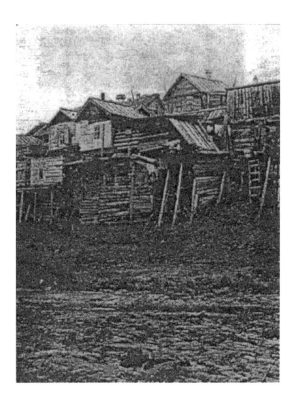

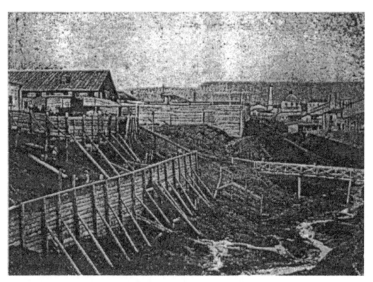

Figure 2 Glebuchev ravine, N.I. Matveev, *Gorod Saratov v sanitarnom otnoshenii* (Saratov, 1906).

by an English company in 1874–75.[55] The reservoirs of the water system were located on the Tarkhanka, one of the arms of the Volga on which Saratov was built. The Tarkhanka ran parallel to the Volga, separated from it by a sandbank. It was linked to the Volga by a canal. In the northern part of the city, where the Tarkhanka formed a kind of bay, the city's water pipe found its source. The water flowed into basins where it was filtered by six sand filters. Thereafter it was collected in a bigger basin (with 'clean' water) from where it was distributed through the city in water pipes. The inhabitants could obtain their water either through taps in the courtyards or – for those whose houses were not connected to the water pipe – through water stalls on the streets.[56]

Apart from the fact that only the city centre was provided with water pipes, the major deficiency of the water supply system was that it supplied the city with notoriously foul water.[57] The water was already severely contaminated at its source. The bay proved to be a very convenient boat yard and during the fall and winter, roughly 150 boats used this place as a wharf, with some of them even staying here for the whole year. As a result, the opening of the water pipe was often obstructed by the boats, which severely polluted the water right from the beginning. Fish-ponds located 50 metres further up the pipe were another source of contamination. The river banks right at the water pipe also provided space for wood piles, all sorts of garbage, and for the washing of linen in the same water which later flowed through the water pipe; finally, notwithstanding the existence of six filters, the city was far from receiving filtered water, since six filters were simply not enough. Moreover, filtering capacities were significantly reduced in the spring and autumn when the water in the Tarkhanka was most severely polluted.[58]

To the vast majority of Saratov's population, which was not provided with any water pipes, the major sources of water supply were either water wells or the Volga River itself. Wells played a fatal role in the health of Saratov. As their surface was commonly on the same level as the soil, they were directly surrounded by sludge and refuse. Usually, they were not covered and cleaned only once or sometimes twice a year; they served as receptacles for dead animals and other filth. Not surprisingly, chemical analyses of the water wells in the *Beloglinskii* ravine in 1905 showed that the water was laden with ammonia and nitric acid. A bacteriological investigation from the same year identified between 2,000 and 3,000 bacterial colonies in the water.[59]

By the end of the nineteenth century, the Volga had long stopped meeting the needs for clean water. The city's contribution to polluting the river was as well known as their unsatisfactory sanitary state itself. Saratov, an official report stated, could compete with Nizhnii Novgorod in its ability to pollute the Volga.[60] But it was not only urban waste which heavily polluted the river. The most alarming agents of pollution at the end of the nineteenth century were oil and mazut, which were commonly transported on barges. The yearly losses of their cargo as a result of accidents were estimated to be 400,000 pud.[61] Breakage and flooding of barges were such frequent events that Saratov's urban population swiftly invented a new handicraft from it. It skimmed off the oily film from the surface of the river, let it stand and thereafter sold it or used it itself.[62] As national and local health officials were quick to point out, the new substances not only damaged the river's fauna but also generated new diseases. One Volga physician observed among his patients gastro-intestinal diseases which reminded him of cholera. As it turned out, the disease was caused by too much use of Volga water. At first, only nine patients were affected by it, but in 1898 the number already ran up to 62. The increase stood in a striking parallel to the increase of oil freight conveyed along the Volga.[63] At the end of the nineteenth century, the enormous significance of the river in spreading epidemic diseases became uncontested by contemporaries. The cholera epidemic would prove their point in dramatic fashion.

Migrants, peasants, sailors

Cholera is a water-borne disease, the transmission of which is facilitated by human communication. Its very rapid spread across Europe during the nineteenth century was closely linked to the development of a modern transportation network. Russia illustrates the point perfectly. The epidemic in 1892 spread with unprecedented rapidity due to the construction of a new railway network stretching from the Caucasus to Poland.[64] The opening of the Transcaucasian railway in 1888, the main route through which cholera entered Russia, replaced transportation through camels and cut the journey between Samarkand and the Caspian Sea to 60 hours.[65] Once arrived in urbanising Europe, the *vibrio*'s spread was promoted by over-crowded housing conditions in the rapidly expanding cities. In the case of western Europe, historians have therefore concluded, cholera was a result of the Industrial Revolution.

In Russia, the industrial boom reached its height between 1895 and 1900. It presents one of the most essential features of the period under consideration. As elsewhere in Europe at earlier times, a particularly critical aspect of the ongoing economic and social transformation was the massive migration of peasants in search of work.[66] Swamping the city's urban infrastructures and opportunities for employment, they confronted urban authorities with major health and sanitation problems. In late-nineteenth- and early-twentieth-century Saratov, peasant migrants formed an essential background to the health hazards the city was exposed to. Moreover, these ever journeying hordes of people carried diseases rapidly from Saratov up and down the Volga and across the country. Any outbreak of cholera in one of the Volga cities thus directly threatened the empire. In fact, the migrant movement played a fatal role in the epidemic history of Saratov, the Volga, and the empire in general.

Saratov was a 'migrant-city' (Brower 1990). Through peasant migrants, the city expanded rapidly during the second half of the nineteenth century. Between 1850 and 1900, its population had more than doubled, rising from 59,400 in 1850 to 143,431 in 1900. Yet further frenetic urban growth – and the urban problems involved in it – still lay ahead following the boom years of Russian industrialisation in the late 1890s. With 235,700 inhabitants in 1914, Saratov exceeded in size any other provincial capital on the middle and lower Volga.[67] Being the ninth-largest city of the empire it ranked among the big urban centres in Russia and compared with other major European cities such as Oslo, Prague, Bordeaux and Genoa.[68]

Migration was the major factor behind these numbers. With urban fertility rates beginning to be slightly higher than rates of mortality from 1895, Saratov's annual natural rate of increase between 1897 and 1911 stood at only 0.643%. This figure fell far behind the average natural increase rate of other cities within European Russia (1.58%).[69]

The large majority of these peasant labourers came from a narrow radius of surrounding provinces, particularly Penza, Simbirsk and Tambov, but also from the northern districts (Khvalynsk, Kuznetsk, Vol'sk) of Saratov province itself.[70] They were joined by peasants from the provinces of Viatka, Kostroma and Nizhnii Novgorod.[71] Furthermore, Saratov was an important stop for a massive migration movement which floated from the Central Black Earth Zone and northern Ukraine to the south and south-east. The commercial grainbelt which offered these peasants the prospect of additional income extended across the steppe from Kherson, Tauride and Ekaterinoslav provinces in the west through the Don Cossack region and up to Saratov and Samara provinces in the Volga River Basin to the east.[72]

Table 2.1 Population of the 10 biggest Russian cities, 1863–1914

City	1863	1897	1914
St Petersburg	539,500	1,264,900	2,118,500
Moscow	462,500	1,038,600	1,762,700
Riga	77,500	282,200	558,000
Kiev	68,400	247,700	520,500
Odessa	119,000	403,800	499,500
Tiflis	60,800	159,600	307,300
Khar'kov	52,000	174,000	244,700
Saratov	84,400	137,100	235,700
Baku	13,900	111,900	232,200
Ekaterinoslav	19,900	112,800	211,100

Figures are from A.G. Rashin, *Naselenie Rossii za 100 let (1811–1913gg.)* (Moscow, 1956), p. 93.

Peasants were compelled to find additional income as wage labourers in either agricultural or non-agricultural sectors. Russia's south and south-east were heavily affected by the growing depression of Russian agriculture that accompanied industrial growth. In addition to general low productivity peasants faced shortages of land and steadily increasing tax burdens. In comparison to other regions in European Russia, taxes reached the highest levels in Saratov and Samara provinces.[73] Rural overpopulation placed additional strains on the resources of the Russian countryside. And, according to Aleksandr P. Engel'gardt, governor of the province from 1901 to 1903, the most important reasons for the decline of agriculture and rising rural poverty in Saratov province were droughts and increasingly frequent crop failures.[74] Significantly, Saratov was one of the most hard-hit provinces by the famine in 1891–92.[75]

On the whole middle and lower Volga the city of Saratov was the main magnet for these impoverished people. In 1892, it concentrated 43% of the industrial production of the whole province.[76] Saratov also had the highest demand for unskilled labourers. In 1901, the local hiring market recruited up to 3,000 people on Sundays and holidays.[77] The nearest industrial centre was Tsaritsyn, which underwent a remarkable industrial boom in the late 1890s and became a serious competitor to the provincial capital. Yet most importantly, Saratov and Tsaritsyn provided the main gateways to the rich grain supplies of the southern steppe. The large majority of the newly arrived seasonal workers embarked in Saratov for hiring markets in Samara province. Those who could not find work there during the harvest went back to Saratov and set off towards the Urals, the Don Cossack region, the Caucasus as well as booming cities such as Baku and Astrakhan'.[78]

Precise quantification of these wandering people is hardly possible. By the 1890s literature as well as statistical investigations on the newly emerged migrant question were rare and difficult to carry out. The Russian government imposed a policy of strict control on the migrant movement through an internal passport system within the village communes.[79] Yet leading a nomadic existence and drifting from job to job, this was a population in permanent flux which evaded any geographical and social definition. A study carried out on behalf of the Ministry of Agriculture in 1896 estimated the number of peasant workers journeying through Saratov city in 1895 at approximately 60,000. According to a commission of the province's sanitary congress (*sanitarnyi s"ezd*) in 1900, the number of peasants travelling through Saratov city twice a year – before and after the harvests – came to 50,000.[80]

Municipal and provincial physicians frequently pointed to the danger these vagrants posed to Saratov's health even at normal times. Peasant labourers were at high risk of catching the most various types of diseases on their way to the city. Saratov received the first migrants at the beginning of February. Long journeys of 200 to 300 verst on foot exposed the wayfarers to intensely cold weather, hunger, diseases and death. A telling document on the sanitary aspects of the *chernorabo-chii vopros* (the question of black, i.e. unskilled labourers) in Saratov city is a study by A. Ershov, who was appointed sanitary physician in the city in 1907. His investigation provides a detailed picture of the seasonal workers in Saratov province and its capital, their reasons for migration, and their life on their way to as well as in the city. His report left a vivid account of the social, economic and hygienic conditions a peasant from Kazan' endured on his journey:

> I left home on 7 January and went along the Volga all the time, sometimes alone, sometimes in peasants' co-operatives (*artely*) with fellow-countrymen and other travellers. Ate whatever came into my hands. Spent the nights in the villages, they have nightshelters everywhere nowadays wherever you go. They are afraid of letting our brothers in peasant houses. It is dirty in the nightshelters, dark. . . . There you drag on the damp floor. In the morning you take your knapsack and again with the Lord to the next shelter. There, you see, again fifty people, some of whom sleep on the floor, and some upstairs. Everybody driven by the need. Well, so am I. I am going for the seventh time. When I was fifteen I started as a fishmonger. I used to earn five to six rubles but now I get 20–25 a month. I look after the workers. That is sort of an overseer. People are from all ends of the earth, from Saratov, from the

north, and from Astrakhan', kalmyks, cossacks, other fellows, my brother –
Kazanets – many of all of these. Up to 30,000, they say. We work until
November, until the frost starts, up to the weather. We start on 15 March and
go for seven to eight months. We hardly live. Money, 150–200 rubles, all
goes to the family. You only keep eight rubles for the way in the next spring.
And that's that. And it would be enough if diseases didn't catch you. And
now the food is finished. Obviously, I get through like this![81]

Sanitary anxieties depended heavily on the ebb and flow of migration. Despite its
many forms and patterns, migrant labour (*otkhozhii promysel*) followed definite
routes and took place in stages. Scholarship on migration in the Central Industrial
Region has shown that migrants went to the cities in the winter and returned to the
villages during harvest-time.[82] By contrast, on the Volga the movement depended
on navigation schedules and lasted from late winter until late autumn. It reached
its peak in June and July when masses of people flocked into the cities for work
on the docks. Like most Volga cities, Saratov grew especially during the summer
– just when cholera was approaching. Most peasants travelled on foot, but many
also used the railways or came by waterway on barges and ships. Boats and ships
were foci of infections. Work on the ships as boatsmen or cooks was a popular job
for unskilled labourers.[83] In 1902, an investigation revealed that 50% of the boatsmen had contracted diseases.[84] Typically they were afflicted by typhus, gastro-
intestinal disorders, dysentery, skin and eye diseases. More importantly, they also
transported malaria and syphilis, Russia's chief communicable diseases. Malaria
most strongly affected the provinces adjacent to the Volga.[85] Saratov province
also took a prominent place in Russia in terms of syphilis with 21.1–21.7 cases
per thousand.[86] District physicians found that the disease was spread in the
villages by soldiers and peasant migrants.[87] As the ship companies rarely provided
any medical care, barges and steamers launched a huge number of sick people into
the municipal and zemstvo hospitals. Thirty per cent of the peasants in Saratov's
zemstvo hospital came from other provinces.[88] In order to manage its available
personnel and medical resources, the hospital had to discharge the sick and send
them home before they had actually regained their health.[89] In 1906, almost a
quarter of patients seeking stationary help were completely rejected.[90]

The majority of peasant migrants preferred agricultural to industrial labour. A
lot of workers alternated between the two, with many returning to the countryside
during the winter. Transient peasants posed one set of problems. Those peasants
who stayed in Saratov to constitute the bulk of the urban labour force posed others.
The estate structure of the city in 1897 as depicted in Table 2.2 illustrates the
unprecedented demographic change the city underwent beginning in the 1890s.

At the top of the social ladder was a privileged minority of nobles, merchants,
industrialists and functionaries in the city and zemstvo administration as well as
members of the free professions. Yet the vast majority of the city's population
were migrant peasants whose living conditions were stark. Only the most fortunate among them were able to find work in one of the city's factories. In 1891, out
of 130,000 people, only 2,945 were occupied in the city's industrial enterprises.

Table 2.2 Estate structure of Saratov's population in 1897

Estate	Estate figures
Nobility	8,069
Clergy	1,678
Honorary citizens	1,959
Merchants	2,051
Townspeople	52,885
Peasants	61,938

Figures from I.V. Parokh, *Ocherki istorii Saratovskogo Povolzh'ia (1894–1917)*, 2 vols (Saratov, 1999), vol. 2 (1894–1917), pp. 27.

Factory employment rose to 9,529 in 1902.[91] Most of the labourers worked as loaders or hack-drivers in Saratov's food processing industries, especially the mills.[92] Other major employers were the railway workshops and small concerns producing miscellaneous ironworks.[93] Yet factory labour was the exception. Far more numerous were the artisans and service personnel. Artisanal work was highly developed. Tailors and shoemakers proliferated; likewise, blacksmiths, bricklayers and joiners took advantage of the new opportunities in construction.[94] In 1895, 11,852 artisans had settled in the city. Their number increased to 16,767 in 1900 and to 20,903 in 1904.[95]

Factory workers lived in squalor, poverty and ill-health.[96] Standard 10–12-hour workdays in dilapidated buildings lacking any light, fresh air and heating ruined their health. An average daily salary of 1.50 rubles allowed them to buy three pasties or three pounds of fish. Yet despite their strenuous living conditions, factory labourers and artisans were in a favourable position. They could make use of the new opportunities in the growing city. Frequently, they were skilled workers enjoying the privilege of more or less permanent employment and the approximation of a living wage. They could settle in Saratov and live with the same landlord for a long time.

At the bottom of the social ladder was the casual labour force. Masses of people wound up working as day labourers at the river banks. Filling a bewildering variety of occupations, they supplied Saratov's vast demand for low-paid and unskilled outdoor labour. Most of them were dockers, carriers, hack-drivers, clerks and sailors. A large contingent also subsisted as vendors, peddlers and huxters. Ubiquitous sellers of berries, sunflower seeds, fresh and salted cucumbers, pasties with meat, rice or berries were an integral part of Saratov's economic life at the banks during the summer. *Limonadchiki*, wandering newspaper sellers and haberdashers, completed the picture. It is impossible to arrive at even approximate numbers for these people. In 1906, a medical report estimated them to number nearly 4,000 but admitted that this figure was much too small since it did not include the most abject stratum of all: the unemployed.[97]

These were Saratov's *Lantsarony*. They were despised by the local population because they were poor, dirty and illiterate; the middle classes described them as an uneducated and culturally backwards army of beggars.[98] Being unskilled, they were useless to the local economy. Yet they presented competition for the urban working forces by driving wages down.[99] At the same time they did not earn enough money to sustain themselves. Socially uprooted, they filled first the doss-houses and then went on to the hospitals, a refuge to the poor and unskilled. Often, they ended their career as *galakhi*, a popular and contemptuous term for 'a creature without definite occupation and of no fixed abode, always in ragged clothes, hungry, often drunk, wandering from one doss-house to the next'.[100]

These day labourers in particular posed a dual threat to Saratov's population: they imported diseases and were particularly susceptible to them. Earning their living from day to day, and poorly paid, they led an insecure and precarious existence. They lived in the worst slums, if lucky in the *Glebuchev* ravine, yet commonly in temporary barracks on the banks or simply in the open air. As autumn approached they filled the doss-houses, the chief strategic place in the spread of typhus in the typhus-stricken city.[101] Their typical diet consisted of cabbage soup (*shchi*) or a salted cucumber with bread and a mug of *kvas*.[102] Usually, their food was dirty, covered with filth and flies. *Kvas*, in particular, caused frequent gastro-intestinal disorders among the workers.[103] Moreover, these labourers were in daily contact with the polluted river water. They thus became ready candidates for the *vibrio*. In typical fashion, cholera entered Saratov in 1892 by means of the boatsmen on the ships. The *vibrio* ravaged the banks where people fell ill in alarming numbers. From there, the disease quickly spread to the ravines where it raged ferociously through the slums in which the labourers lived.

According to local physicians, it was the migrant population which accounted for Saratov's high disease and death ratios and which was particularly predisposed to contracting cholera in 1892. Moreover, local and national authorities alike were aware of the strategic significance of the migrant movement in times of epidemics. To improve the health of the city and of the nation it was indispensable to guarantee medical control over this movement. It was obvious, therefore, that the enormous sanitary problems caused by the social phenomenon of seasonal work could not be solved by Saratov city alone. This needed a provincial, unified organisation. Yet in contrast to Samara or Simbirsk provinces, the province of Saratov did not establish any sanitary organisation to observe, regulate and control this movement until 1904. In medical terms, the migrant movement was out of control. The final section of the chapter will ask how the effects of rapid population growth on diseases could have been mitigated on the eve of the cholera epidemic in 1892.

Local authorities and public health

When cholera threatened Saratov as late as 1892, the city was badly prepared to cope with any medical emergency. Even worse, despite many years of experience with the epidemic Saratov was struck much heavier in 1892 than in any other preceding year. The explanation for such a disastrous visitation involves more than the all-encompassing problems resulting from unprecedented population growth in a rapidly urbanising city. In the end, Saratov's medical fate corresponded to the national experience. To understand why Saratov and the empire were hit by one of the most devastating cholera epidemics of the century at a time when epidemics in western European countries had abated as a result of dramatic sanitary improvements requires an examination of public health policies as conducted at both the national and the local levels.

As contemporaries and historians have argued, the cholera onslaught of 1892 proved so fatal chiefly because Russian health administration was confused, unco-ordinated and thus inefficient. Entangled in its struggle for political dominance and power the Russian government had sloughed off financial responsibility for public health to the local governments without granting them the necessary political autonomy. Furthermore, the central institutions and officials were unwill-ing, incompetent and inept to meet the country's massive health needs.[104] In Russia, as Nancy Frieden has noted, 'health administration had failed to keep pace with advances in Western Europe'.[105]

In stark contrast to this negative evaluation, others have emphasised that the government was much more active and on alert than commonly assumed. Thus, the English contemporary observer of the epidemic Frank Clemow, a member of the Epidemiological Society of London, who worked at the English Hospital at Kronstadt at the time of the epidemic, came to a different conclusion about Russia's medical authorities at least during the epidemic.[106] He maintained 'that the Russian government was fully alive to the danger which threatened the country as soon as cholera was announced from Persia, and that on its part no effort was spared to minimise the effects of the epidemic in every possible way when once it had passed the frontier'.[107]

In fact, a look at the course of the epidemic at a particular locality offers a highly complex picture. There were huge gaps between the legislation of public health measures and their actual implementation, leaving areas of confusion as well as of autonomy. One needs to account for the severity of the epidemic at one place and its mildness at another. Tiflis, for instance, with a population of more than 100,000 inhabitants and located 18 hours by train from Baku, the centre from which the epidemic spread across the Caucasus, suffered comparatively lightly.[108]

The following section analyses the foundations of the regulatory, administra-tive and institutional system to which Saratov's municipality could resort at the end of the nineteenth century; it looks at the available medical facilities and resources the municipality could resort to during the epidemic and asks for the reasons for the city's continuous neglect of medical services; it also describes the state apparatus of anti-epidemic measures. Out of the richness and variety of late-nineteenth-century Russian medicine and public health, the section focuses on the main administrative and organisational lines which are important to understand the course of the epidemic in 1892.

The details of the history of Russian medical administration should not detain us here, but the main lines of its direction and the major difficulties which deter-mined its evolution need to be sketched. Starting with the formation of the nation state in the fifteenth century, Russia developed a highly centralised system of medical organisation.[109] State medical control was institutionalised for the first time in 1620 through the establishment of the Pharmacy Department (*aptekarskii prikaz*) under Tsar Mikhail (1613–1645).[110] Forged by continuous warfare and recurrent epidemics, medical reforms throughout the seventeenth and eighteenth centuries consolidated the state's strong role in the area of public health. Reshuffling the *aptekarskii prikaz* into the Medical Chancellery in 1721, Peter I guaranteed the state's purview over quarantine policy and military medicine as well as the development of medical education and medical science. The work of the institution suffered from chronic financial and personnel shortages, yet the decisive point to be made here is that it firmly consolidated the state's dominant role in medical administration.

Peter's successors rationalised and expanded his legacy for the whole empire. Thereby, a system developed which maintained the overall legislative and financial power at the centre while increasingly assigning the implementation of public health policy to local officials.[111] Frequent and devastating outbreaks of epidemics, in particular the Great Plague in Moscow in 1771, demonstrated that the sheer size of the empire precluded any effective epidemic control and prevention without local involvement.[112] The beginnings of an organised local health administration dated to Catherine the Great's reign. Influenced by the works of German Cameralism, the German-born Empress put public health on a broadened, civilian-oriented basis.[113] Following provincial reorganisation in the 1780s, medical boards (*vrachebnoe otdelenie*) were established in each province in 1797.[114] Operating under the auspices of the governor's or military governor's provincial administration they were mainly responsible for supervising medical personnel and institutions such as apothecary shops and hospitals as well as assisting the medical police.[115] At the central level, Catherine had replaced the Medical Chancellery by the Medical Collegium already in 1763. It was entrusted with directing the advancement of medical education, elaborating precautionary measures against epidemics and infectious diseases and expanding medical facilities for the civilian population. This also included the dispatch of practitioners to the provinces, where hospitals and pharmacies were to be built as well.[116] By the end of the eighteenth century, a highly developed apparatus of medical administration as well as an elaborated system to combat epidemics were thus in place.[117] As a final step, the Ministry of Internal Affairs, in the form of the twin institutions of the Medical Council (*Meditsinskii Sovet*) and the Medical Department (*Meditsinskii Departament*), gained authority over all aspects of civilian medical administration in 1803.[118] Both bodies remained the chief state authorities for medical affairs until 1917.

Yet despite all efforts and positive developments, especially in the field of medical science, medical care remained inadequate already in normal times, not to mention during times of epidemics. Effective and successful state supervision over the country's health was far beyond the realities of available manpower, financial resources and geographical conditions.[119] When the Crimean War exposed Russia's deplorable state of health, the Russian government embarked on a fundamental structural reform to overcome the country's deplorable state of health provision: medical care was delegated to local centres of medical organisation as manifested in the provincial zemstvo and the municipal duma.[120]

Scholars to date have studied a number of aspects of Russia's post-reform medical organisation, either on the national or on the zemstvo, i.e. provincial, level. By contrast, the development of urban medicine has been almost completely neglected.[121] A partial explanation for this neglect lies in the fact that urban health-care remained in a deplorable state until the beginning of the twentieth century – as opposed to zemstvo medicine, which witnessed a rapid development in the 1870s and 1880s. Yet if we are to understand the course of the cholera epidemic in Saratov city in 1892, it requires us to identify the role and function of municipal medicine within the net of national public health organisation during the last decades of the nineteenth century. It is beyond the purview and possibilities of this study to provide a complete survey of the functioning and development of munici-pal public health after the reforms. But it is important to sketch the complex set-up of national, regional, provincial and municipal authorities and institutions within which Saratov's public health organisation functioned. This apparatus was also activated to combat the 1892 epidemic in Saratov. Saratov's municipal administra-tion played only one (and not always the deciding) role among a number of national and provincial agencies. In analysing the institutional framework which determined the city's state of health, the following pages will also describe the medical facilities and resources in the city on the eve of the epidemic.

Legally, the municipal reform of 1870 had transferred a broad range of tasks to the newly established city councils (*duma*) and the municipal boards (*uprava*).[122] In analogy to the zemstvo statutes from 1864, municipal authorities assumed responsibility for the maintenance of urban amenities and for the provision of the population with educational facilities and public health institutions.[123] Local institutions and officials were thus to play a major role in guaranteeing the nation's health. In turn, as Nancy Frieden has argued, it was precisely in the sphere of public health where local governments could gain most authority and independ-ence. The provincial zemstva established a whole system of rural healthcare across the country. They built an extensive net of small hospitals in the provinces; they developed sophisticated medical statistics to investigate the country's health needs and to suggest necessary reforms; they conceived plans for the prevention of diseases and popularised hygienic knowledge among the peasantry. And they were most successful in the fight against epidemics. In recognition of their achievements, an additional law from 1879 authorised the zemstvo and equally the duma to take temporary and preventive measures against infectious diseases and epidemics.[124]

Notwithstanding the progress of zemstvo medicine in the 1870s and 1880s, urban local initiatives in the field of medical care and sanitary renewal remained weak. Like most other cities, Saratov saw the responsibility for public health as a financial burden in the first place. In fact, the new legislation had restricted the competence of local institutions to financial management yet had not empowered them with the responsibility for medical services.[125] Additionally, expenses for public health were considered to be optional (as opposed to the obligatory financial expenses for the maintenance of the police, for instance), with the result that medical facilities and medical care in Russia's cities were in shambles even 20 years after the reforms. In 1899, out of 50 provincial cities, 16 invested 10 kopeeks per capita for medical care, 19 between 10 and 50 kopeeks, and 6 between 50 kopeeks and 1 ruble. To compare, Petersburg invested 2.33 rubles per person.[126] Saratov financed a municipal hospital built in 1878, but otherwise, it did not establish any permanent system of medical organisation until the 1890s.[127] Instead, physicians were temporarily employed during epidemics mainly to disinfect and isolate the sick. Only in 1889 did the duma finally employ two permanent sanitary physicians who, however, were simply too few to provide medical care for a population of over 100,000 people. For the most part, therefore, medical care lay in the hands of feldshers. Vaccination, one of the tasks assigned to local authorities, was conducted in a careless and brutal manner by people who were medically untrained and inexperienced. Moreover, instead of four people for vaccination, as was officially proscribed, the city only employed two. The municipal hospital, equipped with 80 beds, served as a last resort for the destitute and was permanently overcrowded. At the same time, many poor people shied away from it, as the monthly costs of 7–15 rubles equalled between one and three monthly salaries.

Physicians were in low public esteem.[128] City-physicians, in particular, occupied the very lowest ranks within Russia's medical service.[129] Whereas zemstvo physicians had an active voice in provincial administration, municipal physicians were commonly ignored in urban public health politics. As one urban representative stated: 'You hardly ever hear about the invitation of physicians to the meetings of the duma. One is used to looking at them as if they were mercenaries without any right to vote. The opinion of any duma representative is considered higher than the opinion of physicians, even in particular questions.'[130] Municipal physicians had no medical leadership over hospitals. In practice, their activity was highly dependent not only on the decisions of municipal but also of provincial authorities. Appointments of city-physicians had to be confirmed by the provincial medical inspector and the provincial governor.[131] Moreover, city-physicians were ill-paid and overburdened. They earned between 920 and 1,225 rubles monthly as compared to 1,380 to 2,550 rubles earned by zemstvo physicians.[132] Instead of medical care they were preoccupied with forensic medical tasks and police work, such as the sanitary control of schools, markets, almshouses and brothels.

Contemporaries frequently put the blame for cities' state of health on the municipalities themselves. They accused them of general ignorance towards problems of hygiene and sanitation as well as a lack of proper education. But more than ignorance, it was the weak position of municipal health within the Russian public health system that was to blame. Municipal medicine was subordinated to national, provincial and also zemstvo medicine. A major reason for municipal inertia in the field of medical care was political obstacles. In general, local authorities were not supposed to share political power. The supervisory powers of the provincial governors and the Ministry of Internal Affairs were carefully maintained. Binding decrees (*obiazatel'nye postanovleniia*) required the approval of the governor and their implementation depended on the state police.[133]

Moreover, legislation on the local level was kept imprecise and unclear. Municipalities, zemstva and the provincial governments constantly struggled over their responsibilities concerning the implementation of medical programmes. Provincial governments were entrusted with political authority, yet lacked financial means. Zemstva and municipalities, for their part, had financial responsibility, but lacked political rights. To cap it off, the distribution between the financial responsibilities of the zemstva and those of the municipalities, for instance in cases of epidemics, was simply left open.[134] However, legislative uncertainty did not only provide room for misunderstandings and conflicts. It could enhance ever-limited resources. Saratov city, for instance, had a second zemstvo hospital with 350 beds. As provincial capital the city also was the residence of zemstvo physicians.

Administrative confusion on the local level only reflected the lack of coordination between the national agencies. While full authority over public health was not granted to the local institutions, the national government gave its civilian medical organisation low priority. Despite all the changes which had taken place in Russia since the middle of the century, state medical legislation dated back to the introduction of the aforementioned *Meditsinskii Departament* and the *Meditsinskii Sovet* within the Ministry of Internal Affairs in 1803. Whereas the *Meditsinskii Departament* was mainly an administrative institution concerned with the definition of medical ranks or the dismissal of physicians, the *Meditsinskii Sovet* was the highest body for civilian medical administration, which supervised all medical and scientific aspects of public health.[135] Yet it was only an advisory organ which could neither initiate nor execute any policies. Furthermore, as one critic remarked in 1882, it was preoccupied mainly with forensic medicine, the supervision of apothecaries or the recognition of foreign physicians.[136] Physicians had only an advisory function.[137] The influence of the institution on the state of public health in the empire, it was remarked, was therefore 'trifling' (*nishtozhno*).[138]

It is scarcely surprising that the resulting medical organisation chiefly created the impression of an uncoordinated, spontaneous product of incompetent bureaucrats. At the same time, this judgement does not do full justice to the overwhelming difficulties posed by the vast expansion of the empire's territory. Certainly, it was not the intention to create legislative confusion. Considering the country's poverty, it was impossible to create modern state structures. The development of an efficient medical organisation in view not only of very limited resources but also of enormous geographical and local disparities required an administrative master plan. What could an organisation look like that would provide rigorous unity in combination with flexibility on both the national and local levels in order to guarantee efficient information about diseases as well as a swift supply of personnel and medications?

The central government initiated several measures in response. First, it distributed medical jurisdictional authority over a number of ministries and institutions. Important governmental institutions which issued decrees in 1892 included the Ministry of War, the Ministry of Ways and Communications, the Ministry of Finance, the Ministry of Foreign Affairs, naval authorities, and also the Governor General of the Caucasus.[139] In fact, due to the multitude of responsible institutions, medical organisation was cumbersome and hampered any concerted effort to combat diseases, and especially epidemics. Yet given the highly complex social, ethnic and religious composition of the Caucasus, for instance, and its particular vulnerability to diseases and epidemics, it was essential to empower the local state representative with far-reaching rights and authority. Likewise, the investment of the Ministry of Ways and Communications and the naval authorities with special jurisdictional power was an attempt to secure the nation's health in view of the lack of local power and resources on the one hand and the enormous river and railway transportation networks along which diseases and medical supplies spread across the country on the other.[140]

Second, a frequently applied measure especially in the combat of epidemics was the dispatching of high-ranking officials from St Petersburg to disease-stricken places. These delegates were endorsed with unlimited authority over state power and played a crucial role in eradicating epidemics. The first precedent of the practice had been the cholera commission under Count Zakrevskii in Saratov in 1830. During the plague at Vetlianka, General Loris-Melikov departed to the lower Volga. He was equipped with medicaments and accompanied by physicians; furthermore, in order to fulfil his task he was appointed temporary Governor-General of the provinces of Samara, Saratov and Astrakhan'.[141] In 1892, Sergei Witte, Minister of Ways and Communications at the time, would be sent to combat cholera at the Volga. Five years later, Senator Likhachev was ordered to the Volga for a sanitary investigation of the cities along the river. Finally, in 1897, a Special Commission for Measures against Plague was set up under the head of prince Aleksandr Ol'denburgskii, the founder of the Imperial Institute of Experimental Medicine.[142]

The Achilles' heel of this system was its reliance on short-term measures. Temporary commissions endorsed with temporary authority implemented temporary measures. Epidemic control, therefore, often came too late and was haphazardly planned. Moreover, such emergency actions were expensive. Repeatedly, all ministries and institutions put large amounts of money at disposal for the immediate combat of epidemics, yet not for preventive measures.

Finally, a third important means for the advancement of medicine at the end of the nineteenth century were semi-official medical societies and their medical congresses. The most prominent example is the Pirogov Society, which was nationwide at the forefront of promoting public health. Medical societies were also established on the local level where they unveiled a strong commitment to public affairs. In Saratov the concern for the city's public health was most actively promoted by the above-mentioned sanitary society (*sanitarnoe obshchestvo*). Founded in 1877 and refounded in 1886 on the initiative of a group of five physicians, veterinary physicians and apothecaries, the society was joined by members of the provincial and municipal administration, by merchants, advocates as well as members of the press. In 1893, 200 members were involved in its activity. The society's task was threefold: it advocated the investigation of local environmental factors which fostered the spread of diseases and epidemics; it aimed at educating the population in hygienic knowledge by conducting public lectures and organising a public library; finally, it intended to cooperate with state, provincial and municipal institutions as well as private individuals when questions of public health needed to be decided or sanitary measures implemented. In practice, the society elaborated a full project for the rebuilding of Saratov's slaughterhouses after the plague at Vetlianka, which were built in 1888; it enforced sanitary inspections of hospitals, schools, bakeries, hairdressers, printing presses and the theatre; it urged for proper vaccination; and it elaborated numerous articles and talks on Saratov's most vulnerable places in sanitary respect.[143]

Notwithstanding its vital activity, the society could not balance the desolate state of public health in the city. Clearly, Saratov was understaffed, underfinanced and undersupplied with medical personnel, facilities and resources. Neither of the hospitals offered the possibility to isolate the sick or to conduct laboratory investigations. In 1892, when the country was afflicted by a severe typhus epidemic, all the typhoid-stricken people had to be carried out of the hospital before cholera cases could be taken care of. Once the epidemic started, the city's municipality had to cooperate with and to react to decisions taken by the zemstvo, the central government and the ministries. Predictably, a major defect in the state apparatus would be proper coordination among the various agencies which, however, would be vital for getting the *vibrio* under control. Generally, medical and administrative resources were highly strained by the consequences of the famine in 1891 and the severe typhus epidemic which afflicted Russia in the spring of 1892. Only against this background can it be explained why Ivan I. Molleson, "the father of zemstvo medicine" and sanitary physician in Saratov's zemstvo, stated in December 1892: 'Cholera took Saratov by surprise.'

Conclusion

In 1892 Saratov was an ideal place for an epidemic of Asiatic cholera. At the brink of rapid economic transition, the city served as a receptacle for a huge contingent of peasant-labourers who brought mass poverty, malnutrition, economic misery and the susceptibility to illness. Saratov's public health system was not keeping up with the modernisation of life. Local administrative and medical authorities were ill-prepared for an epidemic disease of a modern, urban dimension. The legal and administrative framework within which public-health policies were conducted created organisational confusion and inertia on the local level. The city administration did little to extend and improve the quality of medical facilities and confined its combat against epidemic onslaughts to temporary measures. Being notoriously unhealthy, Saratov's quality of medical care was in a deplorable state. Compounding the problems of medical, sanitary and administrative shortages was the fact that the famine in 1891 as well as the typhus epidemic following the famine in the winter of 1891–92 had absorbed and exhausted the available financial, personnel and medical resources. When the *vibrio cholerae* approached the city in the summer of 1892, it therefore found perfect conditions to produce a local medical, social and economic disaster.

3   Cholera in Saratov, 1892

Russia's cholera epidemic in 1892 was a major medical and social catastrophe. From its onset in May until 1 December 1892 cholera is said to have caused 555,010 cases, 267,880 of which proved fatal. European Russia counted 331,077 cases and recorded 151,626 deaths.[1] In absolute numbers of sickness and death the 1892 epidemic was only exceeded by the outbreak in 1831 (466,457 cases and 197,069 deaths) and in 1848 (1,742,439 cases and 690,150 deaths).[2] With a mortality rate of 45.8 per thousand population, however, the outbreak in 1892 proved to be the most virulent and fatal of the cholera epidemics that had visited Russia in the nineteenth century.[3]

At a uniquely late time cholera set an entire nation on the European continent in turmoil. In addition to the unparalleled medical onslaught one of the most shocking aspects for contemporaries was the massive social disarray which erupted in the epidemic's wake. In late-nineteenth-century Russia, cholera provoked popular responses which bore close resemblance to the reactions known from the first pandemic in Europe: poisonous hysteria, panic, flight and, eventually, open rebellion paralysed local and national authorities. They became as great a danger as the epidemic itself.

For most contemporaries the disastrous course of the epidemic provided further evidence that the tsarist autocracy was too backward and too inefficient a government to relieve the epidemic. Sanitary legislation dating back to the beginning of the nineteenth century alongside confusing and contradictory responsibilities within an imploding bureaucratic apparatus, according to the general critique, prevented any successful effort to control the germ and to protect the population.[4] Moreover, the brutal and repressive policy pursued by the central government aggravated the medical crisis and provoked the massive social disturbances which overtook the country.[5]

Yet it is important to note that the epidemic affected various parts of the empire in different ways.[6] The countryside, as Nancy Frieden has shown, was especially heavily hit as opposed to the cities, which were, after all, equipped with apothecaries and physicians.[7] Other factors influencing the course of the epidemic were the specific ethnic, social and religious characteristics of particular areas.[8] The reactions to the disease, too, varied from place to place. While Russia's south-east was shaken by popular rebellion, other regions remained stable and withstood the epidemic without social disturbances.[9] Certainly, the policy followed by the Russian government significantly contributed to creating a national calamity in particular by resorting to military measures to contain the *vibrio*. Yet in order to account for the diversity of the Russian cholera experience in 1892, it is necessary to dissect the notion of the "backward tsarist autocracy" in concrete terms.[10]

The international historiography on cholera has examined the epidemic as a "disease of society" (Asa Briggs).[11] Wherever it occurred, cholera 'exposed political, social as well as moral shortcomings'.[12] It tested the functioning and efficiency of governmental, administrative and financial structures; it exposed the relations between rich and poor, between authorities and subjects; it challenged medical arrangements and medical knowledge; and it revealed popular attitudes and mentalities towards medical science as well as towards religion.[13] Only by looking at all these aspects can one discuss the question of how much the nation's medical fate in the summer of 1892 was determined by the fact that Russia was still an autocratic state. Conversely, an analysis of the epidemic will illuminate the degree to which late Imperial Russian statecraft and society functioned effectively.

This chapter examines the cholera outbreak of 1892 as experienced in the city of Saratov. Once again in Russia's cholera history, Saratov ranked among the places most heavily hit. Between 15 June and 31 August, the city recorded 4,461 cholera cases and 2,270 deaths.[14] With a death rate of 52.6 per thousand population the city even exceeded the high national average mortality rate (45.8 per thousand population) caused by cholera. Moreover, Saratov became the scene of some of the most violent cholera riots witnessed in the empire in 1892. And, as a key centre during the epidemic, the city's cholera experience conformed to the general pattern as it evolved in Russia's south-east. Saratov's story is representative of the events as they happened at the lower Volga, a region which made headlines in June 1892.

It is impossible within the purview of this study to analyse the cholera epidemic in Saratov in all its aspects. This chapter is divided into three parts, each of which focuses on a particular perspective. The first part analyses the role of the national government in the epidemic. It traces the course of the cholera from its arrival on Russian soil to the Caspian Sea and the Volga delta; it discusses the measures taken by the national government to prevent the *vibrio* from crossing the Persian–Russian border and places them in the context of contemporary medical theories on the disease; it analyses the reasons for the failure of the national scheme of defence; finally, this section describes the arrival of the epidemic at Baku and Astrakhan' as the decisive centres from which the cholera spread across European Russia. By discussing the efforts of the central government to contain the disease, this narrative about the cholera's arrival in Russia also places the epidemic in Saratov in its national and regional context.

The second part of this chapter examines the cholera in Saratov city by probing the function and role of local authorities in the epidemic. It analyses the administrative machinery which was supposed to counter the cholera and describes the responses to the disease by local administrative and medical officials; it further follows the course of the epidemic in the city with respect to various districts and social groups. In so doing the section addresses questions about the relationships between local and national governmental authorities, between administrative and medical officials, and between official authorities and the city's residents.

Finally, the chapter looks at the epidemic from the perspective of Saratov's inhabitants and investigates popular responses and reactions to the disease. The riots which overtook the city (and the lower Volga) in the course of the cholera are one of the most distinctive features of the epidemic in 1892. The final part of the chapter looks at the economic, political, social and medical reasons for public resistance towards official authorities; it follows the course of the cholera riots, examines the underlying social tensions and conflicts which erupted in the disturbances, and places the uproar in its historical context.

Government and epidemic: the arrival

By 1892, cholera had long been awaited in the Russian Empire. The fifth pandemic, which had started its journey from India in 1881, had reached Egypt in 1883; by 1884 it had spread to large parts of Europe, the North African coast, and some parts of North and South America as well as Asia.[15] Russia, with the exception of an isolated outbreak in Vladivostok in 1888, had been spared throughout the decade.[16] As the germ's traditional entrance gate to Europe, however, the Russian government carefully followed the progress of the epidemic during the 1880s. In fact, the Medical Council had discussed the danger of a cholera outbreak in Russia for the first time on 5 July 1883, since it was thought that the epidemic might enter the country from Austria-Hungary.[17] Between 1884 and 1892, the council had prepared an elaborate set of anti-cholera orders which, by and large, were then put into effect in 1892.[18] In 1889, when reports reached Petersburg about cholera outbreaks near Tauride, some 100 verst from the Persian–Russian border, the Medical Council began to take the first precautionary measures against the epidemic.[19] It instructed local medical authorities to organise facilities for the isolation of the first cholera cases and to immediately inform the Ministry of Internal Affairs about them; it ordered the establishment of medical observation points (*nabliudatel'nye punkty*) along the frontier in order to control those who entered the country from Persia and to disinfect their belongings and clothes; physicians and feldshers were sent to the border to reinforce the supply of medical personnel; local authorities were supposed to print brochures in Russian as well as in Turkic languages on measures for the personal protection against cholera; finally, troops were dispatched to the frontier in order to secure its complete closure if necessary.[20] Yet in 1890, a very dry winter prevented the epidemic from crossing the border and in the following year cholera did not occur in either Turkey or Persia. Thus, to everybody's surprise, no widespread epidemic of cholera occurred in the Russian Empire between 1873 and 1892.

But the onslaught was still to come. On 28 February 1892, the first reports reached Petersburg on the revival of the epidemic in Herat.[21] As had already been the case during the famine in the preceding year, the first institution to become apprehensive was the Ministry of Finance.[22] The information prompted it to set up a special commission in order to assess the latent threat approaching the Persian–Russian border and to devise a plan to safeguard the nation. The commission consisted of representatives of the Ministry of War, the Ministry of Internal Affairs, and the Ministry of Finance, and was headed by Aleksandr Kuropatkin, at that time also head of the administration in Transcaspia. It met for the first time on 1 April and took the initial steps well in time before cholera reached the frontier.[23]

In their efforts to combat the epidemic governmental authorities followed the latest developments of epidemiology. The medical establishment in St Petersburg in the 1890s was strongly inspired by the recent work of Robert Koch.[24] It is indicative that the Military-Medical Academy, when appointing a chair of bacteriology in 1896, preferred Sergei Botkin, who had studied with Robert Koch at the Institute for Infectious Diseases, to Nikolai Gamaleia, who had visited Koch's rival Louis Pasteur in Paris and had established the second Russian Pasteur Institute in Odessa in 1886.[25] In 1898, Vassilii Isaev, who had worked with Koch during the Hamburg cholera epidemic of 1892, became director of the Plague Laboratory at Kronstadt, a branch of the Imperial Institute for Experimental Medicine.[26]

Koch's discovery of the *vibrio cholerae* in 1883 heralded a breakthrough in the fight against cholera. In St Petersburg, medical and official authorities were fully aware of the new science of bacteriology and its significance for the containment of the epidemic. Koch's works had been translated in major contemporary Russian medical journals such as the *Journal of Social Hygiene, Forensic and Practical Medicine*, the *Military-medical Journal* and the *Journal of the Society of the Protection of Public Health*.[27] One of the earliest directives issued by the Medical Council in 1892 described the methods of detecting and cultivating the cholera bacilli and provided a list of authorities to be consulted on the subject.[28] The disease was not considered to be contagious in the ordinary sense of the term, i.e. transmitted by touch, by infected clothing or goods, or the inhalation of an infected atmosphere; yet it was accepted that the spread of cholera was facilitated by human communication; a major role in the spread of the epidemic was ascribed to contaminated drinking-water.

Based on this medical position the government drew up a plan of defence which, in theory, stood up perfectly to contemporary international standards. In practice, however, it was unfeasible as it also required the administrative capacities and medical resources of a modern state. Russia's sanitary movement was in its earliest infancy; even major cities, as could be seen by the example of Saratov, lacked an adequate public health infrastructure of medical laboratories, hospitals, medical supplies and medical personnel. Once the germ had crossed the border, the country was defenceless.

Consequently, the state's first official measures were directed at preventing the epidemic from crossing the frontier. As soon as news arrived in St Petersburg on 26 April that the epidemic had advanced north from Herat, the commission authorised the commander of the military in Transcaucasia to seal off the Afghan–Russian border.[29] A few days later a squadron of Cossacks was sent to the Persian frontier in order to establish a *cordon sanitaire*. Those who crossed the border at the observation points were quarantined for three days and had to undergo medical observation. The sick were to be isolated in barracks or hospitals and their belongings disinfected. This way, the government hoped to be able to localise the epidemic as soon as it manifested itself on Russian soil and to eradicate it before it could spread further into the country.

Notwithstanding the timely measures of prevention, the documents reveal that from the outset the 460-verst-long Persian–Russian frontier was not under surveillance. Geographically, the eastern part of the land frontier (where the epidemic eventually entered the country) had no landmarks such as rivers or mountains to aid in controlling the course of an epidemic. A paper given at the Society for the Protection of Public Health (*obshchestvo okhraneniia narodnogo zdraviia*) in 1889 underlined the pointlessness of any quarantine at the Transcaucasian frontier:

> As early as 1845, his highness the prince Vorontsov wrote (. . .) that a quarantine at the Transcaucasian line, in the actual meaning of the word, does not exist, that proper quarantines cannot exist there and that the state will spend the enormous sums of money on their establishment in vain, since they would never be completely established and fully secure the protection of the Transcaucasian region against the intrusion of the epidemic. Even if we doubled or tripled the guards who surveille the Transcaucasian border, Prince Vorontsov further noted, we are not going to achieve satisfying results. Prince Vorontsov bluntly said that even a whole corps of military troops would not be enough to stop the secret communication across the border.[30]

The speaker concluded: 'This way, it is obvious, that the complete closure of the Russian–Turkish–Persian border is out of the question at the present, too.'

Apart from geographical conditions and obstacles, the aforementioned commission itself had dismissed the option of the complete closure of the border on the grounds that this would be too difficult as well as too expensive.[31] However, it decided to close the border in its whole length up to the Caspian Sea on 28 May – when it was already too late.[32] In addition, an acute shortage of medical personnel prevented any efficient observation of the epidemic's progress. The Medical Council in St Petersburg had opened an investigation of the border after the appearance of cholera in Meshed on 14 May. On 17 May, it instructed only six physicians, at the time serving as military physicians in the Caucasus, to go from Tiflis to Transcaspia in order to observe the movement of the epidemic more closely.[33] At the same time, two physicians were sent to follow the further course of the germ in the whole Khorasan province and to make sure that the Caucasian administration would be informed in time as soon as the germ approached the Caspian Sea.[34] One of them, Dr Verbitskii, went to Astrabad and investigated the sanitary conditions of the Persian coast along the Caspian Sea. Leaving the city at the end of May, he had found that the city as well as its surrounding and the whole coast from Astrabad to Persian Astara were completely free from cholera. Thus, he informed the Caucasian administration that it could consider itself secure from a cholera outbreak.[35]

The doctor was badly mistaken. Long before Verbitskii's departure from Astrabad, the germ had arrived on Russian soil – at the opposite side of the Caspian Sea. Considering the structure and protection of the border the disease could easily overrun the sanitary cordon. Consequently, the precise identification of the first cholera case in Russia in 1892 is impossible. From the epidemic's onset, and in a pattern repeated everywhere, the first cholera case escaped medical and official attention. The reports agree, however, that the epidemic entered Russia from Meshed, the religious as well as commercial centre of the Khorasan province, which was linked by a road with Askhabad. Some have speculated that the *vibrio* passed the frontier through pilgrims who – from both sides of the Russian–Persian border – visited the mosque and tomb of the holy Imam Riza, a highly venerated saint among the Shiite Muslims.[36] Others have surmised that the germ reached Russia through Russians and Persians fleeing the outbreak of the epidemic in Meshed.[37] Alternatively, it could also have been imported through merchants.[38] However the disease arrived, the first officially acknowledged cholera case occurred in Kaachka, a village 130 verst north from Meshed, on 18 May 1892. Popular belief held that it had been brought four days earlier by a Persian who had been seen suffering from diarrhoea and vomiting at the marketplace.[39] Located on the recently (1888) opened Transcaspian railway, Kaachka became the starting-point of the epidemic in Russia.

From this point onwards, the government's plan of defence failed. Efficient control of the *vibrio* would have required the timely disclosure of the disease, a rapid medical response and swift and accurate exchange of information between medical and official authorities, local as well as national. Regrettably, nothing of this sort was pursued by the authorities in the Transcaspian region. Although the local physician had identified cholera on 19 May, it was deemed necessary to confirm the diagnosis through a bacteriological investigation, the results of which were revealed only on 25 May.[40] Vital time was lost. Meanwhile, rumours that the epidemic had passed the frontier caused the population in Askhabad to jam the Transcaspian railway, trying to escape the medical threat. In spite of popular perception Major General Fisher von Al'bakh, the governor of the region, denied the existence of the epidemic.[41] On 24 May, he sent a soothing telegram to the governor of the Caucasus dismissing the information about the occurrence of cholera as false. To avoid the propagation of disquieting rumours he asked to announce, that 'in the Transcaspian region everything is all right, cholera cases did not occur here and the existing disease is endemic, generally characteristic for the summer time'.[42] Only on 26 May, one day after the laboratory results were disclosed, did he inform the administration in the Caucasus about the occurrence of cholera in Kaachka;[43] two days later, he finally pointed to the necessity of observing everybody arriving from the Transcaspian region, including the military.[44] By this time, however, the germ was already on its way to infecting the whole empire.

Along the railway the disease travelled eastward to Bukhara, Samarkand (21 May) and Dzhizhak (28 May). On 7 June it appeared in Tashkent, the capital of Russian Turkestan. The province became one of the most severely affected parts in Russia, with numbers of cases and deaths only exceeded in certain districts of the Caucasus and in the province of Astrakhan'. From Fergana the epidemic spread further to the northern districts of Central Asia and Siberia. It passed Ural'sk (8 July), the provinces of Tobol'sk (17 July) and Tomsk (12 July); at the beginning of August it was finally reported from Irkutsk (2 August) and Eniseisk (4 August).[45]

Following the Transcaspian railway westward, cholera travelled through Ashkhabad and reached the port of Uzun-Ada on the eastern coast of the Caspian Sea on 25 May 1892, the same day the bacteriological analysis was finished in Kaachka.[46] Between the ports of Uzun-Ada and Baku, located on almost the exact opposite side of the Caspian Sea, was intense ship traffic. Thus 19 days after cholera had appeared on Russian soil at Kaachka, on 6 June 1892, the first cholera cases were reported in Baku.[47]

The government hastily confirmed medical events. Along the Transcaspian railway it set up isolation barracks supplied with medical personnel and medicaments. It imposed stringent measures of quarantine, isolation and disinfection on the Caspian Sea. A decree issued on 27 May by the Ministry of Internal Affairs ordered that all vessels which had been infected with cholera were subjected to medical quarantine.[48] All cases of cholera occurring on a ship or in any port of the sea had to be reported to the governing authorities at Baku, Astrakhan' or Uzun-Ada, the three major ports representing the western, northern and eastern coasts of the Caspian Sea. Observation points (*brandvakhternye punkty*) were established at the ports of all three cities to carry out the medical observation and control of any incoming ship. If the ship was declared to be free of disease, and no one on board was found to present any suspicious symptoms, it was allowed *free pratique* and received a certificate to that effect. Vessels which were affected had to raise a yellow flag and were detained in quarantine at the observation points for 14 days. Every passenger ship had to have a physician on board to control the state of health of the passengers. The decree further ordered that cholera patients had to be removed to the nearest cholera hospital. Their belongings were either thoroughly disinfected or fumigated. The ship and the remaining passengers also underwent a strict process of cleansing and disinfection. Clothes, linens, rugs, pillow-cases, and everything else which constituted the personal belongings of the passengers, had to be disinfected, preferably with a chloride-lime solution. At the beginning of June, additional instructions regulated in detail the disinfection of freight which had passed a place affected by cholera.[49] After the unloading of the freight, the ship itself was cleaned with hot water and disinfected.[50]

An evaluation of these preventive measures along the frontier needs to place them within the context of medical discoveries and debates as conducted since cholera's first appearance in Europe in 1831. According to medical scientific findings, precautionary measures against cholera were highly contested during the nineteenth century.[51] The important issue of quarantine policy had undergone several phases. In the general uncertainty surrounding cholera during the first pandemic, governments throughout Europe had responded to the disease by resurrecting the same defence system which had originally been developed in the seventeenth and eighteenth centuries to combat plague.[52] Based on the premise that cholera was a contagious disease, the British, Austrian, French and Russian monarchies had deployed troops to maintain quarantines, lazarettes and sanitary cordons around infected areas. Yet whereas isolation and detention had success-fully eradicated plague from Europe by the mid-eighteenth century, they utterly failed to do so with regard to cholera. Instead they significantly contributed to the further spread of the epidemic largely by virtue of the terror and fear they evoked among the population. Throughout Europe, sanitary cordons and quarantines missed their medical aim of halting the disease and were ultimately rendered obsolete through the breakdown of public order. After the experience of the first pandemic, medical authorities widely agreed that the disease was not contagious. Accordingly, most European governments rejected the employment of military measures against cholera.[53]

The new consensus was articulated at a series of International Sanitary Conferences between 1874 and 1892.[54] The idea of military cordons was dismissed by Britain, France, Germany and Austria-Hungary. Italy, which did not join the international agreement, only illustrated once again in 1884 that military defence measures against cholera were medically useless and socially disrup-tive.[55] From the medical-scientific standpoint, as we have seen, this position had found its basis in the miasmatist approach best associated with the name of Max von Pettenkofer.[56] His theory – that the cholera was transmitted through the polluted air – meant that any measures of quarantine were ultimately pointless against the epidemic.

Yet Pettenkofer's medical doctrine was again seriously challenged with the discovery of the *vibrio cholerae* in 1884 at the latest. Pettenkofer's rival Robert Koch found out that the bacillus survived best in water, including drinking water. His experiments further illustrated that infection occurred through the pollution of water by infected individuals and the drinking of this water by others.[57] Koch consequently advocated strong state intervention imposing strict controls on river traffic and stringent quarantine and disinfection measures. As Richard Evans argued: 'The triumph of Robert Koch in 1884 brought the immediate resurgence of contagionism in a new, infinitely more powerful form, and mobilized the resources of the state to a degree unknown since the era of the cordons sanitaires in 1831.'[58] The decisive, modern element in Koch's interventionist approach was that the fight against cholera was directed and surveyed by medical specialists and not organised by troops. Professional medical science thus came to play the primary role in preventing the epidemic.

When medical experts came together in St Petersburg in December 1892 to discuss the epidemic during the preceding summer, one representative of the Volga region pointed out that Russia's quarantine measures of disinfection and isolation doubtless stood at the height of contemporary scientific knowledge and that they deserved full attention. Medical authorities in Hamburg, Berlin, Paris and Budapest, the same physician went on, had resorted to the same medical remedies as in Russia's heartland two months before.[59] Nevertheless, the overwhelming majority of the conference participants evaluated the quarantine policies as carried out in 1892 as a complete failure, in particular along the frontier.

In reality, Russia's quarantine practices at the Caspian Sea did not correspond to Koch's ideas of preventing cholera. The establishment of an effective maritime quarantine as devised by him would have required a strong naval and bureaucratic presence to isolate ships and passengers, to guarantee their provision with food, water and medical care, and to prevent any attempts at evasion of the quarantine instructions. With regard to the last point in particular Saratov's public had no illusions about the permeability of the sanitary defence on the Caspian Sea. On 23 June, six days after the official outbreak of the epidemic in Astrakhan', the *Saratov Journal* (*Saratovskii Dnevnik*) proclaimed that:

> the sanitary observation in Astrakhan' seems not in the least trustworthy to us in view of the possibility of the steamships as well as smaller ships to evading the observation point through one of the many arms of the main riverbed of the Volga. Besides, the medical observation point in Astrakhan' was only established a couple of days after the disclosure of undoubted cases of cholera.[60]

Movement was actually relatively free both on and around the Caspian Sea. Russia's physicians were well aware that ship owners, passengers and fugitives showed little respect for whatever regulations existed.[61] From the first rumours about the disease, a terrified population used every opportunity to evade the sanitary regime and to escape the epidemic's progress. The fishermen in the Volga delta knew the arms of the river better than any government institution and were willing to take people far into the sea for some remuneration.[62] At Baku, thousands of people, in particular Persians, managed to secure themselves a place on a ship after its medical observation and left the city unnoticed at night.[63] Jammed on the ships, a report stated, 'they were dying like flies and only the waves of the Sea counted the victims'.[64] As passengers from Persia were not allowed to be taken on any ship, people passed the Russian frontier post of Astara (circumventing medical observation there) to get on board on the Russian side of the border.[65]

Quarantine legislation itself also left much latitude for evasion. A crucial problem of the sanitary policy as practised throughout the country in 1892 was the splitting up of the authorities responsible for issuing quarantine instructions. According to the medical statutes (*ustav vrachebnyi*) quarantine measures generally were the responsibility of local authorities, i.e. the governor or *gradonachal'nik*.[66] For the ships on the Caspian Sea, however, sanitary instructions were issued by the Ministry of Internal Affairs. At the eastern shore, sanitary affairs were under the auspices of the Ministry of War; at the western shore, under the Governor General of the Caucasus. Finally, the implementation of the quarantine depended on local authorities in Uzun-Ada, Astrakhan' and Baku. As a result, medical officials were confronted with both contradictory and unknown rules.[67] The situation turned out to be highly profitable for the shipping companies, to whom the restrictions were economically detrimental in every aspect. A particular nuisance to them was the obligation to hire a physician on every passenger ship at the company's expenses. As soon as this rule had been lifted by the Ministry of

War for the eastern shore of the sea, ship owners from Astrakhan' (which was under the auspices of the Ministry of the Internal Affairs) claimed the right to staff their ships only with feldshers or not to provide any medical observation at all – as it was practised in Uzun-Ada.[68]

Quarantine authorities were further weakened because legislation was imprecise and fragmentary. No instructions were made as to the penalty the lawbreakers had to face.[69] While the omission encouraged some ship owners to break those laws, it annoyed those who obeyed the rules. Furthermore, the regulations failed to specify clearly the tasks and status of the ship-physician, defining their duty only as 'medical-sanitary observation on the sea as well as on the road'.[70] As physicians were hired by the companies, they had no authority on the ships.[71] Captains and agents looked upon them as subordinates and maintained prior authority even in sanitary-medical questions. Declarations about excess passengers from the physicians were frequently ignored. Moreover, hiring the most energetic and active physicians was not in the interest of the companies. One physician summarised the all too frequent reality: 'Physicians frequently existed only as a piece of furniture, providing the ships with the right to carry passengers.'[72]

The most fatal flaw of the government's scheme of defence, however, was the reliance on local authorities and resources for its implementation. In Russia's south-east, the medical instructions sent from thousands of miles away were far beyond local administrative and medical realities. Local personnel were responsible for registering the sick, for medical examination and treatment, for taking care of the quarantined, for informing neighbouring authorities as well as for calming down the public. Capacities around the Caspian Sea were pitifully inadequate to achieve what the anti-cholera campaign ordered. Scientific laboratory training, modern hospitals, a strongly organised medical profession, the necessary prerequisites of Petersburg's fiction, were lacking.[73] In Baku and Astrakhan' available medical personnel were unfamiliar with carrying out bacteriological investigations or the techniques of preparing disinfection means – provided that these were available at all.[74] At the border, disinfection was passed on to untrained customs officers due to lack of physicians.[75] The cholera hospital in Astrakhan' was 80 verst away from the observation point, which meant an eight- to nine-hour transport of the sick on barges usually accompanied by people who were untrained in sanitary matters.[76] Medical and personnel shortages were accompanied by lack of food and water. At the beginning of the epidemic, more than 3,000 people were detained at a time on the roads outside Astrakhan', which had imposed a quarantine of seven days on all vessels. Cases of death occurred not only because of cholera but because the quarantined were not provided with food and fresh water.[77] While the government sent medical instructions it hardly remedied the critical shortages of medical supplies and personnel. The surveillance of the frontier could only be the first response to the crisis. Almost no preparatory steps followed to prevent the epidemic from entering European Russia and progressing northwards. State initiative along the Volga, Russia's traditional highway for epidemics and diseases, was taken only at mid-July when Astrakhan' and Saratov were already dealing with the consequences of violent cholera rebellions. The campaign as envisaged in the capital simply took no account of the practical problems at the local level. An effective fight against cholera would have required that precisely these were solved beforehand.

Although the government's legislation was contradictory and quarantine policies came too late, local authorities around the Caspian Sea were also not blameless. Their initiative and cooperation was weak. Although the cholera epidemic was presaged by outbreaks in Meshed and Kaachka, Russia's south-east in general made no preparations against its coming. While the approaching germ had sounded alarm in government circles since its first announcement on 28 February, it was generally ignored in public thinking until the summer. Moscow received the information on the epidemic only at the end of June when reports about cholera riots at the lower Volga swept the newspapers.[78] The famine and the typhus epidemic still presented more urgent issues on the nation's public health agenda; besides, even in the age of modern transportation, the Persian border was far away. On 6 May, eight days before cholera appeared in Meshed, the convention of the Ministries of Finance, of Internal Affairs, and Ways and Communications had officially acknowledged that the epidemic in Persia presented a serious and imminent threat to Russia. Yet the first report of cholera appeared in the *Government Herald* (*Pravitel'stvennyi Vestnik*) only on 14 June 1892.[79] By this time, the germ had already passed Astrakhan', Tsaritsyn and Saratov and the government had issued its first cholera decrees. Russia's south and south-east were going to pay in full measure for this lack of far-sightedness.

From the very beginning, then, local authorities failed to respond to the disease with the necessary speed. The disclosure of the epidemic in Transcaspia as well as the sending of information to the neighbouring authorities took too much time. Yet regardless of the delay in Transcaspia, local authorities in Baku and Astrakhan' acted with a criminal disregard to the cities' – and, in fact, the nation's – health. Not without justification did the *Saratov Journal* complain about the passivity of Baku's local authorities at the end of June, stating that: 'The population on the whole Volga suffers from the inactivity in Baku.'[80] Whereas the central government assigned 17,000 rubles to the administration in the Caucasus and in Astrakhan' province in May, municipal authorities in the two capital cities made no effort to prepare hospitals, disinfection means and health staff. This was all the more negligent as both cities had traditionally been the most vulnerable points for the entrance of the cholera into the Caucasus and into European Russia respectively. Moreover, Baku, as late as 1892, was highly susceptible to epidemic diseases. As a result of its extraordinary development in the trade with naphtha the city had grown feverishly during the 1880s.[81] Its population had risen from 14,500 in the 1870s to 111,904 in 1897.[82] Dynamic growth severely affected the city's urban environment. A journalist commented that, 'The city contains gardens without grass, trees without leaves, sea without water, and steppes without air, for it is as impossible to call air that derosene vapour which blows round Baku for many verst as it is to call water that mother-of-pearl tinted, heavy mud which creeps into the harbour, taking every colour of the rainbow in the sun.'[83] Additionally, Baku was in a serious state of sanitary neglect. Most favourable for the flourishing of infectious diseases was an Asian quarter inhabited by Tatar and Persian labourers who, according to Frank Clemow, the English observer of the epidemic, lived in 'indescribable Oriental filth'.[84]

As Baku's municipal council had made no provision for the city's protection, cholera immediately assumed epidemic proportions. Mortality figures mounted so rapidly that the population was seized by panic. Faced with inadequate hospitals and insufficient medical supplies, people tried to avoid infection by flight. The newspaper *Kaspii* estimated that approximately 100,000 fugitives poured out of the city during the first few weeks of the epidemic.[85] Although public hysteria did not turn into open rebellion and violence as it would once the germ had arrived in Astrakhan', it nevertheless paralysed the whole life in the city. Shops and factories were closed and business came to a complete standstill. Baku's police chief (*politseimeister*) drew the attention of the municipality to the need to provide the population with food.[86] The *Saratov Journal* gave a dreary picture:

> Baku presents a terrible picture these days. Being a lively and vivid city just a month ago, the city has turned into some kind of ruin. On the streets one hardly sees anyone – everybody takes refuge in their houses because of the danger of getting infected by cholera [. . .] The public is in a terrible panic, trade and commerce has almost come to a standstill, and nobody is on the boulevards and in the parks.[87]

Even worse, however, the general exodus rendered obsolete any belated effort from the side of medical and administrative officials to control the epidemic. Besieging trains and ships the refugees carried the *vibrio* with them, thus undermining whatever effectiveness quarantine might have had. From Baku, cholera rapidly spread across the whole Caucasus. It was reported in Tiflis on 13 June;[88] on 14 June, cases occurred in Petrovsk on board a steamer coming from Baku; in Susha the disease broke out on 16 June and in Elizavetpol' two days later. By the end of the month, the germ had arrived in the northern provinces of Stavropol' and Terek in the north Caucasus, where it raged with greater ferocity than in any other part of Russia, European or Asiatic. Within five months 133,781 cases of cholera were reported in the Caucasus, 68,353 of which proved fatal.[89] Once in the northern Caucasus, the germ entered European Russia in Rostov-on-Don on 28 June. From here, it moved on to the southern provinces adjacent to the Sea of Azov and the Black Sea and thence further to the provinces of Volhynia, Podolia, Chernigov, Poltava and Khar'kov.

While the cholera spread to Tiflis, events at the Caspian Sea culminated at Astrakhan', Baku's neighbour to the north. The epidemic reached the city on 17 June. As in Baku, the disease found the administration unprepared and its initial assault was devastating.[90] Yet at Astrakhan', the inability of local authorities to cope with the emergency led to a different response altogether. Local authorities established a military regime reminiscent of the anti-cholera measures during the first pandemic. Administrative sluggishness on the one hand and harsh measures on the other compounded the general fear of the disease and led to the

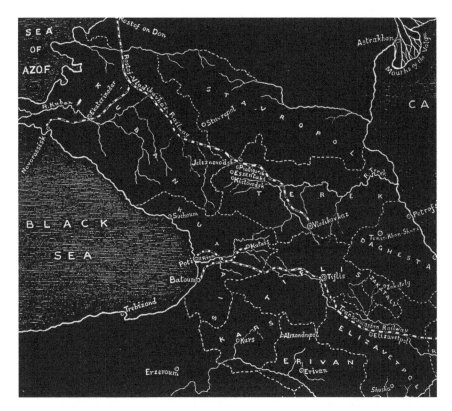

Figure 3 Map of the Caucasus, Frank Clemow, *The Cholera Epidemic of 1892 in the Russian Empire* (St Petersburg, 1893).

complete demoralisation of the public. Resentment and hysteria turned into open rebellion. On June 21, a frenzied mob chased after the cholera wagons and threw itself in fury on the official, the feldsher and physician accompanying the wagon.[91] Once on the move, the crowd spread through the city and stormed the hospital. Cholera patients were moved out to the banks, disinfection means and medical supplies were thrown away. Finally, the whole building was set on fire. The mob tore down tearooms and police stations and, within two days, murdered several physicians and townspeople. As the situation got out of control the governor ordered the military to restore order. Shooting into the crowd, the soldiers killed several people. The injured were brought to the military fortress outside the city, which served as the city's hospital since the cholera hospital had been destroyed.

The detailed factors which contributed to the social unrest and violence at Astrakhan' cannot be discussed here and will be analysed for the case of Saratov. Here, three points are important with regard to the role of the Russian government during the epidemic and to the further progress of the germ towards Saratov. First, whereas quarantine instructions on paper took advantage of the latest developments in scientific medicine, their implementation did not. Quarantine and sanitary practices throughout Russia during the epidemic varied from place to place. Astrakhan' presented a prototype for a frequently practised rigorous isolation policy. Modern medical science justified a stringent but moderate quarantine, led under the direction and observation of medical experts. The sanitary regime at Astrakhan', instead, was coercively enforced by the military and the police and reminiscent of old-style quarantine practices as employed during the first pandemic.

Second, the terror at Astrakhan' heralded a national emergency. It demonstrated that the disease created a potentially explosive situation which threatened public order. Astrakhan' was just the beginning in an unanticipated series of social outbursts which would travel up the Volga alongside the disease. At the Volga delta, the link between diseases and social disorder was established for the first time.

Third, not least through the riots at Astrakhan', cholera posed an immediate health threat to European Russia and, in particular, to neighbouring Saratov. The main channel for the epidemic's spread through European Russia was the Volga and its network of canals. The worst cholera attacks during the 1892 outbreaks were to be found along the river. The westward movement of the epidemic from Rostov was neither as violent nor as fast when compared to the northern route. On the south–north axis, the epidemic covered with startling rapidity nearly 1,200 miles within 12 days.[92] Starting from Astrakhan', the germ attacked, from south to north, the provinces of Saratov (14 June), Kazan' (25 June), Nizhnii Novgorod (7 July) and Tver' (5 August).[93] Generally, the heaviest losses were suffered in the south, particularly in the provinces of Astrakhan', Saratov, Samara and Simbirsk. Mortality lessened, in each succeeding province, as the epidemic moved northward. Before the end of July, cholera had overrun almost all the central provinces. It had appeared in St Petersburg in July and spread in August to the Polish province of Lublin as well as to the northern provinces of Novgorod, Vologda and Olonets. By the end of the year, the epidemic had ravaged most of Russia's European provinces and carried away more than a quarter of a million lives.

When cholera approached Russia in the summer of 1892, the government was fully aware that the epidemic presented a direct and immediate threat to the health of the nation. Long before the disease arrived, the Ministry of Internal Affairs had prepared a detailed plan for a cholera epidemic. It was based on the recent discoveries of the new science of bacteriology and developed a scheme of defence which was completely in tune with the advances of the time. Yet, ultimately, the plan proved unworkable as it presupposed modern administrative and medical state resources. Russia's sanitary movement was in its earliest founding stages, the country lacked an adequate public health infrastructure of medical laboratories, cholera hospitals, medical supplies and medical personnel; moreover, the large majority of cities were not supplied with pure water and waste removal facilities. Once the germ had crossed the frontier, Russia was defenceless.

Facing the emergency, the government resorted to a resolute quarantine policy along the borders carried out by the only instruments available: the military and the police. When medical officials discussed these quarantine practices in

Table 3.1 Deaths from cholera by province: European Russia in 1892

Province	Cases	Deaths
Astrakhan'	21,960	10,980
Don Cossack region	37,680	18,295
Saratov	41,887	21,091
Samara	41,369	18,115
Simbirsk	17,143	7,347
Voronezh	24,046	12,082
Orenburg	10,304	5,339
Tambov	21,284	9,078
Lublin	5,683	2,275
Penza	7,727	3,514
Kursk	10,164	4,274
Kazan'	8,337	3,703
Ufa	7,359	3,511
Viatka	10,307	4,681
Kiev	10,562	3,720
St Petersburg	5,423	1,602
Nizhnii Novgorod	4,347	1,917
Ekaterinoslav	4,281	1,896
Khar'kov	6,280	2,596
Tauride	2,454	1,365
Kherson	4,802	2,224
Bessarabia	3,070	1,285
Podol'e	3,864	1,423
Perm	4,205	2,052
Iaroslavl'	1,241	548
Riazan'	1,752	893
Tula	1,270	368
Orel	1,514	630
Poltava	1,992	863
Chernigov	1,526	484
Moscow	1,515	783
Volhynia	1,162	453
Kostroma	428	212
Olonets	107	52
Vladimir	281	160
Warsaw	170	71
Mogilev	221	99
Livonia	93	48
Minsk	150	70
Pskov	62	31
Grodno	69	37
Tver'	46	15
Novgorod	17	2
Vologda	10	4
Kaluga	7	7
Courland	7	3
Smolensk	4	4
Vil'na	7	4
Vitebsk	2	2
Total for European Russia:	331,077	151,626

Figures are from Frank Clemow, *The Cholera Epidemic 1892 in the Russian Empire*, pp. 36–37.

Table 3.2 Deaths from cholera by province: Caucasus in 1892

Province	Cases	Deaths
Daghestan	23,471	10,457
Terek	27,071	13,114
Stavropol	14,802	7,280
Kuban	28,759	15,100
Baku	11,251	6,876
Zakataly	991	598
Erivan	9,153	5,504
Elizavetpol	9,751	5,690
Tiflis	5,995	3,118
Kutais	613	308
Total for the Caucasus	134,785	69,423
Central Asia and Siberia	89,175	46,831
Total for the Russian Empire	555,010	267,880

Figures are from Frank Clemow, *The Cholera Epidemic 1892 in the Russian Empire*, pp. 36–37.

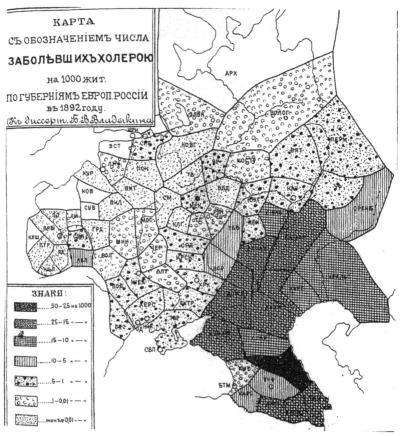

Figure 4 Map of the spread of cholera in European Russia, 1892, B.V. Vladykin, *Materialy k istorii kholernoi epidemii 1892–1895 v predelakh evropeiskoi Rossii* (St Petersburg, 1899).

December 1892 they agreed that the attempt to seal off the country had utterly failed. They pointed to the fact that no *cordon sanitaire* could halt an epidemic if timely information and rapid responses were not provided; they criticised the uncoordinated instructions and initiatives of various authorities, which had undermined quarantine authority and effectiveness; most importantly, they concluded that the chief result of the sanitary zeal was suspicion, fear, resentment and, finally, social unrest among the population.

In fact, the military coercion practised at the frontiers was reminiscent of the anti-cholera campaigns as conducted during the first pandemic. So was the response. Whereas Baku's inhabitants fled in fear of the disease, the sanitary rigour at Astrakhan' resulted in a collapse of public order escalating in major social disturbances and terror. In both cities, the administration lost control of events. Unfortunately, the disorder at Baku and Astrakhan' was itself an uncontrollable means of spreading the disease. From now on, cholera raged unchecked through the country.

City and epidemic: the response

Saratov's first cholera case remains a mystery. Aleksandr Amsterdamskii, a local physician who investigated the course of the epidemic retrospectively in the fall of 1892, dated the epidemic's beginning to 14 June.[94] On this day, medical practitioners assumed the epidemic for the first time when disclosing the dead body of a worker on one of the barges at one of the landing stages.[95] Medical examination revealed that the person had already been taken ill and died the day before. During the following days, suspicious cases spread with increasing frequency along the banks. On 16 June the disease struck a sailor, two workers from the grain depots at the river, as well as the wife of a miller. Three more people fell ill on 17 June. From the banks then, the symptoms of cholera spread quickly along the *Valovaia* and *Chasovennaia* streets to the *gory*, especially to the fourth administrative district of the city, which accommodated the workers at the banks, and also to the *Beloglinskii* ravine, where the workers of the mills were living.[96]

Popular wisdom, however, set the first cholera case earlier. Apparently, one of the workers on the ships had been taken ill by the epidemic already on 12 June. He had arrived on an oil barge from Astrakhan' three days before.[97] Saratov's zemstvo physician E.K. Rosental' retrospectively confirmed this belief. In December 1892 he recalled that the physicians learned at the height of the epidemic about the first cases having occurred among workers on oil barges around 10–12 June (in his version the barges were coming from Baku).[98] Rosental' further mentioned a corpse which was found covered with excrement on 8 June not far from the city and which most likely had been a cholera case. Retrospectively, most other physicians also considered this day the beginning of the epidemic when reviewing its course in the autumn of 1892.[99]

In the general confusion about the *vibrio*'s first arrival in Saratov, the physicians stated one point with certainty: 'Cholera came to us earlier than we started thinking about it.'[100] Indeed, even after the epidemic had been prefigured by the outbreaks in Baku and Astrakhan', it struck Saratov before any preparation was made.

Throughout May until the first week of June the city's medical and administrative officials were strikingly oblivious of the approaching germ. Although it was not unknown that cholera had entered Russia there is no indication that they perceived it as an acute threat. A meeting of the zemstvo physicians and representatives on 4 June, for example, still debated the prevalence of scurvy and typhus in the province.[101] Furthermore, as was the case elsewhere in Russia, the entrance of the germ into the country, the closure of the Persian–Russian border, the progress of the epidemic towards the Caspian Sea, and even its move in the direction of Baku had not stimulated any public or official interest. In Saratov, the first reports on the cholera appeared on 7 June in the *Saratov Leaflet* (*Saratovskii Listok*) and the *Saratov Journal* (*Saratovskii Dnevnik*).[102] The latter sounded the alarm: 'It is necessary to develop the fighting plan in due time, right now; while our societies and assemblies start thinking, gathering, discussing and taking measures on paper, a lot of time passes, in fact so much time, that before the end of the paper production it will be necessary to get to their implementation immediately.'[103] Similarly, on 8 June, one duma representative pointed to the danger of the epidemic and the necessity to take precautionary measures.[104] On 9 June, the provincial governor sent an initial circular to the cities' mayors recommending a clean-up of the cities but for the time being the advice was not heeded.[105] Indeed, from the day cholera arrived on Russian soil until 15 June – when Saratov's physicians for the first time suspected the presence of the epidemic in the city – local administrative authorities, municipal as well as provincial, opted for inaction.

Historical scholarship has argued that the violent social response to the epidemic at the lower Volga cannot be attributed to the type of local administration, for 'the zemstvo province of Saratov had been as wracked with the disease and disorder as the non-zemstvo province of Astrakhan'.[106] Examining the impact of the cholera on the professionalisation of Russia's physicians, Nancy Frieden therefore stressed their argument which ascribed the catastrophic course of the epidemic to limited political power.[107] From the perspective of the physicians, this view was certainly justified insofar as their work was frequently hampered by the general subjection of medical affairs to administrative officialdom. Yet at the same time, their reasoning also reveals a striking lack of understanding of the current organisation of public health. The analysis of the epidemic in Saratov will show that the administration's role was in fact crucial: it was administrative failure that contributed most to human suffering and death. However, it was not only the formal institutionalisation of an administrative apparatus at a certain locality (indeed formal administrative arrangements varied greatly from place to place) but rather the conduct of local officials, their ability to grasp social realities and to make efficient use of medical and personnel resources within the given administrative structure that determined the course of the epidemic. Both aspects need to be looked at in tracing the response of Saratov's officials to the cholera.

To begin with, it is important to recall the administrative machinery which needed to be set in motion to meet the emergency. This is not to repeat the old saying about the inefficient tsarist bureaucracy. Rather, a complicated system of cholera management evolved during the epidemic which in its confusion probably was unique in the whole history of the struggle with cholera. The Great Reforms had set up parallel, overlapping and conflicting institutions in the provinces and in the cities. Control of local sanitary conditions was vested in local authorities through the provincial zemstva and municipal dumas, especially during times of epidemics. In 1890, zemstva were authorised to direct anti-epidemic measures and to issue sanitary regulations.[108] Yet according to the medical statutes (*Ustav vrachebnyi*), which did not incorporate the zemstvo statutes, it was the state which maintained ultimate control over all aspects of public health. At the state level, basic policies were not only formulated in the Ministry of Internal Affairs but also in various other ministries. For railroads and waterways, especially for the Volga, instructions were further issued by the Ministry of Ways and Communications, a position held at that time by Sergei Witte.[109]

Given this dual structure of public health administration, Saratov's municipality competed with the provincial state authorities (i.e. the provincial administration headed by the provincial governor). Their role was further enhanced by the fact that municipal resources alone could not meet the situation and medical and financial support had to be requested from St Petersburg. At the same time, municipal authorities also had to rely on the material and personnel aid provided by the zemstvo administration. The zemstvo, in turn, had to coordinate its measures with those taken by the municipality as Saratov was the focus from which the epidemic spread through the province.[110] One of the decisive questions for a successful combating of the epidemic, therefore, was how all these local authorities and institutions would cooperate, i.e. whether they would achieve an efficient, unified strategy to contain the germ.

In order to overcome the unavoidably confusing and overlapping responsibilities resulting from this double legislation the central government tried to strengthen local agencies. One of the most significant decrees concerning the fight against the epidemic on the local level ordered the formation of Sanitary Executive Commissions (*Sanitarno-Ispol'nitel'nye Kommissii*) in every district and provincial city to direct the cholera fight.[111] The commissions drew their membership mainly from local physicians who were entrusted with planning and carrying out all cholera measures against the spread of the epidemic in a particular district. In theory, they were to control the availability of medical personnel, accommodation in hospitals, the provision of medical aid, organisation of disinfection measures and the arrangements for moving patients to the hospital. Furthermore, their tasks included the implementation of sanitary measures in a particular locality. In conjunction with the police, they had to look after the cleanliness of streets, squares, water supplies and food products. Those refusing the instructions could be punished by the commission. The Sanitary Executive Commission was supposed to come into effect in a specific location as soon as the Ministry of Internal Affairs gave the go-ahead.

This decree aimed to rationalise the management of the cholera campaign by guaranteeing some coordination between the multitude of local institutions. Yet in most cases, it further complicated the administrative problems by adding an additional executive agency.[112] One critic of the Ministry of Internal Affairs commented:

> If a competition was established with the task of how one could make our confused sanitary legislation even more confusing, then, no doubt, one of the most successful solutions to such original task would be the establishment, in addition to the two system of organs, which administer sanitary affairs, of a third one, whereby neither the relations between them nor the responsibilities of each of them are identified.[113]

Although Saratov city itself never established a Sanitary Executive Commission, the institution had an important effect on Saratov as it was formed on the zemstvo and the uezd levels. The network of cholera organisations in the whole province within which Saratov's municipality had to operate thus included: four provincial institutions (provincial medical board, provincial committee on public health, provincial zemstvo assembly, provincial zemstvo board) and two institutions in each of the 10 districts (uezd zemstvo assembly, uezd zemstvo board).[114] The Sanitary Executive Commissions added another 11 institutions. Altogether, there were 35 assemblies, the cities not included, which took care of the province's health during the epidemic.

Inevitably, such a cumbersome administrative construction caused lots of opportunities for confusion and meant interminable delays. But public health administration was also complex and unwieldy in other cities which avoided the eruption of social disturbances. In Saratov, the inability of local officials to assess the medical situation, to perform fundamental social functions as well as to respond sensitively to human fears and needs compounded by administrative problems created a major medical and social disaster.

Having demonstrated their unwillingness to face the threatening reality while the epidemic moved towards Baku and Astrakhan', Saratov's officials entered a second phase of their cholera combat on 16 June. In preparation (and prodded by the provincial governor) the city's mayor, E.N. Epifanov, had convened a meeting of the municipal sanitary commission on 11 and 12 June to develop a plan of precautionary cholera measures. The suggestions of the commission included the division of the city into sanitary districts, the establishment of an observation point and of a quarantine at the river banks and the reinforcement of medical personnel. The meeting also addressed the particularly burning question of the migrant population. It advised the temporary arrangement of accommodation at the banks as well as the opening of soup kitchens at those places where workers were concentrated.[115] These recommendations met with approval two days later in a meeting of the city's sanitary society, which additionally urged that the attention of the provincial zemstvo should be drawn to the epidemic, too.[116]

Once devised, all the measures suggested by Saratov's medical experts still needed the approval of the municipal duma. Yet the duma representatives, when they finally met on 15 and 16 June, did not show any particular sense of urgency.[117] Although the epidemic was the actual reason for the meeting, the sanitary commission's presentation of the cholera measures was postponed to the end and hastily discussed as time was running out. The suggestions of the sanitary society were not presented to the duma at all. Of the actual measures presented by the sanitary commission the most important ones collapsed. The matter of establishing a quarantine and an observation point at the banks was postponed. Likewise, the question of an organisation of permanent medical care for the residents was "left open". Thus, for the time being, the duma only started to organise the sanitary districts within which preventive cholera measures could be carried out. Otherwise, it was agreed that more serious thinking about the epidemic should not be initiated before the cholera had officially been announced in Astrakhan'.

One of the reasons for the municipality's inability to set things in motion was a fatal dependency on bureaucratic formalism. In a statute in 1884 the provincial zemstvo had decided that cholera measures would be taken by the zemstvo only when the epidemic had entered European Russia. As late as 1892, all local authorities, municipal as well as provincial, adhered to this regulation. Epifanov, too, followed the guidelines formalised by the zemstvo – despite the fact that already on 15 June state authorities had urged the municipality to start implementing the instructions on the formation of Sanitary Executive Commissions.[118] Only when notified by the provincial governor on 18 June about eight cholera cases in Astrakhan' did Saratov's mayor convene another duma meeting for the next day to discuss a more detailed cholera plan.[119] By this time, Saratov, too, recorded already seven cholera cases, as Epifanov himself informed the provincial committee on public health the same evening.[120]

In full awareness of the presence of cholera in the city, Saratov's officials continued to deny its existence. At the duma meeting on 19 June, the majority of the representatives were absent. Out of the 72 representatives, only 30 appeared and were prepared to serve as vigilants of the sanitary districts. They went into action the same day. Other initiatives that were going to be taken immediately were imposed on the municipality by the provincial committee on public health (*gubernskii komitet obshchestvennogo zdraviia*), which met in the evening of 19 June. It instructed the municipality to appoint one physician to work at the banks, to establish permanent medical care (*dezhurstva*) in the city, and to establish a cholera hospital with 50 beds.[121] Still, this was no coherent strategy to meet the epidemic.

Unwillingness and lack of initiative, as well as the refusal to believe in the epidemic, were strengthened by the fact that the presence of the epidemic was not as yet officially acknowledged. In Saratov, as almost everywhere in Russia, the official diagnosis of cholera still followed the lines of the pre-Koch era. Individual cases were not considered as sufficient evidence to announce the presence of a cholera epidemic. The practice was partly dictated by medical factors and realities. In 1892 the question of diagnosis was still bound up with scientific and medical disputes and despite the circular issued by the Medical Council on the cultivation of the cholera bacillus, Russian physicians were unanimous about the criteria upon which the epidemic should be identified.[122] Moreover, in too many cases a bacteriological investigation was a hopeless venture as both technical equipment as well as technical and medical knowledge were unavailable. Indeed, Russia's physicians agreed at the St Petersburg conference in December 1892 that cholera should be identified on the basis of the clinical picture as, given the provision of medical care in the country, a bacteriological investigation would only allow the development of the epidemic.[123]

Crucially, the official acknowledgement that an individual place was affected by cholera depended on the administration. As in any other medical question, Russia's doctors had little say in declaring the existence of a cholera outbreak. Administrative authorities, for their part, were reluctant to acknowledge the outbreak of cholera as this meant the implementation of exceptional and costly protective measures for the local government.[124] Instead of relying on its own medical experts, Saratov's municipality, again, left the decision to announce the presence of cholera in the city to far-away St Petersburg. Local physicians had identified the first cholera cases on 15 June.[125] It was only with the official declaration of the epidemic from St Petersburg on 22 June that a more comprehensive cholera campaign was set into motion.[126]

On the provincial level, the response to the epidemic was even tardier. At the meeting of the provincial medical board (*gubernskaia vrachebnaia uprava*) on 19 June, which dictated the first steps to be taken to the municipality, the governor, Prince B.B. Meshcherskii, also made it clear to Saratov's mayor that he should organise the clean-up of the capital and activate the municipal sanitary commission since for the time being no provincial commission would be organised.[127] The zemstvo board met on 15 June in order to debate the anti-cholera measures to be taken by the zemstvo. Lacking as much experience as ideas and initiative, the uprava chose to adopt the cholera plan which had been approved by the zemstvo assembly on 14 December 1884.[128] In addition to the outdated scheme the uprava also discovered that it was actually the task of the provincial administration to organise preparatory measures against the epidemic. So it did nothing – until forced to react by popular rebellion on 28 June. Two days later, the uprava had succeeded in cleaning up one room in the zemstvo hospital for cholera cases and in convening a special meeting of the zemstvo assembly for 3 July.[129]

Provincial medical authorities met for the first time on 25 June. They had no illusions about their timing:

> The cholera in Saratov itself began on 16 June; the fight against it took us off guard, as was the case in all preceding epidemics, and therefore the fight against it has started late; as the disease is already imported it remains only to slow down its steady spread, because to halt it is already impossible.[130]

It took another nine days for the suggestions of the physicians to be presented to the provincial assembly for confirmation on 3 July.[131] The day after, the province established its Sanitary Executive Commission and started to take its first anti-cholera measures.[132]

Not surprisingly, delays, never-ending confusion and hasty improvisation characterised Saratov's defence against cholera throughout June and July. Governing authorities were not only completely unprepared for the epidemic; administrative and medical meetings of the municipal and provincial governments as well as of the district and provincial zemstvo also busied themselves with countless debates about a unified organisational structure to direct a coordinated policy of preventive health. New commissions and sub-commissions were feverishly called into being in order to devise anti-cholera measures at the same time that the first steps were taken to combat the disease. As of 19 June the municipality started its campaign of urban purification and tightened food control on the markets. The sanitary vigilants (*sanitarnye popechiteli*), usually recruited amongst physicians, policemen or educated laymen, began to visit squares, streets and private courts to identify the major sanitary perils. They instructed homeowners to clean their courts and wells, to wash cesspits and disinfect them with lime. On the markets the police inspected the stalls of fruit vendors, controlled the water of *kvas* sellers, and subjected the tradesmen to fines for inedible products or the untidy maintenance of their shops. Once the epidemic was officially declared, the sale of vegetables, raw fruits and *kvas* was heavily restricted. On 24 June all the small shops at the banks were forced to close down completely.[133] To provide a healthy diet to the poor, the municipality set up four soup kitchens and tea stations at the banks which sold cheap tea, soup, as well as bread and meat. Furthermore, the city built two barracks with 50 beds each at the river to provide temporary accommodation for the migrant population.[134]

While cholera was in the city, Epifanov also started to address the shortage of medical supplies and doctors. One of the first measures adopted by the city administration was the removal of all the patients from the Demidov house, which in normal times served as the typhus department of the municipal hospital, to turn it into a cholera hospital for 75 patients.[135] The mayor further asked the medical society for support in organising permanent medical care in each of the police districts in the city.[136] In view of the shortage of medical personnel he also sent telegrams to Moscow and Kazan' to ask for the dispatch of medical students to help with the cholera epidemic in Saratov.[137]

The provincial administration, on its part, confined its activity for the time being to republishing and distributing a brochure written by Ivan Molleson in 1878 about the most important public and individual measures to prevent people from contracting the disease. The brochure described the principal symptoms of cholera and stressed the necessity of cleanliness, a particular concern with diet, moderation and immediate medical care to avoid infection. It warned people to avoid eating raw vegetables, fruits and berries and drinking *kvas* at the market. Water, whether used for drinking or washing, had to be boiled before use. The booklet further recommended dressing warmly: people should especially keep their legs and stomachs warm. An excessive lifestyle (*razgul'naia zhizn'*) and excessive work were to be avoided. If, despite all these precautions, a cholera case occurred, the sick person was to be isolated immediately and a physician called. Until the physician's arrival, the sick person had to be kept warm and given mint or strong tea. Any further treatment as well as the disinfection of the house would take place under the surveillance of the physician.[138]

All these efforts were much too late and insufficient to prevent a medical catastrophe. No short-term sanitary campaign could have removed Saratov's unsanitary conditions. The attempted establishment of even a rudimentary medical infrastructure lasted from 22 June (the opening of the Demidov house) until 18 July (the establishment and equipment of cholera hospitals by the state).[139] Thereby, important medical institutions and organisational structures to combat the epidemic were only established after the cholera riots at the beginning of July.[140] In addition to being late, many of the measures approved were very difficult and often impossible to enforce. Numerous suggestions remained only paper solutions, while the chronic shortage of financial and personnel resources prevented their implementation. Already on 24 June, Epifanov declared at a meeting of the provincial committee on public health that the municipality could not implement the municipal cholera plan approved on 16 and 19 June due to the shortage of physicians and feldshers.[141] Throughout the epidemic the 380 beds provided by the municipality, the zemstvo and the state could not accommodate the thousands of cholera cases;[142] temporary accommodation at the banks was established for 200 people and not for 2,000 as needed;[143] likewise, the available 60 sanitary vigilants were far too few to guarantee an adequate control of the sanitary deficits in the city and to ensure the immediate reporting of cholera cases.[144]

Yet even more fatally, as it turned out, the effectiveness of the cholera campaign was undermined by the social abyss between local governors and the populace. The information about public and individual precautionary measures in newspapers and brochures could not reach the majority of Saratov's illiterate residents. The municipality therefore asked the priests to read and explain the cholera instructions in the services. Priests also opened the tea rooms and soup kitchens with prayers and explanations about the necessity of being concerned about a particular diet.[145] But even if familiar with the instructions, most inhabitants found them impossible to follow, especially the very poor, who were most susceptible to the disease. Again and again the newspapers complained that many homeowners could not afford to buy disinfection means. Despite the fact that the Medical Department had ordered the reduction of prices on disinfection means, the apothecaries, as the *Saratov Journal* noted, 'feeling themselves as lords of the moment, immediately raised the prices (of means of disinfection)'.[146] Not only did the city administration not take action against the apothecaries, it also refused to clean the courts of the poor at the municipality's cost.[147] Many courts, therefore, remained untouched by the cholera campaign as the residents either simply did not know about the instructions or, if they did, they had no possibility to follow them. Moreover, people continued using the contaminated water out of wells and the Volga River since the municipality provided only very few alternative sources for boiled water.[148] By implementing only rudimentary measures, the municipality's attempt to secure the city did not only demonstrate the social gap between local governing officials and the population but actually sharpened the rift. By the beginning of July, Saratov's city administration had failed to convince the population that it actually did something for them.

In contrast to the apathy of local officials, those measures which were implemented were enforced by coercion. As medical personnel were insufficient, the police were charged with reporting the cholera cases, bringing suspected patients to the hospital and controlling the cleanliness of courts, houses and market squares. Cholera was made a crime. Compounding the brutality of the police officials was their incompetence. 'A police official poured cold water into a bucket, some lime and cooking salt and, without letting the salt dissolve, began to sprinkle the concoction in all four corners near the oven, under the oven, on the oven, and even into the oven itself,' the newspapers reported on the typical practice of disinfection procedures.[149] Inevitably, the cholera defence measures by the police aroused distrust and eventually resistance among the population. In the end, it destroyed any chance of success in the cholera campaign.

While municipal and provincial administrative and medical officials established commissions and sub-commissions to discuss measures against the epidemic, cholera ravaged the city. Following official medical statistics, Saratov recorded 4,461 cholera cases and 2,270 deaths within two and a half months.[150] Thus, 27.2 people per thousand contracted the disease and 17.46 per thousand died. This mortality rate exceeded the cholera mortality in Hamburg in the same year (13.4 per thousand) which, as Richard Evans has shown, was not a particularly severe cholera death rate when compared with other places and other times.[151] Nevertheless in Saratov, for the following two decades, the cholera outbreak of 1892 set the ultimate standard for local medical and administrative officials against which all aspects of the city's state of health were measured. A closer look at death rates, numbers of victims and the course of the epidemic can explain its immediate as well as its lasting effect on Saratov's public mind.

Unfortunately, there is no detailed statistical material on causes of death in the city for as early as 1892 to accurately assess the impact of cholera on Saratov's mortality pattern. Yet certainly cholera became the major killer in the city in 1892. The epidemic added an extra 2,000 deaths to the 5,800 lives Saratov otherwise lost on average in one year.[152] From 1895 to 1906 infant mortality, which accounted for more than one-third of the city's annual mortality, took approximately 2,300 lives yearly and thus came close to the number of deaths brought about by cholera within 10 weeks.[153] As Table 3.3 illustrates, cholera raised Saratov's average annual mortality rate from 40.7 per thousand to 56.7 per thousand.

Table 3.3 Death rates per 1,000 inhabitants in Saratov, 1891–1902

Year	Deaths per 1,000	Year	Deaths per 1,000
1891	40.7	1897	36.8
1892	56.7	1898	42.6
1893	32.9	1899	40.8
1894	37.8	1900	40.8
1895	39.8	1901	42.1
1896	36.9	1902	45.5

P.N. Sokolov, "Sanitarnyi ocherk goroda Saratova", *SZN*, 1904, no. 5, p. 53.

In addition, it needs to be taken into account that the real number of cholera cases and deaths was most likely much higher than medical officials suggested. Thus, the police recorded a considerably higher overall mortality rate (66.5 per thousand) for the city in 1892 than the physicians (56.7 per thousand).[154] Aleksandr Amsterdamskii himself had reservations about his cholera figures. Many families concealed the disease for fear of medical treatment and disinfection procedures; frequently, the physicians themselves failed in correctly diagnosing the cause of death on the official forms or did not record cholera cases at all; and finally, the medically established figures only involved the period from 15 June until 31 August while the epidemic lasted until late October. For all these reasons, Amsterdamskii estimated that the actual number of cholera cases ran up to 6,000, and that there was a higher mortality rate as well.[155]

Compounding the high overall mortality caused by cholera was its distribution over time, which also contributed to making the epidemic a shocking experience for those who lived through it. After the scattered, though increasingly frequently occurring cases of cholera between 15 and 28 June, the epidemic suddenly grew to more than 100 new cases every day by the beginning of July.[156] People now witnessed more than 70 deaths daily. On 4 July, the *Saratov Journal* noted that the cemetery recorded almost twice as many burials of adults within one month than during the whole year of 1891.[157] On 5 July, the epidemic reached its peak with 165 new cases and 111 deaths. From then on, the disease gradually abated, yet throughout the whole month of July the average daily death rate ran up to 41 people and the number of new cholera cases to 74.

Other factors need to be considered in assessing the impact of the epidemic. As some of the pioneers of historical scholarship on cholera have argued, by hitting mainly the poor cholera was an expression of social inequality in the face of disease and death.[158] Further research by Asa Briggs and Michael Durey has replaced this view. Both scholars concluded in their works that cholera affected all parts of a given society and therefore gains its significance as a barometer of social cohesion and stability in a time of crisis. More recently, Richard Evans has taken the existing positions under close scrutiny in what is as yet the most encompassing analysis on the "dimensions of inequality" which could be revealed by the epidemic.[159] For Saratov even as late as 1892 there is hardly any reliable material available which would allow one to delineate the distribution of the epidemic in real detail, i.e. the morbidity and mortality caused by cholera as related to the individual districts, to income, occupation, gender and age. General conclusions, however, can be drawn on the basis of the material collected by the municipal and the zemstvo hospital, the latter being both the biggest and the best-administered hospital in the city.[160]

Geographically, certain districts were ravaged particularly relentlessly by the epidemic. Beginning at the banks, cholera first spread to the fourth administrative district in which – in the *Valovaia* and *Chasovennaia* streets – were located cheap apartments for those workers who came directly from the steamships to the city.[161] Between June and July the epidemic significantly intensified from these foci and at the beginning of July almost everybody in these quarters adjacent to the *Glebuchev* ravine fell ill. With a death rate of 80% the area recorded the highest mortality from cholera in the city. At the *gory*, as well, cholera systematically

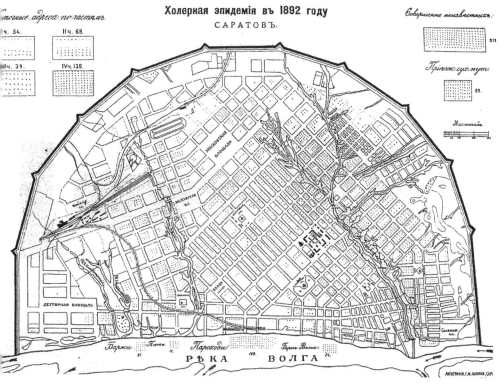

Figure 5 Map of the spread of cholera in Saratov, 1892, N.I. Matveev, *Gorod Saratov v sanitarnom otnoshenii* (Saratov, 1906).

struck house by house. Sometimes, the *vibrio* carried away a whole family within one hour. The epidemic further raged ferociously beyond the *Beloglinskii* ravine where the workers from the mills were living. And finally, at the beginning of July the river-front area where the epidemic had started became another centre of infection as a significant number of people stricken by cholera was coming from the Volga ships and barges. Altogether, the 60% of Saratov's population living at the city's margins accounted for 86% of all cholera cases.[162]

Saratov's physicians linked this geographic distribution of the disease to the possibility of having access to an uncontaminated water supply.[163] Yet as the material collected by the zemstvo hospital reveals the city centre was by no means immune. Places of infection included *Kamyshinskaia, Moskovskaia, Tsaritsyn-skaia, Tsyganskaia, Nikol'skaia, Nizhniaia* and *Astrakhanskaia* streets as well as the Theatre Square. A map created by Amsterdamskii confirms the broad distribution of the *vibrio* across the whole city.[164] Certainly the heaviest concentration of cholera cases was to be found in the city's traditionally weak sanitary spots but the pattern of the epidemic's distribution nevertheless illustrates that Saratov was afflicted everywhere. Sanitary facilities were bad throughout the whole city and nearly everywhere the water sources were polluted.

More illuminating is a look at various population groups. Although the zemstvo hospital only registered the information of its own patients it can be assumed that the data provide a representative cross-section of the population as all the hospitals were located in one area of the city. Clearly, the brunt of the epidemic was borne by people registered as peasants and townspeople (*meshchane*) who accounted for the vast majority of the population. Of the 446 patients recorded in the zemstvo hospital, only 27 belonged to other social categories.[165] The municipal hospital recorded 606 peasants and townspeople out of 641.[166] Most striking is the relatively low proportion of local people who were treated in the hospital. Eighty-five patients out of 434 in the zemstvo hospital were from Saratov city or Saratov district. More than 50% of those affected were registered in the provinces of Penza, Samara, Nizhnii Novgorod and Simbirsk.[167] Partly, the explanation for the preponderance of outsiders lies in the fact that many of the city residents tried to avoid the hospital at all costs and preferred to die at home. But at the same time, these figures also point to the population group most affected by the disease: seasonal migrants constituted the bulk of the cholera patients. This is confirmed by the classification of the hospital patients according to occupational groups. One hundred and ninety patients fulfilled all kinds of jobs on the ships.[168] These people were particularly vulnerable to the epidemic not only because they were poor and lived in unsanitary conditions; they also ran a high risk of catching the *vibrio* because of their work, which brought them in close contact to the river water. The remainder of the patients included workers from the hotels as well as small food and drink businesses; craftsmen working at the mills at the banks; workers from the railway; and finally, shoemakers, workers at the press, tailors and other craftsmen who were, however, not particularly exposed to the disease through their work at the river.

The course of the epidemic in Saratov thus confirms that the better-off residents were much less susceptible to the *vibiro* than the rest of the population. It is noteworthy that seasonal migrants who came for work on the ships and at the banks during the summer actually played a more important role in catching and spreading the disease than local residents. They were followed by a group of small shopkeepers, tradesmen and porters, who appear to have been particularly struck by the cholera. Having little possibility and chance to escape the *vibrio*, these people at the same time had no representation in the duma. They would have to make themselves heard by resorting to violence and rebellion.

When trying to explain the medical and social disaster caused by the epidemic across the whole country, Russian contemporaries pointed mainly to the violent and rigorous policy pursued by the central government. It is true that some of the misguided measures on the national level, especially the harsh quarantine rules imposed at the Caspian Sea and in Astrakhan', played a decisive role in the epidemic's rapid spread up the Volga. Nevertheless, placing the responsibility for the failure to effectively combat cholera solely on St Petersburg is one-sided and too crude. The analysis of local public health policy in Saratov provides a much more complex picture. Admittedly, the contribution of local governing authorities to fostering the epidemic as well as human suffering was significant. Overlapping jurisdictions, a confused chain of command as well as the chronic shortage of funds and personnel seriously hampered the swift distribution of information as well as medical supplies. Yet these were not the primary factors which determined the course of action taken by Saratov's administrative authorities. The truth was that, until forced by popular rebellion, municipal and provincial officials simply did not take the epidemic seriously. Legally entitled to take initiative in times of epidemics, local administrations failed to prepare the population, to develop a contingency plan and to take precautionary measures energetically – despite the forewarnings coming from Baku and Astrakhan'. This cannot be explained solely on the grounds of bureaucratic sterility and formalism, although, as could be seen at some moments, the development of initiative and ideas outside formal frameworks was often beyond local capacity. But the order from St Petersburg on 15 June to implement the decree on the formation of Sanitary Executive Commissions was actually of no real significance to the municipality until the epidemic was officially declared on 22 June (by St Petersburg as well). Ultimately, the decisive impetus for local governing officials to finally take action was the cholera riots.

In conclusion, although constrained by legislation as well as resources, local officials were not at their mercy. Rather, it was economic motives and the concern for public order that dictated the municipality's policy. Financial interests prevented the establishment of a quarantine at the Volga, which – in view of the fact that the migrant workers from the ships provided the highest contingent of the cholera cases – might have proved successful in containing the epidemic in good time. And, despite the shortage of personnel and medical resources, the actual problem during the first two weeks of the epidemic was not the shortage of resources but rather that those resources that were available were not utilised effectively. The cholera riots were a reaction to the ambiguous policy of the municipality which failed to protect the residents on the one hand whilst subjecting them to harsh police surveillance on the other. In fact, since the epidemic assumed its biggest proportions only after the riots, one might argue that it was the policy taken by local authorities that actually caused the medical disaster.

People and epidemic: the riots

In June 1892, before the presence of cholera in Saratov was even officially declared, the Persian consul at Tiflis passed on a cholera legend to Tiflis's population. First published in the *Tiflis Leaflet* (*Tifliskii Listok*), the legend circulated through Russia's newspapers and gained widespread popularity. On 18 June the story was printed in the *Saratov Journal*:

> One day, a mullah rode on a donkey to a city; suddenly, not far from the city, he saw a terrible ghost, moving right behind him. Dumbfounded by horror, the poor mullah almost fainted, but in the end, he overcame his fear and asked: "Who are you and what do you need?" To his surprise, the ghost respectfully bowed and said: "My name is cholera, and I am sent by Allah into the city to exterminate everybody who has sinned against him." To the mullah's question of how many sinners Allah had ordered the ghost to wipe out the ghost replied: "Five hundred people." "Listen", said the mullah, "swear to me that

you won't kidnap more than five hundred victims in this city." The ghost swore an oath, the mullah invited him to sit on the donkey behind the mullah, and they continued their journey. On arriving in the city, they departed after the ghost once more repeated his oath. After two, three days the mullah, having finished his business, left the city and asked how many people had died from cholera. He was told that three thousand had died. "Phooey!" exclaimed the mullah, recalling the oath of the ghost, "you have cheated me." But when, at a further distance from the city, he met the ghost again and started to reproach him with cheating the ghost assured him that he had only taken five hundred people, and that the remainder had died from fear.[169]

According to the interpretation in the *Saratov Journal*, the legend served as an illustration for the necessity to keep calm during the epidemic. Not to lose heart and to maintain one's vitality, the newspaper stated, were the best means to protect oneself against cholera.[170]

The legend was actually a herald of events to come. Fear and panic were the most distinctive features of the Russian cholera epidemic in 1892. They determined the course of the epidemic in Saratov as well as in the empire. Panic was the direct vehicle of introducing the infection into European Russia, and panic was one of the most powerful agents in distributing it throughout Astrakhan', Saratov and then up the Volga and throughout the country. Causing massive social uprising, the terror resulting from the epidemic became as great a danger as the cholera itself.

The role of cholera as a catalyst for social tensions and conflict erupting into full-scale riot has occupied a central place in the international historiography on the epidemic. Cholera, so goes the core of the argument, presented a challenge to society, a test of how its political, administrative and social mechanisms functioned in a time of exceptional stress. To the pioneering scholar in the field, Louis Chevalier, '*par le fait de l'épidémie, attitudes et comportement politiques et sociaux se confondent et se trouvent ramenés aux formes les plus primitives de l'existence individuelle et collective.*'[171] And for Asa Briggs, cholera 'tested the efficiency and resilience of local administrative structures. It exposed relentlessly political, social and moral shortcomings.'[172]

Riots were the most prominent social response, especially during the first pandemic which overtook Europe in 1830. Russia presented the most extreme case. Most legendary in the country's cholera history is the uprising at the Haymarket Square in St Petersburg in 1831.[173] Brought under control by Tsar Nicholas's personal intervention the uproar became a symbol of the tsar's courage and authority. Such was the impact of the riot that it captured the imagination of contemporary artists. It inspired Pushkin to write his dramatic masterpiece *Feast during the Plague* (*Pir vo vremia chumy*) and is further commemorated by the monument at the Haymarket Square.[174] Yet notwithstanding the infamous events in St Petersburg, the most serious cholera riots since the first pandemic occurred at the lower Volga, in particular in Astrakhan' and Saratov. It was at the country's periphery that governmental authorities were most challenged.[175]

During the fifth pandemic, however, social disturbances caused by cholera need to be regarded as the exception to the general pattern. Over the course of the century, the progress of medical science, the implementation of sanitary reforms and the increase of education resulted in a gradual containment of the epidemic. This in turn led to the abatement of cholera riots in western Europe. Still, cholera riots during the fifth and sixth pandemics are known from Italy.[176] Yet Hamburg, for instance, did not experience any social disturbances during the outbreak in the summer of 1892, while Saratov was shaken by them.[177] Moreover, Saratov was not the only case in Russia. Empire-wide, the population exhibited attitudes and behavioural patterns – from panic, flight, poisonous hysteria and the scapegoating of doctors to violent tumults – that mirrored the reactions from the first pandemic in 1830/31.

The final section of this chapter analyses the various popular responses to the cholera outbreak in Saratov in the summer of 1892. It looks at the emergence of public fear and unrest after the arrival of the first cholera rumours; it examines the economic, political, social and medical reasons for increasing opposition to official authorities, both political and medical; it also describes the cholera riot as the culmination of public resistance and identifies the underlying social tensions and conflicts which, prompted by the cholera, erupted into a full-scale revolt. Finally, the section pinpoints the consequences of the riot, both for the city and for the empire.

In stark contrast to official authorities, Saratov's population had been stirred up by the cholera news since the beginning of June. While local authorities were waiting for the officially proclaimed outbreak in Astrakhan', thousands of refugees arriving from the Volga delta foretold the brewing disaster. They brought direct reports about the latest events around the Caspian Sea, including the rigorous measures deployed to contain the disease.[178] First-hand accounts about the epidemic also spread through letters.[179] The disturbing accounts together with the fugitives' very presence had a deeply unsettling effect on the *Saratovtsy*. The local press described the atmosphere in the city as "restless/anxious" (*bespokoinyi*), "alarmed" (*trevozhnii*) and "agitated" (*vozbuzhdennyi*).[180] The prospect of cholera had stirred people's imagination, as one newspaper put it, 'up to colossal dimensions'.[181] Cholera became the topic of the day.

The news from downstream partly raised alarm since it arrived at a time of utmost economic and social strain. Human physical and mental resources were drained. I.I. Molleson expressed a widely held view when awaiting the cholera in June:

> The time we are living through now, of course, will long stay in our memory since the famine with its companions, the epidemics of typhus and scurvy, will leave fatal and indelible marks on the population for a long time. Yet the situation might get even more tragic because while we have still not managed to cope with these two diseases a third, even more terrifying disease approaches us from Persia.[182]

Yet purely economic and material factors do not sufficiently explain the tremendous impact cholera had on the imagination of the population. Other elements compounded public anxiety. The province had been exposed to an outbreak of bubonic plague in 1878, which people still remembered with unease. Strict quarantine measures had successfully contained the epidemic but had also created a situation such as in wartime, by placing serious economic restrictions upon the population and depriving it of basic personal rights. Worst of all, the law stated that any breach of the quarantine regulations, which were usually unknown to the populace, was to be punished with death.[183] The prediction of further economic disruption and personal deprivation in the midst of extreme physical and mental distress could not but provoke popular alarm.

Even more importantly, however, cholera itself had created a horrifying image during the past century. Since 1823 when the epidemic first arrived on Russian soil it had been present during at least 26 years in large parts of the empire. In European Russia it had claimed more than 1,600,752 victims. Saratov province had lost more than 67,859 people during 11 cholera years.[184] By the end of the nineteenth century, the memory of the cholera's medical and social severity, particularly during the first two outbreaks in 1830 and 1848, was very much alive. Those who had survived the first two epidemics in Saratov still remembered the extremely hot weather preceding them, the panic which had gripped the population in the face of the unknown, lethal disease, and the heaps of dead bodies which had been brought to the cemetery.[185] The terrifying impact of cholera on the city's population, Saratov's elderly residents maintained, had been even stronger than that of the plague, which had at least been a disease already familiar to them.[186] Although this comparison most likely does not stand up to historical reality, it reveals the apocalyptic attitude with which cholera was still awaited as late as 1892.[187] As Frank Clemow explained to the contemporary English reader, cholera 'is the modern Russian equivalent of our ancestors' "A plague upon you".'[188]

Fear and anxiety gripped rich and poor, educated and illiterate alike. Most noticeable to contemporary observers, panic dissolved itself into mass flight. Every major city at the lower Volga was deserted by thousands of terrified people who desperately jammed the ships in an attempt to escape the disease. The bulk of the refugees embarked at Astrakhan', where the governor actively encouraged the departure of the city's population by giving free tickets to the poor. Such was the run on the steamers in the south that it became difficult to get on a ship in Saratov. On 23 June the *Saratov Journal* noted that:

> Lately, we are told, huge numbers of passengers are noticeable on the ships coming from Tsaritsyn. Rumour has it that these are *Astrakhantsy* moving to up-river and to other provinces. All classes on the ships are overcrowded by them, so that in Saratov almost no places are left for those who want to take a place at the local docks.[189]

In Saratov, it was especially the well-off citizens who tried to leave the city either by train or by ship.[190] Some of them were so horrified that they sought refuge at Lake Elton which, so the rumour went, had always been spared by cholera.[191] The newspapers even declared that the administrative buildings at the lake, which had been deserted with the closing down of the salt mines, would provide comfortable accommodation for fugitives. Both statements soon proved false. Three weeks later the press had to report that 'the fugitives are bound to return unless they wish to live there in a tent, following the example of the Kyrgyz.'[192]

In this climate of unsettling rumours, fear, panic and mass flight, the administrative confusion in Saratov during the first three weeks of the epidemic further stoked people's anxiety. While fugitives made the cholera public knowledge, the municipality's full anti-cholera "plan" was not set in motion. Yet partial preventive measures went into effect right after the second duma meeting on 16 June. No information or instructions had prepared the population about the public preventive measures that would be taken. The publication of Molleson's booklet as well as the posters which informed about the cholera campaign came too late to prepare the *Saratovtsy* in good time. And when it came, illiteracy and poverty rendered it impossible for the vast majority of the population to follow the important recommendations: scrupulous cleanliness, particular concern with diet, immediate medical care and moderation.

From the very beginning, therefore, the procedures taken by the administration failed to convince the population of their protective mission. At best, people reacted by stubbornly denying the existence of the epidemic. Countless complaints in the press testified the widespread popular refusal to acknowledge the threat. It was only in the second week of July that the *Saratov Journal* finally observed some seriousness about the situation among the populace.[193] Roderick McGrew has shown that such denial of cholera was a common response to the epidemic since 1831 and was itself a reaction to fear.[194] Yet, in addition the denial of the epidemic was also an expression of the growing suspicion of the people towards official authority.[195] The municipality's first cholera measures were not only unpopular but also incomprehensible since the cholera had not yet arrived. Moreover, they clashed headlong with what people had hitherto been used to. Remote lanes and courts which had never received any attention by governmental officials were suddenly visited by police authorities and medical personnel. To cap it off, the same people who had so far neglected to carry out any welfare programmes for the poor now ordered the poorest inhabitants of the city to clean their courts at their own cost.[196] Ultimately, these measures built up popular suspicion towards official authorities, while they did nothing to provide effective control of the epidemic.

Relations between the people and governmental officials deteriorated rapidly as the first cholera cases passed through the city. The municipality switched to a policy of assiduous interventionism. To prevent the population from eating contaminated food the city administration heavily restricted the sale of vegetables, fruit and *kvas*. On 24 June all the small shops at the riverbanks were forced to close down completely.[197] With regard to the events on 28 June this decision proved most fateful. It deeply affected many of the city's inhabitants' very existence since it interrupted their normal economic activities and cut off their major source of income. Also, it spread dissatisfaction on the ships. On 26 June, two days before the riot, the *Saratov Journal* provided the full picture:

On what are the labourers and passengers on the ships to feed themselves? It is already the third day that the arriving passengers on the ships, for whom the ship buffet is inaccessible, are disappointed in their hopes – to provide themselves with food products at our shops at the banks. They are all closed down and the poorest passengers have to leave Saratov hungry, because looking for products in the city is accompanied by the risk of missing the departure of the ship.[198]

Compounding the economic issues at stake, the decision to close down the small shops created and exposed social conflict. For while the authorities restricted petty trade within the city, no effective measures were taken to control incoming goods from the ships. Gathering anger about social inequality in the face of cholera was at the same time exacerbated by the fact that the disease struck mainly the poor. Not surprisingly, most inhabitants started to take not only the municipality's measures but also the epidemic as a whole as a full-scale attack on the people arbitrarily launched by a malevolent government which was aiming at killing the poor.

Civil conflict was stoked by the sanitary campaign which took effect in full form as soon as the epidemic was officially declared. St Petersburg's strategy of coercion set the tone. The 'Instruction on the formation of sanitary commissions' plainly approved the violation of civil rights and Saratov took it literally.[199] What followed after the official announcement of the epidemic on 22 June had little to do with modern scientific medicine. Instead, the city's defence bore close resemblance to the epidemic world which had found its artistic expression in Defoe's and Manzoni's novels on seventeenth-century London and Milan.[200] Since neither sufficient doctors nor health officials were available in Saratov to enforce the municipality's scheme of defence the police were charged with the detection of cholera cases as well as with the execution of the administrative rules. This destroyed whatever trust and confidence people might have had in their government. The police officials lacked the medical knowledge to identify a cholera case and were notorious for the brutal handling of the sick. They dragooned anybody who exhibited suspicious symptoms into the hospital, regardless of whether this was a cholera case or not, much to the resentment of the populace and medical officials.[201] One resident described the atmosphere:

Of course, measures have been taken to put an end to the dreadful epidemic, but the measures taken are most foolish in a way. Imagine, the police administration, in the person of its main representatives, drum into every subordinate down to the last police constable and horse guard, that provided they see people with symptoms of a disease named "cholera" in the city, they should without debate take these people into the police stations. In such a way, it went on for three days, carts drove around the city to collect the sick. Some were caught in a state of complete drunkenness and when they woke up, after the way had shaken them in order, and saw the gates of the municipal cholera hospital they took to flight; and the nurse had to catch the imaginary cholera cases.[202]

While normal life came to a standstill the medical aspects of the epidemic added to people's fear. By the end of the nineteenth century, cholera was still a disease which could attack and kill a victim within hours. Its outbreak was unpredictable, and its causes not yet known. Whereas tuberculosis was a permanent, omnipresent killer, cholera raged through a population rapidly and disappeared leaving the dead behind. This rapidity and temporary nature made cholera psychologically unmanageable for societies which had developed coping mechanisms for long-term killers (such as tuberculosis).[203]

Additionally, the sick exhibited horrifying symptoms. The disease could strike if the *vibrio cholerae*, after being ingested, entered the human digestive tract. The bacillus released a toxic poison which made the intestinal wall porous in both directions. As a result not only were nutrients absorbed from the intestine into the blood stream but the blood fluid could drain backward into the intestine. This unleashed the illness. Massive purging and vomiting of liquid (the "rice-water stools") transformed the human body into a living corpse. A person could rapidly lose up to two-thirds of his body fluids; as a result, the blood coagulated and ceased to circulate properly. With falling blood pressure the victims' skin became blue, their eyes hollow, and their bodies cold as ice. Due to the loss of oxygen and salt, agonising cramps tortured the sick. Within a few days, often even within a few hours dehydration as well as the lack of chemicals and electrolytes could lead to total renal failure, toxaemia and death.[204]

Against such painful and horrifying disease there was still no cure in 1892. Koch's discovery of the *comma bacillus* in Egypt and Calcutta in 1883/4 had inaugurated a new era in the history of cholera insofar as it provided a reliable means to diagnose the disease and to take preventive public health measures against it. However, by identifying the existence of the *vibrio* in cholera-stricken places, Koch had not actually proven its causative role. It was only Koch's further research during the Hamburg epidemic in combination with the course of the epidemic itself in 1892 that led to the decisive breakthrough of his bacteriological model of cholera against Pettenkofer's miasmatist approach.[205] Yet even then, he could not offer any effective remedy against the bacillus.

It is against this clinical background that popular suspicion and hostility towards medical authorities in Saratov in 1892 needs to be seen. Even when taken to the hospitals against their will, there was little chance for the sick surviving inside the buildings. Indeed, the new cholera hospitals and barracks which were established along the Volga River became a major source of fear and horror for the people. Ironically, although it was a centre of epidemic diseases, Saratov possessed no facility at all to accommodate and isolate the victims of an epidemic emergency. The Demidov house, the hastily improvised cholera hospital, could accommodate only 75 patients. Despite the additional temporary barracks which were established along the river banks by the city, the zemstvo and the state, the available facilities were far from sufficient. Even when the epidemic had already abated, the hospitals were so overcrowded that the sick were kept in military tents in the court of the municipal hospital.[206]

Conditions inside the hospitals were appalling. Most of the improvised cholera buildings were crumbling, unhygienic and lacking in fundamental facilities. According to a medical report the cholera barracks at the Volga banks between Nizhnii Novgorod and Astrakhan' were badly equipped and mostly encompassed empty buildings without furniture, dishes, medications and physicians. Saratov's cholera hospitals, the report noted, were in the worst state when compared with any other provincial capital at the Volga.[207] A student working at the zemstvo hospital during the epidemic described a place of horror:

> The hospital was overcrowded, in fact too overcrowded, with too few nurses; nobody could look after the sick. I cannot remember this dark barracks, where masses of sick were piled up, without horror. The place was terribly crowded. Here a patient vomits, there another has diarrhoea, all this falls directly on the floor, the same floor, on which their nearby neighbours roll in agonizing cramps. And the groaning, why all the groaning? What terrible agony must the sick, from whose mouth these terrible groans are heard, experience![208]

Alongside material shortcomings, the inexperience of hastily hired medical students as well as the lack of cure itself exposed Saratov's cholera patients to drastic therapeutic methods and medical experiments. Most universally approved and frequently applied in the city (and in Russia in general) were hot baths to improve the patients' circulation and provide relief from the cramps.[209] They were clearly favoured in Saratov, insofar as medical facilities and resources allowed, for the Demidov house, in fact, had no bath.[210] Beyond harmless baths, however, the city's physicians in 1892 modified treatment strategies which had been handed down since 1831.[211] The most commonly employed method involved depletive therapies, especially the administering of purgatives.[212] By 1892 the international medical community had discarded depletion as ineffective against cholera, yet Saratov's physicians continued to pour calomel and bismuth into their patients, two favourite substances since the first pandemic.[213] Subcutaneous infusions of saline solutions were also made in order to counteract the dehydration. According to the report from the zemstvo hospital this strategy 'yielded no results'. In too many cases, medical treatment was painful and, moreover, had deadly consequences. The zemstvo hospital as the best equipped of the available institutions recorded a death rate caused by cholera of more than 56%.[214] Here was the plausible source for the popular idea that doctors were poisoning people.

One further element massively reinforced people's bitterness towards medical authorities: the state's funerary regulations prohibited any funeral services for the dead and violated traditions of mourning.[215] In no circumstances was the dead corpse to be given to the relatives for the burial. Instead, it had to be wrapped in sheets dampened in disinfectant solution, put into a coffin which was tightly nailed and brought to a special cholera cemetery.[216]

Terrified and frequently illiterate, Saratov's inhabitants took their own view on the cholera campaign. A poisoning phobia overtook the city. People were convinced that the government had invented the cholera in order to exterminate surplus populations.[217] Medical officials and policemen, popular imagination held, acted as state agents who intended to kill off the poor. Modifying the medical theory of the deadly cholera toxin, poisoning became the major killing method. People also figured out how the poison was administered: it was contained in some liquid in small bottles which were carried around by medical and police officials. The deadly substance was simply inhaled as the victims were forced to sniff at the bottle.[218] If not poisoned, the sick were allegedly buried alive in the hospitals. The local press circulated an extreme version of this widely held belief:

> In the city persistent rumours go round about some townsman with the name Kashin, who was drunk yet taken for a cholera case and brought to the hospital where he was laid into a coffin and covered with lime. When he woke up at night, he ran home dressed in a blanket. At his appearance his family got so scared that his wife as yet is close to death. It needs to be noted that many people believe in these tales and it would be desirable that these rumours were refuted in an official way.[219]

Everywhere, the authorities met with a sullen opposition. Although petty trade was forbidden, shopkeepers continued their sales through the backdoors of their shops; countless reports in the newspapers commented on the widespread refusal to report cholera cases to the police; families tried to shield the cholera sick from medical attention and to protect their belongings from fumigation and disinfection procedures; even the dying rejected their prescriptions and preferred to die unattended than to fall into the hands of the doctors.[220] Within only a few days, evasion turned into open resistance.

Forewarnings of an imminent rebellion entered the city by ship. On 25 June an open revolt broke out among the passengers aboard the steamship "Niagara", most of them fugitives from the riots in Astrakhan' on 21 and 22 June. As a few cholera cases had occurred on the ship it had to halt at some distance from Saratov. This agitated the passengers. Up to 50 people, armed with hammers from the engine room, threatened to throw the captain of the steamer into the water and to kill the engine-driver if he halted the ship. Soldiers from Saratov arrived in good time to cope with the rioters.[221] Yet these rumblings were only the first indication that the arrivals from Astrakhan' might not only bring medical but also social disaster. Two days later, on the eve of the riot, isolated verbal threats were hurled at Saratov's physicians and police members. The population threatened 'to prepare them in Astrakhan' fashion' (*razdelat'sia po Astrakhan'skii*), but nobody was actually attacked or hurt. Nevertheless, the provincial administration grew apprehensive about the rising anxiety in the city. To provide a visible presence of governmental authority it sent military troops for a ceremonial march through the centre on the evening of 27 June.[222]

The exercise failed to prevent the riot. In the early morning of 28 June, the spectre of the cholera poison ran its course on the *Verkhovnyi Bazar* – Saratov's main market square and as such the centre of news, gossip and all kinds of rumours.[223] Public hysteria was stoked by a man (said to have been a plasterer) who appeared at the market square smeared all over with lime claiming that he had been collared by the police with pincers, put into the van and sprinkled with lime but managed to escape. Gradually, groups of people filled the streets adjacent to and surrounding the market square. Armed with stones, sticks and axes, they developed into a throng estimated to number up to 2,000 people. According to the newspaper reports, a cholera van sparked off the tumult. It was a widespread belief that the vans carried mainly drunkards to the hospital instead of sick people. As a woman was being taken into the van in front of people's eyes, the populace pounced on the vehicle, beat the driver and tore the van into pieces. This unleashed the violence which quickly spread through the whole city centre.

Deadly scenes marked the upheaval. At the market square, the populace saw a passer-by who was unlucky enough to wear a white jacket. In the mistaken belief that this was a doctor people gave chase. They seized the person at the *Tsyganskaia* street, where they stabbed and stoned him. A friend of the victim, who tried to intervene, was shouted down and took to his heels when attacked and beaten by the populace. Less fortunate was the student who attempted to calm the crowd. People overpowered him and pelted him with stones. Both the pedestrian and the student were stoned and trampled to death. Shortly thereafter, a night watchman was taken for a policeman and mortally wounded.

At the southern side of the market square, knots of people gathered in the adjacent *Nikol'skaia, Nemetskaia, Aleksandrovskaia* and *Gromovaia* streets. On seeing three policemen the crowd shouted 'Hurrah', and gave vent to its fury. While two policemen made their escape the third was seized and beaten until unconscious. Excited and in blind anger, the crowd began a systematic manhunt for doctors and policemen. Street by street it stormed the apartments of all the doctors living in this area, smashed the windows and pillaged their rooms. After that, the police building in the district was broken into. The mob charged the police office, broke the furniture into fragments, destroyed all documents and forms, and covered the surrounding streets with shreds of paper.

Meanwhile, another crowd set off for the recently opened cholera hospital. At around 11 o'clock the building was taken by storm. The physicians made their escape. One feldsher took refuge in the bell tower of the nearby Vladimir church and was rescued by the priest who faced the crowd holding a cross in his hands. Undoubtedly endangering the whole town the rioters released the sick. Some of them escaped, others were taken back to their homes by the invaders. The remainder were laid out on the street. The liberators poured milk and water over them, and rubbed them with ice, all the while reassuring the sick that they were not stricken by cholera. Inside the building all windows were broken and furniture as well as coffins crushed into pieces. Following this, the mob set the whole building on fire. Threats of violence from the crowd prevented the arriving fire brigade from extinguishing the flames and the hospital burned down.

From the cholera hospital people converged on the municipal and the zemstvo hospitals, pillaging an apothecary shop on the way as well as the apartments of all the doctors living close by. Everywhere people broke the windows, smashed the furniture and left the rooms in shambles. Order was only restored with the arrival of two military battalions at the Cathedral Square. The crowd greeted the soldiers with shouting and whistling. When a stone struck a soldier on his head, the troops opened fire. One person was killed and eight people injured. The crowd dispersed and the city was placed under curfew. On the next day, the *Saratov Leaflet* reported:

> The city provided the picture of a military bivouac: on the Cathedral, Theatre, Moscow, and Poltava Squares, at the hospitals, banks and at other locations troops were permanently placed; in the afternoon of 29.6 two cannons were put up at the Cathedral Square, near the *Nemetskaia* street. Military staff and provincial administration took temporary shelter in the hotel 'Rossiia'. On the streets in the city centre as well as in its environs military troops continue to march. All theatre performances in the *Ochkin* theatre are cancelled; all inns, pubs and shops are closed. The public is absolutely calm, orderly walked on the streets and in the *Lipki* gardens. Many suspected participants in the riots are arrested. Order in the city is restored.[224]

Most contemporary observers ascribed the violent tumults on the lower Volga to the 'superstitious ignorance' of the population. Only a few days after the event, Saratov's mayor explained at a meeting of the provincial zemstvo that 'there are many reasons for the riots, but the main reason is the ignorance (*temnota*, lit.: darkness) of the population.'[225] In a similar vein, the *Saratov Leaflet* denounced the people for being as ignorant (*temno*) in 1892 as during the first cholera epidemic 60 years before and soberly concluded that neither reforms nor increased schools had fulfilled their civilising mission.[226] Furthermore, the local press branded the rioters as savage (*dikie*) and mad (*bezumnye*).[227] It was 'bestial envy towards the educated classes' which drove people to resistance.[228]

According to the provincial governor, the riots were something foreign, something that had been imported to Saratov from outside:

> These arrivals, homeless people, who have no relation to the place and its population, and who share no common interests with them, are exclusively guided by their passions, they are not subjected to any kind of order and earning sometimes from day to day a significant amount of money, they give way to drinking and unruly conduct. I allow myself to express my conviction that this element, under the impact of vine, provides a fruitful soil for all kinds of popular uprising. (. . .) No doubt, that after the disturbances in Astrakhan' the representatives of the unsettled crowd moved from there to Saratov with the aim to escape persecution; and by spreading exaggerated and false rumours about the measures taken in Astrakhan', they significantly contributed to the ferment which erupted on 28 June by spreading exaggerated and false rumours about the measures taken in Astrakhan'.[229]

These views have essentially been adopted by historians of late-nineteenth-century Russia. The complex problem of collective violence and social protest has so far mainly been investigated as an important indicator by which to study the development of a growing working-class consciousness and thus the working class itself. Thus, examining labour violence in late-nineteenth-century Russia, Daniel Brower argues that violent riots played an important part in the relations between factory and workers until well into the twentieth century.[230] According to him, Russian factory workers continued to expose an anarchistic, 'primitive' behaviour when defending their interests. However, by adapting violence to the needs of a working-class movement, 'the rise of violent protest late in the century constituted as important a signal as strikes of the emergence of working-class consciousness and a proletarian movement (. . .).'[231]

Brower's article stimulated a heated controversy about an interpretative framework for labour violence in late-imperial Russia and has been sharply criticised for its conceptual simplicity and terminological shallowness.[232] Robert E. Johnson pointed to the necessity to take account of the manifold forms, origins, as well as goals of worker unrest and to the shifting patterns of social protest as related to social and economic change over time. He further suggested that works on social violence outside Russia by Hobsbawm, Thompson, Rudé and Tilly would provide instructive and helpful methodological models to approach the issue. Similarly, Diane Koenker urged historians to analyse the specifics of examples, including the social identity of the participants, their targets, as well as the concrete reasons for violence. Additionally, she suggested posing questions based on comparative examples. Indeed, Friedgut's study of the Iuzovka riots is the exception among the prevailing studies on the Russian workers movement which, again, concentrated on St Petersburg and Moscow.[233] A closer look at the events in Saratov thus offers an instructive example of social protest in Russia's non-industrial periphery.

In addition, Saratov's cholera riots shed further light on the comparative history of cholera. Analysing the riots in Iuzovka, Theodore Friedgut placed his findings within the context of the Russian labour movement, yet simply did not take into account the rich historiography on cholera and cholera riots in particular. He relied on Frieden's analysis of the cholera rumours, but no reference is made to the important study by McGrew, not to mention the works by Chevalier, Durey and Morris. As a result, despite providing a thorough analysis of the social and economic conditions of the Iuzovka labourers, Friedgut did not satisfactorily explain the cholera riots. Following the dubious theoretical concept provided by Brower, he could not identify some sort of class consciousness in the riots and thus conceived them as essentially irrational and blind violence wielded by an ignorant, superstitious and fearful populace whose aim was 'catharsis' and 'plunder'.[234]

This strict juxtaposition of class consciousness versus ignorance and superstition is grossly oversimplified and additionally misleading. Such explanations reduce the rioters to passive Russian yokels and thus render impossible any attempt to place their resistance in its historical, political and social context. Moreover, they ignore the historical significance of the cholera riots themselves. For by 1892 popular violence as a reaction to cholera was anachronistic in most parts of Europe. The progressive scientific understanding of the disease, the sanitary reform movement, increasing medical socialisation and general education had led to a gradual decline in cholera mortality and consequently to the abatement of social disturbances caused by cholera as well. The Russian experience of the fifth pandemic stood out in Europe not only because a whole nation proved susceptible to epidemic disaster when this was not the case elsewhere in Europe anymore. Even more striking, large parts of the country succumbed to violent terror, thereby revealing social and medical attitudes which had basically vanished from Europe long since. The resort to the population's ignorance and madness cannot explain this phenomenon – if solely because it deprives the epidemic of any meaning to the rioters anyway. Yet it needs to be explained why cholera could unleash such violence in 1892, whereas the famine in 1891–92 did not. Examining further particulars of the events in Saratov, such as the protesters' social composition, their objects and behaviour and the underlying reasons for tension and eventually overt revolt might offer a more comprehensible explanation, elucidate the meaning of the rioters' behaviour and place the uproar in its historical context.[235]

To begin with, a closer look at official accounts of the cholera riot in Saratov does not uphold the image of the uprooted peasant migrant prone to revolt and rebellion. One of the most exhaustive articles on the cholera disturbances in the newspaper *Russian Gazette* (*Russkie Vedomosti*) noticed that the crowd mainly consisted of all kinds of tradesmen.[236] This profile is amply attested by the public reports in the same newspaper on the court trial which began on 23 October of the same year.[237] It appears that of the 154 people brought to trial, 50 were registered as townspeople (*meshchane*) and 69 as peasants (*krest'iane*). Seventeen rioters were recruited from the military. The remainder were simply listed as countrymen (*poseliane*). Many of the participants were between 20 and 35 years of age.[238] It emerges from their statements, as well as from the evidence provided by the witnesses, that most of them made a living in the city as small shopkeepers, craftsmen and journeymen. They had stable jobs and abodes and were sufficiently settled to be recognised at the court by local witnesses and policemen. Except for one worker at the Reineke mills, neither factory workers, vagrants nor slum dwellers were recorded in the report.

The immediate motives of the rioters certainly were the heavy economic restrictions implemented by the municipality on 24 June. Yet their assaults were carefully targeted against selected victims (physicians and policemen), while violence was mainly confined to the destruction of their property. Neither shop looting, nor the wrecking of machinery or the invasion of market squares were elements in Saratov's disturbances – a point in which the city's riots differed from those in Iuzovka.[239] It is also striking that the disturbances took place in the most respectable and fashionable precinct of the city, confined by the *Aleksandrovskaia*, *Nikol'skaia*, *Tsaritsynskaia* and *Konstantinovskaia* streets. By contrast, in Naples in 1884 the cholera riots happened in the Lower City, the area which was inhabited by the poorest residents and most afflicted by epidemic diseases. Russian state authorities might have failed in assessing social realities. But they were right in decoding the essence of the uproar: it was a challenge against official authority in the first place.

Without any organisational representation in what was still an autocratic state, Saratov's tradesmen were left to their own devices in defending their economic as well as their health interests. Small tradesmen and shopkeepers were not represented in the duma. A working-class movement was only in its earliest incipience. The first industrial disturbances occurred in 1899 and the era of public demonstrations conducted by political organisations with well-defined programmes and objectives took off only after 1901.[240] When political and medical authorities intervened in the most haphazard and brutal way into people's personal lives and existence, the population had to articulate itself by its own means.

As scholars on the history of cholera have stressed, however, such harsh attacks against medical and administrative authorities would not have been possible without a long history of deep-rooted popular resentment against governmental authorities.[241] A traditional place of exile for religious dissidents, conscripts and serfs since the seventeenth century, Saratov could boast to be most famous for its spirit of independence and rebelliousness as well as its centuries-long tradition of peasant revolts.[242] Not accidentally, the province and its capital had proved most susceptible to cholera riots during the first two pandemics. In 1861, the province had counted 120 peasant rebellions, 64 of which were militarily suppressed.[243] In the capital the ground for social discontent and political protest had been well prepared at least since the 1850s when Chernyshevskii, the later editor of the *Contemporary* (*Sovremennik*), worked as a teacher at the local gymnasium (1851–52). Whereas peasant resistance waned in the 1870s, populists (Land and Liberty, People's Will, and the Party of People's Rights) were attracted to the province in the hope to find a fertile soil for revolutionary propaganda. Throughout the 1880s and 1890s the province abounded with former members of the populist movements, the most prominent among them Stepka Balmashev, Vera Figner, M.A. Natanson and G.V. Plekhanov. In 'circles', 'salons' and 'evenings' they gathered the local working population, predominantly craftsmen and often shop owners.[244] Clearly by 1892, the soil was prepared for the articulation of social discontent. Saratov's wage-earning inhabitants were clearly aware about their economic interests even though these were not as yet organised in political parties and programmes. Not surprisingly, the Party of the People's Rights created the bridge between the movements of the 1870s and the agitation that led to the formation of the Socialist Revolutionary Party in Saratov.

The riots in Saratov in 1892 confirm the more recent research on cholera by Michael Durey (Britain), Roderick McGrew (Russia), Francois Delaporte (France), Richard Evans (Germany) and Frank Snowden (Italy), to name just a few, who have demonstrated that the origins of the social responses to cholera involved more than the eruption of class antagonisms. In addition, they demonstrate that social violence in Russia at the end of the nineteenth century cannot be reduced to the issue of class consciousness. Furthermore, they dismiss the stereotype of the fickle Russian peasant prone to violence and irrational destruction. Saratov's inhabitants responded to the epidemic by means of open rebellion for a series of identifiable reasons. Faced with a deadly disease people could not feel protected by the rigorous, yet at best half-way and belatedly implemented measures of their local governors. Unaccustomed to medical attention, the sanitary measures they were subjected to were unfamiliar, incomprehensible and economically threatening. At the same time, medical procedures were brutal and inhuman. Furthermore, the riots were the social response to those authorities who had neglected the welfare of the majority of their subjects. Creating the conditions under which cholera could flourish, local governors had fostered deep-rooted suspicion and hostility among the population against them. By 1892, those who were most affected by the lack of water supply, poverty, illiteracy and cholera still had no voice which represented their interests against local government.

The social tumults in Astrakhan' and Saratov had demonstrated that popular unrest could become as great a menace as the disease. The government was thoroughly alarmed and immediately took drastic measures. On 2 July, the Ministry of Internal Affairs responded with further repression. It declared that any social disorder and violence caused by the cholera would be cut off by military means. Arsonists and murderers would be court-martialled according to war-time laws.[245] In Saratov, the declaration was pasted all over the city. As its direct result, more than 200 people were arrested.

Violence fostered the spread of the epidemic. Trying to escape the disorder in Saratov, many people carried the disease across the province and up the Volga. Saratov's fugitives were reported from places as far as Perm and the Kama region.[246] Along with the disease they spread social unrest. By force of example, a series of riots overtook the whole province and affected Khvalynsk, Petrovsk and the Pokrovsk settlement. In Balakovo, a district city in Saratov province, people took the only just finished cholera hospital to pieces.[247] Most famous became the brutal murder of the physician A.M. Molchanov in the district town of Khvalynsk.[248] In the villages, too, physicians encountered innumerable difficulties as a result of the cholera rumours which spread from the capital to the countryside. In Viazovko, Nikolaevsk and Popovko, the doctors had to depart under threats from the population.[249] Yet the unsettling effects of Saratov's riots extended far beyond the provincial borders. When a townsman (*meshchanin*) brought news of the events from Saratov to Nizhnii Novgorod, a general put him into a cholera barrack so that he could convince himself as an involuntary assistant about the reality of the cholera and the caring role of the physicians.[250] In Kazan' peasants were sentenced to one to two months' imprisonment as they stirred up public opinion against physicians.[251]

With the breakdown of public order in the south, local and central governing authorities started to take the epidemic more seriously. State, zemstvo and municipality finally caught up on what needed to be done. On 4 July, the *St Petersburg Gazette* (*St. Peterburgskie Vedomosti*) noted:

> In the fight against cholera one can notice some animation. The medical personnel in the cholera region has been strengthened by 50 physicians, 22 students and 37 feldshers. Petitions from the cities, zemstva and various private institutions about the dispatch of medical staff of various ranges are

followed without hesitation [. . .] The efforts are mainly directed to halting the further spread of the epidemic along the Volga.[252]

State authorities got down to establishing medical observation points along the Volga River. On 18 July the Ministry of Ways and Communications sent a delegate from St Petersburg down the Volga in order to provide the hospitals with medical supplies and linens. For the first time since the outbreak of the epidemic the zemstvo met on 1 July to discuss its contribution in combating the cholera.[253] It decided to provide extra space for cholera cases in the zemstvo hospital and to organise more medical personnel. And the municipality established permanent medical care at the banks.

Furthermore, as a result of the cholera riot Saratov had a much higher mortality rate caused by cholera as compared to any other city at the middle and lower Volga. The immediate medical consequence of the disturbances was a sharp increase in cholera cases. Whereas the zemstvo hospital recorded between three and five cholera cases in June, numbers abruptly rose to more than 20 cases daily at the beginning of July.[254] Aleksandr Amsterdamskii reported eight cholera cases in the whole city on 28 June as opposed to 164 cases on 6 July, the day the epidemic reached its peak.[255] The explanation for this dramatic development involved more than just the fact that the population had carried the sick out of the hospitals; people had also collared the hospital linens, pillows and sheets and taken them home. Parts of the hospital fittings were also pawned.[256] At the same time, the rioters had destroyed the all too scarce medical facilities. Many physicians were no longer willing to work in the hospitals without armed guards.

Conclusion

Cholera, as R.J. Morris has put it, 'was a test of social cohesion. To follow the cholera track was not just, as some observers have claimed, to follow the track of filth and poverty, it was to watch the trust and co-operation between different parts of society strained to the utmost.'[257] The question of how and to what degree cholera challenged and exposed the strengths as well as the weaknesses of a given society has occupied a central place in the historiography of epidemic. Richard Evans suggested that cholera experience might tell us something 'about the abilities of . . . state structures to adapt to the challenge posed by disease and its associated discontents.'[258]

The Russian cholera epidemic of 1892 presents a perfect case with which to test this hypothesis. At the end of the nineteenth century the only autocratic state in Europe experienced a cholera epidemic which devastated the whole country and created violent social reactions in its wake. Examining the factors that led to the catastrophe is not only significant for the comparative history of cholera; it also allows one to probe the viability of the tsarist regime at the dawn of the revolutionary era. Who was responsible for the death of almost a third of a million people during the summer of 1892? Were the government and Russian society working together or were they already falling apart?

In his analysis of the famine in 1891, Richard Robbins concluded:

The Imperial government's ability to deal effectively with the famine in the face of its acknowledged political and institutional problems indicates that at the beginning of the 1890s the old regime had considerable reserves of strength. Its officials, while no doubt inefficient and venal by present standards, were capable of creative and imaginative response to a serious domestic crisis. Nor had the government so far alienated the public that it could not rally broad support for its activities. [. . .] Surely the ability of a state to mobilize its human and material resources to meet an immediate challenge is a token of its capacity to survive. In 1891–92 the Russian government accomplished this task. The story of the famine year suggests that the Tsarist regime was more resilient, its grip on life firmer, than its critics, past and present, have maintained.[259]

This view is not uncontested. Historians have widely argued that both famine and cholera plainly exposed the weakness and ineptness of the tsarist government and thus significantly contributed to fostering a process of growing alienation and conflict between the government and the population.[260] The analysis of Saratov's cholera epidemic in 1892 can shed further light on Russian statecraft at the end of the nineteenth century. Indeed, the course of the epidemic suggests that common assumptions about the backward, inefficient and repressive tsarist regime need to be differentiated and modified. Certainly, the central government did not ignore the epidemic, and as early as April 1892 it took the first steps to counter the approaching menace. Moreover, Russian state authorities launched what might be considered the largest anti-cholera campaign in the European history of the epidemic. In addition to the measures along the Persian–Russian border and on the Caspian Sea, the state established 77 cholera hospitals along the Volga River and in the Kama Basin within two weeks and staffed them with medical supplies and personnel.[261] Barracks for the reception and treatment of cholera patients were also built along railway lines;[262] a stream of decrees and orders regulated in detail the provision of disinfection means, the supervision of food and drink on boats and at landing docks, the arrangements for moving patients to hospitals, the dispatch of immediate medical aid, the general sanitation measures in the cities and much more.

However, the epidemic did plainly expose and magnify serious institutional and political deficiencies of the old regime. Russia had not as yet embarked on the sanitary reform movement which protected most western European countries from the *vibrio*. The major reason for this deficit was a partially modernised legislative and administrative framework which devolved the financial responsibility of public health to local authorities while maintaining the final authority over all medical affairs in St Petersburg. As a result, the best protection against the *vibrio*, the sanitary achievements of the modern state, were lacking empire-wide. In addition, the confused and contradictory medical jurisdiction hampered the swift supply of information, medical and personnel resources during the epidemic itself. State measures within the country were simply enacted too late to prevent a national medical and social catastrophe.

Yet the crucial weakness of the national policy to combat cholera was the reliance on quarantine measures which were coercively enforced by the police and the military. This strategy set the Russian experience of the fifth pandemic apart from western Europe, where most governments had rejected the use of militarily controlled quarantine procedures. Imposing the quarantine instigated the violent terror that erupted among the population at the lower Volga.

However, the fight against cholera conducted on the national level does not sufficiently explain the disastrous course of the epidemic in Saratov. Here, it was above all the weakness of the anti-cholera combat by local administrative officials which contributed most to the medical and social catastrophe. Local authorities failed to make use of their autonomy during the epidemic crisis, to develop precautionary measures in good time, to prepare the population and to mobilise available medical resources on suspicion of a cholera outbreak. Lack of initiative and imagination, an adherence to bureaucratic sterility and the unwillingness to face the menace compounded institutional obstacles and allowed the *vibrio* to flourish long before local authorities started to act.

Having neglected to protect the population medically, the city futilely resorted to brutal measures in order to control the epidemic once it had erupted. The populace, terrified by the disease itself, unprotected by its local governors and subjected to incomprehensible and inhumane sanitary and medical procedures, responded with suspicion, malevolence and, finally, violent resistance. The uprising, which was the product of local conditions, demonstrated the deep abyss gaping between administrative officials and the population. The cholera epidemic clearly revealed social and political antagonisms and ignited an explosion. Moreover, the riots that overtook the lower Volga signalled an atmosphere of widespread distrust, disregard and resentment towards the state and its representatives at the local level. Most importantly, the fact that governmental authorities resorted to military force in order to bring the rebellion under control indicated not that the tsarist regime was strong but that its authority was precarious.

4 Sanitised politics and the politics of medicine

The nation was dismayed by the cholera epidemic of 1892. That such an outbreak claimed more than 200,000 victims at a time when western European countries had already successfully overcome the *vibrio* belied the claim that Russia was a powerful, modern state. Public outrage at administrative bungling and brutality filled the newspapers, the medical press and the numerous congresses, both local and national, which were summoned in the epidemic's wake.[1] Compounding the high mortality figures, the violent uprisings accompanying the disease also pointed to deep-seated social cleavages and revealed the failures of Russian state-craft. On balance, the epidemic had exposed Russia's existing state structures as archaic and served as a massive indictment of the country's political, social and economic foundations.

Since Asa Briggs's and Louis Chevalier's early works on cholera, historians have been intrigued with the question of cholera's impact on society. Not only did cholera epidemics reveal the political and social shortcomings of a given society; that society's response, as Michael Durey put it, could also disclose 'much about its character which is not easily observable during periods of peace and relative harmony, or at least when underlying social tensions are hidden by the crust of formal social relationships'.[2] Briggs's and Chevalier's initial inquiries have inspired a number of monographs on the epidemic's impact on Western societies. Although their position has not gone unchallenged, most notably by Charles Rosenberg and Margaret Pelling, Briggs's and Chevalier's claims still determine the key themes addressed by the historical literature on the subject. Even Rosenberg noted that 'an epidemic provides a convenient and effective sampling device for studying in their structural relationship some of the fundamental components of social change'.[3]

Historical studies on cholera to date have discussed the epidemic's significance by focusing overwhelmingly on Europe's first encounter with the disease. The dramatic mortality brought about by a still unknown and exotic killer naturally led historians to assume that the impact of the first cholera epidemic on local popula-tions and society was far greater than that of subsequent outbreaks. After the first two pandemics, the epidemic became less lethal and the shock of the disease wore off. Declining mortality rates played an important role in minimising cholera's power to disturb society.[4]

Yet as the two existing studies on cholera's latest visitation to western Europe demonstrate, the historical significance of a cholera outbreak cannot be assessed through the number of victims left in the *vibrio*'s wake alone. The examples of Hamburg in 1892 and of Naples in 1884 suggest that later cholera epidemics in the two cities had a longer lasting influence when compared with the preceding outbreaks.[5] Both Naples and Hamburg were the only major cities in western Europe to suffer a medical crisis caused by cholera in 1884 and 1892 respectively. Governing officials and medical professionals were shocked to learn that their communities were still so susceptible to the disease at a time when medical discoveries had already led to the *vibrio*'s containment and control at most other places. It was 'timing rather than the sheer numbers of cases and deaths', Frank Snowden writes of events in Naples, that 'underpinned the extraordinary impact of the events of 1884'.[6]

Russia's cholera epidemic of 1892 is widely regarded as an important turning-point in the country's history. The epidemic's historical significance is usually related to the famine of 1891–92, which Orlando Figes has characterised as nothing less than the 'moment when Russian society first became politically aware of itself and its powers, of its duties to "the people", and of the potential it had to govern itself. It was the moment, in a sense, when Russia first became a "nation".'[7] Likewise, Frieden has argued in regard to the cholera epidemic in particular, that it heralded a 'new era of rising political consciousness and social activism'.[8] She has also demonstrated the decisive impact of the epidemic on the physicians' process of professionalisation. Overall, the twin disasters of famine and cholera are evaluated as events that marked the start of a significant social and political transformation which eventually threatened to corrode the very foundations of the tsarist regime.[9]

This chapter discusses the significance of Saratov's cholera outbreak in 1892 by examining the city's long-term response to the epidemic. It analyses the means and strategies by which the municipality addressed the major causes of the tragedy: lack of sanitation and medical facilities, overcrowding and poverty. In two sections, the chapter looks into the most important projects of reform undertaken in the city during the two decades following the epidemic. The first part describes municipal initiatives in the field of urban renewal, specifically the attempts to regulate sewage disposal, water supply and housing; it also discusses the state's interest in and support for Saratov's sanitary reform; it examines the reasons for the city's failure to carry out major public work projects, which the cholera demanded; finally, this first section outlines the role that cholera played in the development of philanthropic work, which became the city's primary way to tackle the newly emergent problem of the urban poor.

The second section analyses the cholera's impact on Saratov's medical profession. It discusses the alterations to local public health administration made by the central government in the immediate aftermath of the epidemic and the resulting changes in power relationships between physicians and governmental authorities on the local level; it examines the new spheres of influence for the medical profession in both municipal and zemstvo administration; and it analyses the interplay of scientific and political agendas which made the alliance between the doctors and local governments possible.

Miasma and urban renewal

Saratov weathered the epidemic crisis. Municipal and provincial strategies to contain the disease collapsed due both to the gravity of the cholera onslaught and the violent opposition of the population. After the breakdown of public order and medical services, the epidemic reached its greatest intensity in early July.[10] From mid-July onwards, the number of cholera cases and deaths declined and in August the disease subsided to approximately 10 new cases per day.[11] As summer gave way to autumn, the epidemic abated. Sporadic cases of cholera continued to occur throughout the winter months, but by November, the first of a series of four cholera years was over.[12] Life in Saratov returned to normal.

Yet the effects of the summer's events occupied the city for decades to come. Saratov's cholera outbreak was a public scandal. Throughout the epidemic, extensive reporting in local and national newspapers conveyed a detailed picture of the tragedy. The terrible mortality figures brought more into public view than just the dismal technical failures of local administrative authorities who were completely unready to meet the challenge, organised inefficiently and deficient in facilities. By launching a blind assault upon the *vibrio* with weapons of brutal force and coercion, Saratov's officials had exhibited an inability to understand medical needs as much as political and social realities. As medical disaster was transformed into a social one, the population became even more estranged from its governors. Explosive violence and public unrest provided the shocking lesson that administrative failure endangered the foundations of the state itself. Saratov's misfortune was a national misfortune. Such a fiasco called for a response.

The impact of cholera on nineteenth-century society remains a key aspect of the historiographical controversies about the subject. As Michael Morris has pointed out, 'cholera injected a new and disturbing element, for it tested received attitudes and mentalities, probed society's resources and resourcefulness, and exploited its weaknesses and shortcomings, structural, political, social and moral.'[13] As a challenge to political and social systems, the argument continues, cholera served as a stimulus to change. With regard to sanitary improvements and public health administration, many historians have claimed that cholera served as a decisive catalyst for reforms.[14] These views have not been uncontested. In fact, the extensive literature on Europe's first experience with the disease, considered to have been the most dramatic and most challenging, generally stresses the very limited impact of the disease on sanitary reforms. Britain's first cholera epidemic, for instance, did not instigate any reform activity. 'The 1832 epidemic failed miserably to generate amongst the middle-classes a recognition that public health reform was necessary. After 1832 they seemed to have forgotten everything and learned nothing.'[15] Rosenberg denied a direct link between cholera and public health development and environmental reform.[16] And Pelling took as her starting point the assumption that 'probably on all levels, cholera was a distraction rather than an impetus to reform.'[17]

However, more recent research on the final major cholera experience in western Europe has significantly expanded our knowledge about cholera's reforming potential. In Naples in 1884 and Hamburg in 1892, cholera had a tremendous impact on sanitary reform efforts. Hamburg's epidemic outbreak in 1892 set into motion a series of wide-ranging reform projects involving the reorganisation of poor relief, of water supply, sewage disposal, slum clearance and overcrowding, and, most importantly, a reform of the city's suffrage law.[18] Even more far-reaching was the impact of cholera on Naples. As a direct result of the epidemic, Naples underwent a comprehensive process of rebuilding and renewal (known as *risanamento*). In its plan for redevelopment, the city actually followed the larger European pattern famously embodied in the rebuilding of Paris under Georges Haussmann. Yet whereas Haussmann's vision was guided by motives of prestige, aesthetics and political control, Naples's *risanamento* pursued the single purpose of making the city immune to cholera. Vast sums of money were spent on preventing the recurrence of the disease.[19] Despite all intents and purposes, however, reform impulses in both Hamburg and Naples proved short-lived and eventually failed to meet their objectives. Hamburg's projects fell victim to powerful mercantile and industrial interests.[20] In a similar manner, Neapolitan renewal, a national symbol for the solution to Italy's 'Southern Question', was compromised by local vested interests.[21]

In Russia, the first four epidemics had not brought about any significant sanitary reforms. The cholera of 1830–31, just as in Britain, did not stimulate any reform activity.[22] Russia's sanitary movement, which took its earliest beginnings in the 1870s, was not called into being by the cholera epidemic of 1872, but rather by the gradual establishment of a basic public health infrastructure (the zemstva), which sought to combat all sorts of diseases and epidemics.[23] The new emphasis on public health, hygiene and sanitation gained momentum in the 1880s. The Pirogov Society was founded in 1883 and the publication of what became the most widely read medical journal in pre-revolutionary Russia, Viacheslav Manassein's weekly *The Physician* (*Vrach*, 1880–1901), put out its first issue.[24] Concurrently, Russia's leading authority in the field of urban sanitation and public health, the Swiss-born physician Friedrich Erisman, was appointed professor of hygiene at Moscow University in 1882.[25] But these developments, too, were not a result of a cholera epidemic: in the 1880s, Russia had escaped the disease. Moreover, the new medical ideas scarcely influenced public health administration. The work of the Botkin Commission, appointed by the Medical Council in 1886 in order to examine the possibility of reforms in national public health administration, ceased with the death of Botkin in 1889. It was taken up again only by Georgii Rein as a result of his experience with cholera in the Donets Basin in 1910.[26] For the sanitary movement to be executed at the local level, the country needed a fundamental change in the relations between state and society, between central and local power, and in particular a more influential position for the medical profession.

In stark contrast to previous cholera outbreaks, Russia's epidemic of 1892 stirred up the entire nation. The shock of such an onslaught at such a late time impelled governmental officials, medical experts, scientists and the educated public to reflect on the causes of the disaster. Hundreds of thousands of deaths accompanied by violent public disturbances built up pressure for social and medical reform. In Saratov, the epidemic's history had exposed the city as being particularly at risk. In 1892, doctors, municipal authorities and government officials set out to reduce Saratov's vulnerability to the disease.

As did the vast majority of Russia's physicians outside St Petersburg, Saratov's medical profession generally explained the frequent occurrence of cholera in the city on the basis of the miasmatist model. In their proposals for reform, local doctors drew inspiration mainly from the works of Pettenkofer and his mediator in Russia, Friedrich Erisman.[27] The theory, as we have seen, combined climatic, meteorological and geological factors with sanitary considerations. Under certain environmental conditions, a damp subsoil allowed the cholera germ to create a miasma which in turn carried the disease through the air. It followed that living on high ground was beneficial to immunity against the disease while living in damp, overcrowded dwellings, with limited circulation of air, was not.

In accordance with Pettenkofer's theory, local authorities first turned their attention to Saratov's densely settled *Cloaka Maxima*, the ravines. Such a move was unusual. 'In normal times,' Saratov's first tourist guide explained to the visitor, 'the ravines cannot serve as a topic for conversation, since they usually do not demon-strate their existence in the world in any way.'[28] Only when the city was disturbed by something, the guide continued, was the population at the ravines and the *gory* brought to the forefront. Cholera's appearance in 1892 confirmed the rule. The exceptionally high incidence of cholera cases and mortality within the ravines relentlessly exposed them as a health hazard for the entire city. Constituting 60% of the urban population, the ravine inhabitants accounted for 86% of cholera cases in the whole of Saratov.[29] The immediate impression was that of 'some human murrain, like the biblical plague'.[30] Soon, local and national newspapers supplied their readers with vivid portraits of the living conditions in the ravines. The *Saratov Leaflet* reported on the small courtyards, crammed with wretched hovels 'on chicken legs' and continuously railed against the mass of refuse and rubbish which had not been removed 'since time immemorial'.[31] And the newspaper *Russian Gazette (Russkie Vedomosti)* portrayed the *Glebuchev* ravine as an 'ideal anti-sanitary location' where people's sheds 'infect the whole surrounding place with miasmas'.[32] Local medical experts joined the chorus. They pointed to the 'murderous air' in the ravines and stressed the overcrowded, dark and damp living conditions;[33] they complained about the lack of fundamental hygienic and sanitary standards; and they pointed to the absence of clean water.[34] From the medical point of view, the *Glebuchev* ravine provided ideal conditions for the development of miasmas and the spread of diseases across the city. The epidemic created pressure to sanitise this area.

The city's governors sought to attack the problem at its roots. On 2 October 1892, directly in the wake of the disease, the duma decided to install an entire sewage system.[35] Local physicians had harshly criticised the practice of carting off Saratov's refuse to the overflowing municipal dump outside the city as early as the 1880s. Yet only the cholera epidemic provided a sense of urgency in the matter. A specially set up sewage commission, including urban architects, engineers, physi-cians and administrative officials, got down to work in order to delineate the area where the sewage system was to be built, and to elaborate initial estimates of the city's water consumption, as well as the expected costs involved in the project.[36] Only after three years, a Berlin company, *Narun und Petsch*, sent its representative Moritz Knauf to Saratov for two months in order to inspect local conditions for the construction of the system. Apart from the project devised by *Narun und Petsch*, other proposals were put forward by a second company from Berlin (*Seelmeyer*), a firm from Amsterdam (*Liernur*) and by the municipal engineer-architect A.M. Sal'ko.[37] By this time, however, the duma's interest in solving the city's sewage problem had already faded and the project collapsed amidst endless correspondence between numerous sub-commissions. In 1897, the merchant G.V. Ochkin, founder of Saratov's summer theatre, pointed out to the mayor that there was no sign for the intention of the municipal administration to introduce a sewage system and he repeatedly urged the municipality to resume the sewage question.[38] The following year, a presentation to the duma summed up the current situation: 'obviously the question about the sewage system in our city is now at that stage of development, at which it was before Mr Knauf visited us.'[39]

In the end, the state itself sparked local inertia. True, St Petersburg judged the provision of basic public services to be a local affair. Municipal legislation placed the responsibility for funding and carrying out public work projects affecting the health and education of local residents into the hands of individual communities. At the Volga, however, the central government intervened directly. Already during the plague at Vetlianka in 1878/79, the state had demonstrated its interest in instigating long-term preventive measures to improve the state of health at the Volga. Thirteen years later, the cholera epidemic exposed even more dramatically how the empire's health depended on medical conditions along the river. Improved communication and increasing traffic during the previous decade had made the Volga's sanitary circumstances of vital importance to the whole country. To sanitise the Volga was to protect the whole empire.

Powerful economic motives gave leverage to the project. Epidemic outbreaks were costly affairs. National and local governing authorities and medical experts unanimously regarded the implementation of temporary ad hoc measures to contain the disease as too expensive.[40] Long-term investment into solid sanitary improvements would pay off because the enormous expenditures brought about by having to maintain quarantine procedures or finance relief measures could be avoided. Moreover, epidemic outbreaks also halted ever-increasing trade and economic activity along the river, thus causing further financial losses. The state's desire to remedy the situation therefore involved more than preserving the nation's health. Most fundamentally, as state senator V.I. Likhachev pointed out: 'To bring the entire Volga region, from Nizhnii Novgorod up to the northern coast of the Caspian Sea, into proper sanitary conditions, by means of systematic measures, is a matter of national importance having enormous economic significance.'[41]

With memories of cholera still fresh, state authorities leapt into activity in 1897. That year, an outbreak of bubonic plague was reported from Samarkand, which threatened to invade the empire. The government immediately dispatched a commission of scientists and public health experts to the Volga. Under the leadership of state senator V.I. Likhachev, the expedition was to inspect sanitary conditions in the Volga's urban centres.[42] It was only the first in a series of scientific enterprises. Over the next decade, delegations of the country's most renowned medical specialists, hygienists, chemists, engineers and state officials travelled up and down the river in order to examine the cities' weak sanitary spots, to report on them to the government, to come up with proposals for improvements and not least to control the implementation of large-scale public works programmes. Not surprisingly, considering the river's medical history, state authorities kept particularly close tabs on the lower Volga. Faced with the renewed cholera outbreak in 1907, the Ministry of Internal Affairs established a special commission for sanitising the cities of Astrakhan', Tsaritsyn, Saratov and Samara in October 1908.[43]

To the experts from St Petersburg, Saratov's major sanitary evil was all too obvious: its system of refuse disposal. In 1901, the government charged N.K. Chizhov, a member of the technical-construction committee of the Ministry of Internal Affairs, with the task of planning a sewage system. His proposal was presented to Saratov's uprava in 1904.

Yet state assistance involved more. The major problem to be solved was money. Like most Russian cities, Saratov was starved of capital and credit. The municipal statute that placed the financial responsibility for public health upon local governments also heavily restricted possibilities for raising levies.[44] In 1901, the year when Chizhov began to elaborate his 1.6 million scheme, Saratov's financial budget amounted to 2.4 million rubles.[45] Admittedly, over the next decade revenues increased almost threefold to more than 6 million rubles in 1914.[46] But so did expenditures. Between 1881 and 1907, as Table 4.1 shows, Saratov's

Table 4.1 Saratov's municipal expenditures, 1880–1907

Category	1880	1905	1907
Maintenance of various government agencies, military, police and fire service	217,017,04	444,839,44	351,135,50
Maintenance of municipal government	73,342,32	129,782,22	135,707,43
Maintenance of various urban buildings and enterprises	20,473,86	342,298,49	386,745,92
Health and sanitation	84,387,42	258,428,52	301,468,03
Municipal services	51,045,00	110,149,04	221,791,81
Education	91,108,61	285,801,76	374,353,07
Charitable services	27,974,30	35,714,57	52,647,05
Others	39,633,46	61,817,94	61,644,12

Figures of the municipal financial commission in 1880 are reprinted in S. Gusev, A. Khovanskii, *Saratovets*, pp. 73–74; for figures from 1905–1907 see *Doklad gorodskoi biudzhetnoi kommissii v gorodskoi uprave* (Saratov, 1909), pp. 141–142.

investment into the provision for health, welfare and education of a rapidly growing population almost quadrupled. In addition to the increased expenses for social needs, the city was required to make large annual payments (amounting to about 20% of the budget) to the state, in particular for the maintenance of the police and the quartering of military troops. Eventually, the Russian–Japanese War in 1904–05, the revolution, combined with bad harvests and epidemics, profoundly shattered the city's financial balance. At the end of the decade, the municipal budgetary commission was bound to state that the historic year 1905 also marked the 'beginning of the era of municipal debts'.[47] In fact, as the century progressed, the gulf between Saratov's growing social problems and the financial resources available to meet them had become insurmountable. Underfinanced and in debt, Saratov was unable to defend the public welfare of its population.

The state acknowledged the quandary. Nothing signalled the national importance of Saratov's sanitary renewal more than St Petersburg's willingness to assist in raising substantial funds for the sewage project. As Valeria Nardova has shown, sources for state financial credits or other loans were scarce and almost inaccessible to municipal governments.[48] By 1904, the central government had deemed only a few major urban public projects worthy of state subsidies. Odessa, for instance, had received loans worth 12 million rubles for the improvement and modernisation of its port.[49] Other examples included Riga, Khar'kov, Kiev and, above all, the two capitals.[50] At the lower Volga, Saratov and Astrakhan' joined the ranks of those cities to receive state credits for the build-up of their sanitary infrastructures. Saratov received a credit of 1.6 million rubles in 1904.[51]

The state, however, left the actual work on the sewage system up to the city. It took the threat of another cholera outbreak in the summer of 1907 for Saratov's municipality finally to decree the start of the construction of sewers for the same year.[52] And even this decree produced no results. On their arrival in Saratov in 1909, the delegates of the above mentioned commission for sanitising the lower Volga cities convinced themselves that the decree from 1907 had remained a 'dead letter' and that construction had not yet begun.[53] Of even more concern, it turned out that, out of 3,853,875 rubles, which the city had received in the form of other loans between 1904 and 1908, and out of which 2,580,000 rubles were supposed to be spent on the sewage system, only 1,215,000 rubles were left.[54] The report of the commission soberly concluded:

> Astrakhan's municipal administration has used the loan, which was given to the city by the government for the purpose of sanitary constructions, for building the townhall and other necessities, which have nothing to do with any sanitary infrastructure. Likewise, Saratov's municipal administration has used part of the loan, given to it for the construction of a sewage system, for other needs and has not begun the construction of a sewage system up to the present time.[55]

Money, as the commission was quick to suggest, was only part of the problem. As in most other Russian cities, Saratov's electorate was restricted to but a tiny fraction of the total population: fewer than 1% of the city's residents were eligible to vote at the end of the nineteenth century.[56] In its social composition, Saratov's duma was dominated by merchants (58.1%), followed by members of the nobility (29.7%), and townspeople (*meshchane*, 12.2%).[57] These delegates represented the elite of the city's residents who inhabited the city centre. Out of 74 deputies, only two delegates spoke on behalf of Saratov's impoverished and densely populated periphery. Catering to the interests of the better-off citizens, the municipality gave little if any consideration to Saratov's most insanitary areas. From the outset, construction of a sewage system was envisaged only for Saratov's centre, i.e. the first, third and parts of the second administrative districts.[58] Even among the physicians, only two objected that a sewage system in the city centre would not affect conditions in the ravines and thereby reduce Saratov's overall mortality rates.[59] Yet this was not actually the aim of the undertaking. As late as 1907, the local physician and deputy mayor V.I. Almazov, while taking up the sewage question in a major presentation to the duma, admitted during the discussion that the high mortality figures in the ravines had been unknown to him.[60] In reality, the municipality viewed the disposal of urban sewage as an economic venture to increase municipal income, not as a basic public service to improve the city's sanitation.[61] Only if the landlords paid for the pipes from their houses to the mains themselves, the duma figured, would individual houses be connected to the sewage system.[62] Such sums (280 rubles) generally were beyond the means of most of Saratov's homeowners, but the beneficiaries of the service were also expected to pay a permanent subscription fee.[63] Given these conditions, construction on the sewage system finally began only in 1912.[64]

In a similar way, the duma addressed a complementary project: the expansion of the city's aqueduct. Following the miasmatist model of explaining diseases, Saratov's city fathers were less concerned with the provision of pure water than with flushing the sewer system.[65] Admittedly, the municipality invested in improving water pipes and filters in 1901 and 1902. Yet again, the ravines and outlying districts did not benefit at all from the new services. Distribution of water remained far from complete and Saratov's exorbitantly high water prices further restricted the usage of clean water to the better off. The poor continued to take water from notorious wells and the Volga River.

Yet nothing demonstrated municipal indifference to the plight of the poor more clearly than the city's failure to improve housing conditions for them. Concerns about the housing crisis in the *Glebuchev* ravine had already been raised before the epidemic. In fact, the urban building plan of 1812 had explicitly prohibited settlement in the ravines. Saratov's duma had taken some first steps to control settlement in the area from its earliest beginnings. In 1871, it put forward a clearance scheme entailing the demolition of the buildings in the ravine and the resettlement of 435 displaced families.[66] The programme required an individual court process on each house to be pulled down and, more importantly, the costly provision of financial support and building and land for the house owners. Thus, with the exception of three house owners who were resettled, 'the project was not fully carried out and therefore had no success'.[67] The outbreak of the plague at

Vetlianka in 1878 for the first time brought state authorities on to the scene. Loris Melikov, appointed temporary general-governor of Astrakhan', Saratov and Samara provinces, ordered Saratov's duma to expedite the clearance process of the ravines and to establish a park in its place.[68] Throughout the next decade, however, financial constraints and budgetary priorities (such as building the Radishchev museum) prevented the project. When in 1887 the duma decided instead to allow alterations to and the reconstruction of current buildings in the ravine, a mistake by the municipal secretary, mixing up 'rebuilding' (*perestroika*) with 'new building' (*postroika*), legalised the building activity in the ravines.[69] Even though the cholera epidemic had once again drawn public attention to the unparalleled living conditions in this area, it did not stimulate any discussion about housing reforms. Here, too, it was only the arrival of the Likhachev Commission, the result of the anticipated outbreak of bubonic plague in 1897, which put new life into the debate.[70] Municipal authorities seized the opportunity to present a petition to the senator asking for financial subsidies from the state for the clearance project. To support the application, the municipal engineer A.M. Sal'ko came forward with a tangible scheme for the implementation of the clearance plan in 1899.[71] Yet having hit on the idea that the state should pay for the undertaking, Saratov's reforming zeal faded as soon as the plague threat had passed. As was the case with the sewage question, debate about the resettlement of the ravine inhabitants was only renewed under the impact of revolutionary upheaval in conjunction with the pressure of the renewed cholera threat in 1907 – without achieving any results. In 1909, G.V. Khlopin reported to the government that:

> No serious real attempts for sanitising the ravines from the side of the municipal administration are made; the whole question is limited to paper production and the calculation of vast expenses, which the project requires. Meanwhile, not a single exact technical plan for sanitising the enemy has been devised, and consequently a sound basis for the calculation of the required costs does not exist.[72]

As the fate of Saratov's rebuilding projects shows, the city's sanitary infrastructure cannot be seen as a direct result of the cholera epidemic in 1892. Initial impulses for urban renewal were short-lived and were inevitably only reanimated in the face of other epidemic onslaughts. Even then, however, Saratov's municipal authorities did not display any serious concern about preventing the recurrence of epidemic outbreaks. To them, instead, the cholera epidemic of 1892 had demonstrated the national significance of sanitising the city and thus relieved the municipality of dealing with the task and, most importantly, its financial burden.[73] Even more remarkably, just as in other Russian cities the municipality's rebuilding programme gave no thought to the poor. Urban renewal was clearly not intended for their benefit. Failing to improve housing and hygiene for those who were most directly affected by the epidemic, Saratov's city fathers ignored one of the chief reasons for the onslaught of 1892. In so doing, they violated the most important lesson that could have been learned from the cholera riots: an effective defence against future cholera attacks had to give top priority to remedying the problem of poverty and solving social antagonisms.

As it turned out, the social question was to be dealt with by other means and strategies. Provision for the poor was the task of charities, not of urban renewal schemes.[74] Because the municipal rebuilding programme suffered from incompleteness and substantial defects, which undermined any intention of making the city immune to cholera, voluntary initiative stepped in to make a vital contribution to improving the health of the population. Public welfare, in fact, presented one domain where the epidemic effected an important transformation. Given the absence of any coherent official strategy to fight the disease plus the frightful scarcity of financial, medical and personal resources, voluntary work had already played a decisive role in taking up the epidemic's challenges. Charitable initiatives unfolded as soon as the epidemic was officially acknowledged. In one of its first moves, the municipal duma appealed to local individuals and institutions for their support in contending with the crisis. It asked the owners of commercial enterprises, workshops, hotels and inns to provide boiled water for free;[75] it called upon volunteers to transport urban refuse out of the city;[76] it requested that apothecaries distribute medication to the poor for a reduced price;[77] and, above all, it asked local medical societies to assist in reinforcing medical services to the residents.[78] A variety of philanthropic enterprises stepped in where municipal and provincial officials had failed. Individuals, charitable institutions, the church, religious societies, medical professional organisations, shipping companies, urban enterprises and factories joined in a concerted effort to organise a minimum of medical assistance and welfare for the sick and their families. Their commitment involved a wide range of activities, including, most basically, the provision of food and boiled water in soup kitchens and tea rooms, which were hastily set up and opened at the banks, the landing docks and across the city.[79] Other activities sought to organise relief for survivors.[80] Probably the largest sphere of voluntary support, besides fundamental material welfare, entailed medical help. As has been seen, the two local medical societies, the sanitary society (*sanitarnoe obshchestvo*) and the society of physics and medicine (*fisiko-meditsinskoe obshchestvo*) had already played a decisive role in elaborating anti-cholera measures and advising governing officials on the efforts to be taken to combat the disease. Once the epidemic was in the city, the societies established voluntary night shifts to improve medical provision.[81] And they organised public lectures so as to explain the disease to the population.[82] These initiatives sought not only to mitigate the economic hardship that accompanied the epidemic but also to alleviate social distress and anxiety which disturbed the entire city. In terms of medical provision and care, they constituted virtually the only resource for the municipality in the first two weeks of the epidemic.

However, voluntary relief measures could hardly bear the burden of protecting the population. On balance, in view of the gravity of the epidemic, the immediate impact of charitable activity was very limited. One local physician highlighted the situation: 'In Saratov one cannot gather as many volunteers as are necessary for the work.'[83] Moreover, philanthropic efforts were restricted by the fact that the famine had already fleeced available resources. At the height of the cholera, on 7 July 1892, Saratov's provincial charity institutions, which had been set up to assist the population during the famine, were closed.[84] Likewise, the municipal bureau for the poor recorded that incoming private donations in June had ebbed as compared with the preceding winter months.[85] Apart from limited resources, many charitable initiatives were not particularly successful since they were avoided for fear of the dreaded disease.

Yet the actual significance of voluntary initiatives went far beyond immediate emergency measures. Their importance needs to be assessed on a long-term basis. As Adele Lindenmeyr has shown, the Great Reforms had hardly effected any improvement in the provision of adequate public relief.[86] Only private charitable societies, individual reformers and the church stepped in to aid the poor.[87] Yet unlike western European countries, which came to consider poverty and relief as problems of utmost importance during the course of the nineteenth century, Russia lacked any comprehensive state poor relief system up to 1917. Existing legislation ascribed the responsibility for public welfare, just as for public health, to local authorities, to peasant communes and estate bodies.[88] Since zemstva and (later) dumas usually lacked the means to finance philanthropic activity and since, moreover, jurisdiction over poor relief was highly confusing and contradictory, sharing as it was between several local bodies and state institutions, most local governments passed the burden on to other institutions or simply left it to private charity.[89] Despite a significant upsurge in organised private charity in the post-emancipation era, therefore, provision for the poor was overwhelmingly neglected and hardly adequate to meet the need.

Any substantial efforts at poor law reform were not only obstructed by formidable financial difficulties and legislative conflicts, involving, most crucially, the battle between central authority and local autonomy; there was an additional factor which sanctioned the official position and existing practices: a widespread tolerance for begging. Until the late nineteenth and early twentieth century, Russia's charitable ideal perpetuated the image of the poor as the incarnation of Christ. Poverty was generated by misfortune. As Lindenmeyr points out: 'Fire, famine, illness, death – these, not unemployment, taxation, or other social ills, or the habits of the poor themselves, were the misfortunes of life that produced poverty.'[90] Such a view, to be sure, had not gone completely unchallenged. Since the beginning of the nineteenth century, economic and social changes had begun to erode the prevailing religious understanding of poverty and its underlying social structure.[91] Yet in striking contrast to western Europe, Russia's poor at the end of the nineteenth century were not as yet perceived as social pariahs. Accordingly, relief was not a field to be socially policed and controlled by state governmental institutions.[92]

The twin crises of famine and cholera impelled a fundamental shift in relief attitudes and practices. The cholera epidemic, in particular, brought the country's destitute into public view as never before. Cholera not only killed disproportionate numbers of the poor, the undernourished, ill, illiterate and unskilled; cholera also maximised the economic and social misery which had caused it. The *vibrio* not only exposed a yawning social chasm, but actually created and exacerbated it.

And most importantly, the disease enabled social conflicts to explode. In dramatic fashion, the medical havoc redefined poverty as much a breeding ground for disease as a threat to political stability, public order and economic progress.

Official explanations for Saratov's cholera riots, as has been seen, most clearly reflected the acute sense of panic and alarm at the pressure coming from below. Depicting the poor as envious, bestial, savage, ignorant and mad, governmental authorities not only absolved themselves of any responsibility for the riots but also emphasised an urgent need for the policing and control of a petulant and unruly rabble. Under the impact of full-scale insurrections, official and medical authorities nationwide began to pay unprecedented attention to the question of poverty and destitution. Significantly, in late 1892 the government established a commission (known as the Grot Commission) to reform the Statute on Public Assistance.[93]

In Saratov, the devastating experience of famine and cholera instigated a dramatic change in the commitment of provincial and municipal authorities to poor relief. To begin with, self-governing institutions started to collect basic knowledge and information on a vast array of social problems. In Saratov, the 1890s witnessed a proliferation of articles and statistics on, and depictions of, the poor and all their relatives – beggars, prostitutes, criminals, the unemployed and homeless.[94] Detailed investigations into their living conditions confronted government officials and the educated public for the first time with the profound consequences of urban growth, in particular with the germ-related problems of overcrowding, poor sanitation and lack of medical facilities. The information amassed in these studies presented an important accomplishment in itself and established the necessary factual basis for further municipal efforts in the field of sanitary reform. Beyond that, however, expanding knowledge about the destitute also went along with an increasing perception of the poor as a distinct subculture marked by its own social conditions, work habits and daily life.

On the basis of the new knowledge, zemstvo, duma, voluntary associations and individuals set about establishing a network to organise some basic provision of aid to the poor. Charitable societies flourished. A tourist guide to Saratov of 1898 listed 24 charitable associations, 15 of which were founded after 1891.[95] Fundamentally, their activities entailed arranging the supply of the needy with food, clothing and money. Saratov saw a remarkable increase in the number of almshouses from 8 in 1890 to 28 in 1898.[96] Voluntary institutions ran soup kitchens, homeless shelters and orphanages. Other initiatives aimed at improving medical care for the poor by providing rudimentary medical facilities and supplies or setting up medical institutions such as schools for nurses or maternity hospitals.

More was involved, however, than purely humanitarian concerns. A crucial aspect of philanthropic work was the mission to reform the poor morally and to improve their working skills and habits. Houses of industry (*dom trudoliubiia*), kitchen schools (*kukhonnaia shkola*), trade schools for children and other forms of educational facilities set about transforming the destitute into educated, industrious workers. The moralising attack against the urban poor took off in full form in 1898, when the city duma founded the 'society for the aid of the poor of Saratov' (*obshchestvo posobiia bednym Saratova*). Intended to serve as an umbrella organisation that would coordinate the otherwise isolated welfare activities in the city, the society's work was explicitly based on the principles and considerations as manifested in the Elberfeld system of poor relief.[97] During one speech, deacon L.T. Miziakin clearly laid out the reason for its foundation:

> Otherwise, the ragged and hungry army of unfortunate people will never stop to send to us out of its various holes its begging envoys who already now block in such profusion all our pavements, all church entrances, and who never stop troublesome to grab our clothes; otherwise the many representatives of that dark tsardom of begging, desperation and vice will and can never stop to fill our prisons and hospitals; This, the terrible tsardom, will eternally protest with its infected atmosphere against the existing order of things, permanently threaten us with all sorts of possible diseases and epidemics, which can any minute in irrepressible stream pour over us out of the depths of the dark and damp basements, out of impossible nightshelters, and out of all the systematically built cesspits of the Glebuchev ravine.[98]

Here was the real reason why the ravines and their inhabitants received public attention. The health threat of the 'tsardom of the poor' was the threat of social and political disarray. By taking charge of the lives of the needy, Saratov's dominant strata sought to establish and confirm the city's social hierarchy. Philanthropy became an exercise of social discipline and political power as local elites anxiously responded to the pressure rising up from below.

Ultimately, such pursuits accomplished little. Moral reform and social control were partly frustrated by the realities of the poor who mainly sought shelter for the night, something to eat or refuge from the cold. Moreover, institutional facilities were highly insufficient and inadequately equipped to meet the needs of a rapidly growing city. Most importantly, however, philanthropic efforts were discredited by the fact that the city failed to address at the same time fundamental needs of the poor. In fact, as Saratov underwent rapid urban growth, the gap between rich and poor widened. For an increasing majority of Saratov's inhabitants, living conditions were stark indeed. The average monthly income of Saratov's workers was about 15 rubles by the time of the next cholera visitation in 1904.[99] The minimum rent for a room in a co-operative apartment (*artel'naia kvartira*) ranged from 1.20 to 1.50 rubles per month;[100] workers for the shipping companies spent another 6–8 rubles per month for one meal a day at the landing docks. These meals usually consisted of soup containing some vegetables, which Saratov's physicians dismissed as highly insufficient.[101] Typically, a whole family was to be supported from this salary. These conditions precluded any investments in public health. Since a monthly stay in the municipal hospital cost between 7 and 15 rubles, substantial medical care meant the remainder of the family was sentenced to starving and begging during the time of the disease.[102]

Saratov's patterns of morbidity and mortality at the beginning of the twentieth century confirmed that the urban poor were at just as much risk of being infected by the *vibrio* as they had been in 1892. In 1902, the city's mortality rates continued to stand at about 40.53 per thousand inhabitants. As of 1903, mortality sharply decreased, yet still, as late as 1906, the year before cholera revisited the city, 6,023 people died.[103] The decline in mortality was mainly due to the heavy influx of adult population from the surrounding districts (*uezdy*), which began in 1902. Strikingly, it was chiefly Saratov's better-off areas, in particular the first and third administrative districts, which experienced a significant decline in mortality rates. Mortality rates in the sixth and fourth districts almost equalled those in the first, second, third and fifth districts together. Taking into account the inaccuracies in diagnosis as well as municipal statistics, Saratov's pattern of death was highly suggestive of filth, overcrowding and malnutrition. Children constituted the bulk of the high mortality figures: they perished predominantly from diarrhoeal diseases as a result of poor dietary conditions and sanitation.[104] Adults in early twentieth-century Saratov died in particular from respiratory diseases (e.g. pneumonia). The continued prevalence of typhus and typhoid was another infallible indicator of unhygienic living conditions, poor diet and overcrowding.[105] Typhus epidemics, in particular, revisited the city year after year in the first decade of the twentieth century. While projects of urban renewal benefited only the better-off, philanthropic initiative could not minimise social inequality. Neglected and betrayed, Saratov's poorer residents started to articulate their needs in radical manner as the new century began.

Unlike previous cholera epidemics, Russia's outbreak in 1892 brought about a widespread recognition of the country's need for extensive reforms. Accompanied by public unrest and violence, the event called into question existing political and social structures in dramatic fashion. Under the immediate impact of the epidemic, local and state authorities thus stipulated reform initiatives to improve Saratov's sanitary conditions and to alleviate the city's alarming problem of poverty.

Yet reforming zeal soon receded. In Saratov, neither the epidemic of 1892 nor that of 1907 served as a direct inspiration of urban renewal. Rebuilding projects were not only thwarted by financial limitations; rather, they fell victim to various local interests and priorities. Sewage systems, water supply and housing reforms simply were not uppermost in the minds of the duma delegates as civil amenities. The improvement of public health by means of technical infrastructures, the city fathers believed, was a task of state importance and thus had to be financed by the national government. The city could then reap the profits from new economic ventures. In conformity with these aims, none of the reform proposals and city rebuilding projects showed any consideration for the poor, who were most endangered by diseases and epidemics. While the housing reform never got under way, the provision of sewage refusal and pure water supply was intended only for the city centre. From the outset, the major source of the city's vulnerability to the epidemic in 1892 was ignored.

Instead of alleviating social antagonisms, local elites developed means and strategies to counter growing social pressure. Governmental and voluntary organisations set about mitigating economic hardship and social distress by philanthropic efforts. However, public welfare was hardly adequate to meet economic and social realities and was, moreover, compromised by the fact that the poor were otherwise not considered worthy of attention. Nonetheless, reform and developments in the field of poor relief did have some impact. For the first time, local authorities took inventory of the needy as a social entity and set about addressing their existence. More importantly, the development of public welfare significantly effected improvements in public health provision in Saratov during the 1890s and 1900s. This, however, can only be understood in conjunction with the reforms in medical administration which followed the epidemic.

Cholera and Saratov's doctors

As it turned out, cholera's most important and long-lasting legacy affected the city's physicians. Already during the summer of 1892, their role offered a bright spot in an otherwise dismal cholera record. True, at first glance doctors all over Russia convinced neither themselves nor their contemporaries of their capabilities in diagnosing and treating the disease. The medical profession itself was terribly aware of its failures. In his report on the cholera epidemic, Dimitrii Zhbankov criticised 'the mass of all kinds of mistakes and negligence on the side of the physicians, the mistrust and sometimes the emergence of dangerous misunderstandings from the side of the population'.[106] Yet at the same time the physicians deserved recognition for not having spared themselves in their efforts to save human lives in the face of immense obstacles. Even Saratov's mayor was compelled to acknowledge their courage and determination. At the height of the epidemic he expressed his appreciation for the physicians' work and stressed the fact that in the midst of violent pogroms against the medical men, Dr S.A. Markovskii had been the first to look after the sick on the streets after the mob had burned down the cholera hospital.[107]

The cholera demonstrated physicians' utility while forcing them to re-evaluate their position in society at the same time. As Nancy Frieden's works have documented, Russia's physicians had embarked on the process of professionalisation since the Reform Era. Yet in contrast to most Western medical professions, which established their autonomy against the background of a history of corporate rights and self-governmental institutions, Russia's physicians operated as 'servants of the state'. At the end of the nineteenth century, the state still maintained highest control over all their professional responsibilities, their education and licensing, their social position and professional status.[108] The cholera epidemic had exposed the physicians' peculiar stand within the country's social and institutional milieus. Their enormous efforts, risks and not least the deaths of their colleagues during the crisis contrasted unfavourably with their lack of rights. If the government needed medical expertise and efficient cooperation, they claimed, it first of all had to vest the medical profession with decision-making powers. In return for their professional knowledge and sacrifices, physicians expected a more influential role in public policy and pressed for reform, in particular in local administration.

Government officials appeared to corroborate this claim. In the immediate aftermath of the cholera, state authorities seemed to open up new prospects for more autonomy and initiative in local governmental institutions. From 13 to 20 December

1892, the Medical Department of the Ministry of Internal Affairs organised a national conference to examine the summer's medical catastrophe and to develop plans for future epidemic relief. For one week, high-ranking state officials from the Ministries of Internal Affairs, of War, Finances, Ways and Communications, and from the Medical Council convened with local administrators and more than 160 physicians and medical students who had been working in cities and villages, on railroads, ships and in factories all over Russia during the epidemic. Participants included some of Russia's most outstanding scientists, medical experts and public health pioneers such as Vassilii Grebenshchikov, Viacheslav Manassein, Dmitrii Mendeleev and Ivan Molleson.[109]

In a very unusual move, the state resorted to non-governmental specialists and zemstvo representatives and heeded their knowledge and expertise. The physicians examined the wide range of problems that had prevented a successful fight against the cholera. They reported on the inadequate policies of preventive health (sanitary control of cities, landing docks, factories, almshouses, shops, etc.), the effect of quarantine measures on rivers and railways, and the control and protection of migrants. Medical issues such as the problem of identifying the first cholera case, the registration of the sick, disinfection measures and funeral procedures were closely scrutinised. Moreover, the physicians devised stringent measures in expectation of a second wave of the epidemic in the following year.[110]

In a similar vein, local government authorities quickly convened provincial medical conferences so as to benefit from the physicians' experience and advice. In Saratov province zemstvo physicians met already on 4 and 8 December 1892 to suggest preparatory measures for a possible cholera outbreak in 1893. They elaborated a detailed plan which addressed all major problems and deficits that had cropped up during the summer. A thorough timetable regulated the tasks to be tackled: the popularisation of knowledge about the disease (to be started instantly); the improvement of sanitary conditions, especially of the ever-contaminated water supplies; involvement of priests for the registration of the sick; preparation of buildings for isolation and treatment; organisation of courses to teach disinfection measures to lower medical personnel; and the increase of medical personnel (on 1 March and 1 May), preferably with physicians and feldshers who were already familiar with the province.[111]

But physicians gained much more than just a strong voice. The government's changed attitude went far beyond an increased recognition of their expertise and work. For the first time, it actually provided the medical profession with an influential, decision-making role within local institutions of government. The most important recommendation made by the participants of the conference in St Petersburg concerned the continuation of the Sanitary Executive Commissions in order to coordinate and control the measures taken by individual commissions and institutions.[112] This suggestion was instantly approved by the Medical Department.[113] To avoid the confusion caused by the Sanitary Executive Commissions in 1892 their competencies were significantly enlarged. In essence, they were established as the highest institution in provinces, districts and cities in directing public health measures. They received the right to dispose of the financial means of existing public health institutions and, likewise, about any financial resources and any donations derived from other state and public sources.

This regulation, as historians have pointed out, was a tacit admission by the state that the current organisation of public health had failed.[114] Gathering local governmental officials, zemstvo and city representatives, and numerous physicians into a single body, the central government sought to overcome the dual structure of medical affairs administration that had hampered progress in the past. Inevitably, however, the instruction radically shifted power structures on the local level.[115] Since the decree explicitly stated equal rights for all members of the commission it also complied with the physicians' demands for more influence.[116] From now on, physicians could take over the responsibility for planning and implementing anti-epidemic measures.

In Saratov province, the medical profession made full use of this new opportunity. When the Sanitary Executive Commission assembled in February, Molleson had only to explain the medical plan elaborated in December.[117] His points were approved by the administration without much further discussion. In addition, he was asked to go to St Petersburg and Moscow in order to persuade physicians and medical students there to come to Saratov the following summer. More importantly, under medical guidance the commission developed an impressive activity list during the following months in order to prevent a repeat of 1892. Every physician who had worked in the province during the cholera was called upon to record in detail his observations and experiences with it. Their reports were rapidly collected and published in a volume of 500 pages, which provides one of the most insightful available sources for the epidemic in the province.[118] In addition, the doctors prepared for the next summer. They enforced medical personnel; they organised facilities for the isolation and accommodation of the sick; they purchased disinfection means from Moscow and other countries; and they gave public lectures about the disease. When the country witnessed an impressive (and unexpected) decline in cholera mortality in 1893, the doctors were quick in taking the credit. Certainly many factors contributed to the containment of the epidemic in its second year, yet one of them was the successful work of the Sanitary Executive Commissions.[119]

The cholera tragedy came to mark a watershed in the physicians' professional development. Armed with a sharpened sense of their vulnerable position in society, an impressive record in fighting the epidemic in 1893 and not least with governmental support, Saratov's physicians began their fight to enhance their social status and to assert their professional interests and rights.

Medical-scientific theory powerfully supported their case. Miasmatist theory explained diseases as complex socio-medical phenomena caused by social, economic and environmental influences. Curative medicine, Russia's advocates of preventive medicine maintained, did not take into account the conditions that bred diseases.[120] To improve people's health it was necessary above all else to create a healthier environment. This view, with its emphasis on sanitary science, social hygiene and preventive medicine, found strong support among the vast majority of

Russia's medical profession. Throughout the 1890s, Russia's physicians profoundly refuted the achievements of laboratory medicine.[121] Given the country's existing medical and sanitary services, modern science as developed in St Petersburg was utterly unconvincing to them. The cholera epidemic had proven their point.

Yet much more was at stake. In practical terms, Russia's sanitarians believed one had to begin with the systematic collection of empirical statistical evidence as a theoretical basis upon which the diseases could be analysed and explained and preventive measures be taken. In addition, the advocates of sanitary science pressed for cultural change. Medicine, as Nikolai Pirogov, Russia's major medical reformer of the nineteenth century stated, 'has to fight against the ignorance of the people and to alter their whole world outlook'.[122] Physicians had to become educators. They were not only to propagate elementary hygienic knowledge but also to reduce illiteracy and to raise the cultural level among the population. Russia's physicians confirmed Erwin Ackerknecht's stated view that 'miasmatic theory could easily become a social programme'.[123] Russia's environmentalists placed medicine at the centre of a programme for social reform.

It was at this point that Pettenkofer's and Erisman's medical theories met the scientific and political agendas of both the medical profession and ruling elites. To the physicians, as Frieden has shown, the disciplines of hygiene and sanitation, as scientific approaches to public health, also served as strong conceptual bases for the profession's commitment in community welfare programmes.[124] Since these offered the only field of work where the profession could gain recognition and some public influence, social service became a means by which the profession could redefine its social role as distinct (and independent) from the position ascribed to it by the Table of Ranks. The 'servant of the state' was replaced by the ideal of the public servant. After the Great Reforms, the endeavour to fulfil its new service ethos increasingly enabled the Russian medical profession to form corporate bonds and to strengthen its professional autonomy.[125] Against this background, the intrusion of laboratory discipline, which was strongly supported by St Petersburg's medical establishment, did not only threaten to render the sanitary reform movement obsolete. In Russia, the new science of bacteriology challenged the foundation of the medical profession's conception of itself.

The cholera epidemic in 1892 even sharpened the professional-political dimensions of miasmatism. For at the same time that miasmatist theory strengthened the aspirations of the medical profession to attain a more influential position in society, anti-contagionism offered a scientific underpinning for the strenuous endeavours by ruling elites to control the lives of the poor. In Saratov, where the epidemic had brought the violent potential of the population into plain view, medical men, who demanded cultural change and social reform, could be of use to those in power. Medical science seemed to offer a solution to the problems of social control and disorder. The scientific justifications for advancing hygiene and sanitation confirmed the claims of local elites to appropriate urban space and to redefine the urban environment. Over the next two decades, the municipality rewarded the doctors for their expertise by opening new spheres of influence, which involved increased medical authority, employment and prestige.

The first crucial initiative was a large-scale organisational effort by Saratov's municipality to sanitise and 'medicalise' the population. Painfully aware of the pointlessness of temporary sanitary measures during the cholera epidemic, Saratov's governing authorities acknowledged the need to invest in a permanent medical-sanitary infrastructure to effect long-term improvements in the city's state of sanitation. In 1894, for the first time, public health became an integral part of municipal governmental affairs through the creation of a sanitary commission (*sanitarnaia kommissiia*) operating at the uprava.[126] As the key institution giving fresh direction and inspiring new initiatives in urban sanitation and medical provision, the commission instigated a number of public health activities enhancing status, employment and the authority of local doctors. Most crucially, the commission also ensured better medical services for the poor. For this purpose, the city was divided into four districts. Each opened a surgery (*ambulatoriia*) staffed with one physician, a feldsher, one vaccination expert and two disinfection specialists.[127] Large parts of the population, for whom a hospital visit in the city centre was far beyond financial means, were now offered access to medical treatment for free at the city's margins. Apart from medical provision, an important component of the new service was educational. After the cholera epidemic had brutally revealed the destructive alienation of the population from the medical profession, the surgeries' mission was to familiarise the poor with medical care and to build up trust between them and local doctors. The physicians were instructed to convey to their patients fundamental hygienic knowledge. They were willing to treat patients at home, and they tried to gain the trust of Saratov's women by distributing free milk for newborn babies.[128] These strategies proved successful. By 1906, physicians could report that the surgeries were respected, trusted and well visited by the poor.[129]

In addition to creating a basic medical network for the poor, the sanitary commission hired extra sanitary inspectors (*sanitarnyi vrach*) to examine and regulate the sanitary conditions of schools, almshouses, market squares, factories, bath-houses, the banks and other public institutions and places.[130] Already equipped with legal authority, the physicians were granted comprehensive police authority in questions of cleanliness and sanitation. A newly established medical-police commission officially institutionalised the physicians' enlarged power.

Alongside municipal recognition, Saratov's medical profession gained further prestige from the expansion of provincial public health services during the 1890s. Prior to the cholera epidemic, the cooperation between zemstvo deputies and medical employers, in Saratov as elsewhere, was tense. While most zemstva regarded the responsibility for public health above all as a financial burden, their medical employees had little power and were in no position to affect the priorities of the new institutions.[131] In Saratov province, the situation had been especially difficult. In March 1892, three months before the cholera, the entire contingent of zemstvo physicians had quit their jobs to protest the dramatic reorganisation of the medical board by the administration, which virtually abolished any participation in public health matters on the part of medical personnel.[132] Yet once the Sanitary Executive Commission (later renamed the *sanitarnoe biuro*) endowed the physicians with decision-making authority, the situation changed. While the zemstvo now seemed to open a practical perspective for the medical profession to change its position within society, the zemstvo deputies supported the physicians' cause on the grounds that medicine offered one of the few, yet important opportunities to regain political power over local affairs.[133] Under the powerful leadership of Ivan Molleson, Saratov's zemstvo thus undertook most energetic efforts to unify and coordinate medical services across the province. Medical work flourished in the 1890s. Saratov's sanitary office (*sanitarnoe biuro*) organised professional conferences in the province to plan and regulate medical work; it made improvements in the field of medical statistics; it implemented a series of sanitary measures across the province; it advised and controlled the work of the multitude of institutions and offices involved in tasks such as the construction of hospitals, the provision of medications or the hiring and firing of medical personnel; and it began to publish the results of its investigations and activities in its own journal, the *Saratov Sanitary Review* (*Saratovskii Sanitarnyi Obzor*), which became an empire-wide acclaimed professional medical journal.[134] Time and again, however, its work was hampered by disputes between the zemstvo and medical personnel. Thus, Molleson resigned in 1896 after arguments with the administration. His departure temporarily led to the closing down of the medical-statistical biuro at the zemstvo and the *Saratovskii Sanitarnyi Obzor*. Yet by then, Saratov's sanitary society (*sanitarnoe obshchestvo*), which was based in the provincial capital, was already too vital. It took over the work formerly directed by Molleson and successfully petitioned at the provincial zemstvo assembly for the reestablishment of a province-wide executive medical body.[135] In 1901, the zemstvo assembly decreed the establishment of a department of public health (*otdelenie narodnogo zdraviia*) under the auspices of the zemstvo governing board. With the appointment of Nikolai Teziakov as head of the new institution, provincial medical affairs, once again, were directed by an authoritative, high-profile public health scientist who continued the fruitful work started by Molleson. By the early twentieth century, the doctors from Saratov had gained respect nationwide and acclaim for their professional activity.

An important result of these developments was the active involvement of zemstvo and duma physicians in the deliberations of the municipality. In Saratov city, the activities of the municipal Sanitary Executive Commission went far beyond strictly medical affairs and public welfare in practice. The commission was the central body deciding over the entire process of urban renewal. Alongside the municipal architect, engineer, several duma representatives and the mayor, the commission was predominantly composed of the city's leading physicians. As has been seen, their medical opinion convinced the municipality to concentrate on the sewage question after the cholera epidemic; in subsequent years, doctors participated in elaborating crucial proposals and plans for the construction of a sewage system; they analysed and commented on the sanitary conditions across the city; and they were the experts in identifying and analysing the city's social question. So successfully did local physicians offer their expertise for the exercise of local power, that Saratov's deputy mayor in 1907, V.I. Almazov, was a physician.

Yet nothing proclaimed the enhanced prestige of Saratov's doctors more than the striving by local authorities to open a university in the city. On 1 December

1906, Saratov's duma decided to support the petition for its foundation.[136] At the cost of other projects of urban renewal, the municipality supported its application by expressing its readiness to provide 1 million rubles for the construction of and equipment for the university buildings; it further offered the entire Moscow Square, a territory of 26 *desiatin* (28.34 hectars) right in the city centre, as building ground for the new institution; it allowed municipal hospitals to be used for teaching and work; and it made temporary facilities available until the newly constructed buildings were ready to take up academic activity.[137] After two years of negotiations, in the spring of 1909, the State Council and State Duma in St Petersburg gave their approval to the new academic foundation.[138] Six months later, on 6 December 1909, a ceremonial act opened Russia's tenth university in the city of Saratov. The institution, as conceptualised in St Petersburg, was to maintain a single faculty of medicine. Over the next few years, Saratov's doctors acquired their own university campus. The complex which arose at the Moscow Square consisted of four separate buildings accommodating an institute of experimental medicine (two buildings), an institute of physics and an institute of anatomy. Yet this was only the centrepiece of the project. A separate building on the *Nikol'skaia* Street came to hold an academic library; other facilities accommodated laboratories, clinics, a student dormitory and administrative staff. A botanical institute and botanical garden completed the picture. At the same time that the construction process was under way, renowned medical scientists were appointed to draw up the curriculum: V.I. Razumovskii, an authoritative surgeon from Kazan', took up the post as rector of Saratov's university; also from Kazan' came I.A. Chuevskii, head of the physiology department, V.V. Vorms, head of the department for physiological chemistry; and A. Ia. Gordiagin, head of the department of botany; furthermore, V.D. Zernov and B.I. Birukov from Moscow were charged with taking over the departments of physics and zoology respectively; finally, N.G. Stadnitskii arrived from the university in Novorossiisk to direct the department of anatomy.[139] Saratov became a centre of modern medical science.

Nancy Frieden has pointed to the 'paradox that at a time of rapid scientific advance, when other medical professions used that progress as a key to improved status, the Russian profession stressed its social service role as a means to gain prestige'.[140] She explained the phenomenon as the result of the 'tradition of public service, the ideals of the sixties, the attractions of zemstvo medicine, and the direction of the Pirogov Society'.[141] In a similar way, Alexander Hutchinson argued that the opposition of the vast majority of Russia's physicians towards the new disciplines of bacteriology and microbiology until the early twentieth century had its roots in the physicians' fear that their 'long struggle to reduce poverty and improve education might be abandoned in the headlong rush to the laboratory'.[142] Strikingly, both Frieden and Hutchinson ignore the direct connection between scientific and political agendas which influenced the doctors' medical position. As Evans has so clearly laid out for the German case, even Robert Koch's success with his bacteriological cholera model in fact owed more to social and political factors, such as the emergence of nationalism, protective economic policies and increasing state intervention, than to its intrinsic scientific contribution.[143]

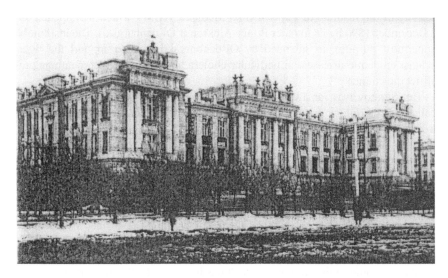

Figure 6 Imperatorskii Nikolaevskii Saratovskii Universitet, V.A. Solomonov, *Imperatorskii Nikolaevskii Saratovskii Universitet. Istoriia otkrytiia i stanovleniia (1909–1917)* (Saratov, 1999).

The analysis of Saratov's local response to the cholera epidemic allows one to go further than Frieden and Hutchinson have done in order to explain the predominance of localist theory in Russia. In fact, the stress Saratov's doctors laid upon Pettenkofer's medical theories until late into the twentieth century, an emphasis typical of Russia's physicians as a whole, is remarkable in view of the ascendancy of bacteriology as even more beneficial to enhancing the medical professions' status elsewhere in Europe.[144] Even more striking, in Russia the hegemony of Pettenkofer's medical philosophy went alongside triumphant successes in the field of microbiology and bacteriology which, for the first time, established Russian medicine as a national science gaining international recognition and acclaim. For in St Petersburg, the cholera epidemic of 1892 had inaugurated the era of Russia's most celebrated achievements and medical discoveries, in particular in the field of microbiology. Here, the most dedicated young scholars, who were cast in a modern scientific mould following the innovations at Russian universities in the 1860s and 1870s, were ready to plunge into studying the biological causes of epidemics. Educated in the laboratories of Sergei Botkin and Il'ia Mechnikov as well as in the most prestigious German and French laboratories, they had gained an excellent command of the dramatic changes that had occurred with the great discoveries of Koch and Pasteur. They were fully prepared, in the course of the bacteriological revolution, to place their scientific work in the mainstream of European research.[145] To this generation, the cholera epidemic hit at a crucial moment. Under the impact of hundreds of thousands of deaths Nikolai Gamaleia, Daniil Zabolotnyi, Sergei Vinogradskii and Ivan Pavlov started their careers. Their most spectacular successes became linked to the activity of the Institute of Experimental Medicine (IEM), which was opened on 8 December 1890 by its founder Prince Aleksandr Ol'denburgskii. The institute's uppermost purpose, as intended by Ol'denburgskii, was to support the fight against epidemic diseases, in particular cholera and plague, which continued to afflict the country.[146]

But Saratov was far away from St Petersburg's medical successes. Here, a belief in bacteriology was not the way to enhance the doctors' status. Not only did it contradict the populist traditions of Russian community medicine; outside St Petersburg laboratory medicine also conflicted with the professional and political interests of local doctors. Given the specific political and social context of Russia's individual localities, resulting from an autocratic state structure in which local authorities were nevertheless responsible for public health, Pettenkofer's philosophy was much more useful in validating the doctors' scientific and social status at the local level. It allowed them to accommodate themselves to local governmental authorities, who, for their part, had a vested interest in defending their local autonomy against central authority and power.

Such a compromise was going to have its costs. In Saratov, as elsewhere in Russia, the doctors' decision to adapt scientific stances to political purposes inevitably had profound political consequences for their professional work. The political goals of local self-governments, i.e. zemstvo and duma, became vital for their medical work. And vice versa, the physicians' professional goals, in particular the vision of social reformism, affected their politicisation. As time went on, the original apolitical approach to public health and public welfare became highly political. Within only one decade following the cholera disaster of 1892, it would be political reform, not social reform, which would provide the key to the improvement of public health. It was the cholera's next visitation that shifted the focus.

Conclusion

Tracing the basic stages of Saratov's initiatives in urban sanitary renewal during the two decades following the cholera epidemic, one must conclude that the disastrous record of the summer of 1892 left the city fathers unimpressed. In the field of urban rebuilding, the basic conditions that had given rise to the epidemic were not addressed and went unchanged. Neither did the organisation of proper sewage disposal, purified water supply and housing for the poor get very far; nor did these reform initiatives actually reach the targets defined by the epidemic. The introduction of basic sanitary services in the city therefore did not emerge as a consequence from the cholera. To be properly understood, these innovations need to be placed in the context of a long-term process of sanitary reform, which went back to the 1870s and received its decisive impulses from the accelerated economic, social and political developments of the 1890s and 1900s.

In terms of the effects of urban renewal, as we shall see in Chapter 5, Saratov was not only equally susceptible to the *vibrio* in 1907; in fact, the city's environment had deteriorated. When G.V. Khlopin was charged with the task of investigating Saratov's hygienic conditions in 1909, his findings confirmed that the symptoms of urban pathology had increased. The city, now swollen to a population of 235,000 people, still dumped its urban refuse into the *Glebuchev* and the Volga River; the housing crisis for the poor had become so acute that people filled the almshouses and night shelters where they slept 'side by side, shoulder to shoulder not only on the plank beds but also on the filthy, stinking, and cold floor'.[147] And many areas in the city were still deprived of access to clean water. In particular, it was the city's poor who were most affected by the sanitary neglect of the municipality. After 15 years, they would be just as much of a risk for being infected by the *vibrio* as they had been in 1892.

In one area, however, the cholera epidemic effected important changes. Local doctors, for the first time vested with decision-making authority after the epidemic, could expand their newly gained privileges and in subsequent years enhance their social status and professional prestige. Scientific expertise allowed them to collaborate with local governing authorities and exert considerable influence in the process of urban renewal; they further instigated and conducted wide-ranging programmes in sanitising and medicalising the population; and they successfully fostered the improvement of medical institutions and public health provision in the city. In fact, in the first decade of the twentieth century, Saratov's progress in the field of medical care and public health provision by far exceeded developments in most other Russian cities. Crucially then, in contrast to 1892, Saratov's medical defences were ready when cholera returned in the new century.

5 The revival of cholera: 1904–1910

No sooner had Russia entered the new century than cholera returned. European Russia was first affected in 1904, when once again the epidemic manifested itself at the lower Volga. Yet the germ confined its outbreak to a brief flare-up, causing an estimated 9,230 cases and 6,700 deaths.[1] It subsided during the next two years only to come back in 1907, infecting the whole empire. From then on, the disease did not stop causing trouble. Over the course of four successive years, European Russia witnessed a recorded 262,690 cholera cases and 124,140 deaths.[2] The most severe outbreak hit the country in 1910, when the germ is said to have taken almost 100,000 lives within three and a half months.[3]

Russia's sixth cholera pandemic differed considerably from the 1892 outbreak. During the previous decade, scientific advances had unravelled the mystery about the aetiology of the disease. Current opinion widely acknowledged that cholera was a social disease fostered by economic hardship, sanitary neglect and dietary deficiencies. Medical and governmental authorities, in Russia as elsewhere, knew about the precautionary measures needed to prevent and contain the disease. With cholera's causality identified, the mortality caused by the bacillus had greatly diminished. In fact, for the industrial nations of western Europe the epidemic was almost an anachronism. As Frank Snowden put it: 'In 1904–1910 cholera could even be described as a disease whose time had passed because highly effective means existed to prevent, contain, and treat it.'[4]

In such an altered context, cholera's return to Russia did not unleash the tumultuous popular responses that had characterised the previous outburst. The social impact of Russia's sixth cholera visitation was of a different ilk. Its importance lies in the challenge it posed to the autocratic regime in a time of revolutionary upheaval. Cholera had long had the capacity to stir up the political and social system of a given society and to act as a stimulus for extensive reform. It was only consequent for scholars to ask to what extent the disease contributed to the collapse of social order.[5] Yet this approach to the social history of the epidemic has not gone unchallenged. Charles Rosenberg concluded as early as the 1960s that despite its dramatic emotional impact the disease had no long-lasting direct consequences on the political and administrative structure of the societies it attacked.[6] And Margaret Pelling, more recently, regarded the attention historians have paid to cholera epidemics as generally misplaced. Other epidemic diseases, she argued, accounted for much higher mortality figures and thus presented a more enduring concern for nineteenth-century societies.[7] Nevertheless, as Snowden has shown, questions about cholera's capacity to contribute to revolutionary events still stimulate historical discussion to date.[8]

In a particular historical configuration, Russia's sixth cholera pandemic came to coincide with a political revolution after the aetiology of the disease was understood. The *vibrio*'s return to Russia bluntly exposed conditions of life across the country as unacceptable, nowhere more than in its capital. To the educated public, the germ's enduring presence remorselessly raised questions about the modernity and civilisation of the state. The indictment arrived in troubled times. While the country was waging a war against Japan, precipitous urban growth exacerbated social pressures and discontent, culminating in the revolutionary assault on the autocratic regime in 1905. At the intersection of political, social, economic and scientific developments, which were complicated by the revolution, the disease raised the question of whether the autocratic state was able to defend the most elementary interest of the population: protection against death. Given such a context, cholera came to question the regime's right to rule. And conversely, the outcome of the revolution affected the course of Russia's cholera until 1910.

This chapter examines the course of cholera in Saratov between 1904 and 1910. As in any previous cholera epidemics, the lower Volga assumed its traditional place as one of the country's epicentres. Strikingly, Saratov city was much less stricken by the bacillus throughout these years when compared with its neighbouring cities of Astrakhan', Tsaritsyn and Samara. And yet, despite relatively limited mortality, it was in Saratov city and province that the epidemic most powerfully demonstrated its potential to erode the autocratic state's political legitimacy. Once again, therefore, Saratov attracted nationwide attention because of an outbreak of cholera.

It is not possible, and indeed not the intention, to analyse the sixth pandemic in the same manner and detail as the epidemic in 1892. The sixth pandemic did not produce an equivalent public response and abundance of material to that occasioned by the 1892 outbreak. Even at its peak in 1910, cholera was hardly discussed in Saratov's local press.[9] With increasing medical understanding and decreasing mortality, the disease simply did not capture such public attention any more. Moreover, its significance was overshadowed by political and economic events. The outbreak most likely to be comparable to the year 1892 certainly is the one of 1910. Yet the chapter takes a longer view since the impact of the epidemic in 1910 is incomprehensible without establishing the revolutionary context of 1904–05 within which anti-epidemic policies were formulated and implemented.

The following chapter is divided into two parts. The first section, analogous to Chapter 2, places the sixth cholera pandemic in Saratov in its national context. It delineates the development of the disease between 1904 and 1910, identifies its distinctive characteristics and pinpoints its peculiarities in comparison with the *vibrio*'s course in 1892; it examines how the scientific explanation of the disease altered the government's anti-cholera policies and discusses the immediate achievements of the new strategy; it further analyses the new administrative framework within which anti-cholera measures were to be conducted after the disaster of 1892; finally, by looking at the interaction of medical and political reform, this first section discusses why the new scheme of defence proved incapable of effectively combating the disease and why the Russian state failed to eradicate cholera on a long-term basis.

The second part of the chapter analyses the course of cholera's sixth pandemic in Saratov city itself. It describes the germ's first arrival in 1904 and examines the economic, social and political challenge posed by the disease to governing authorities in a time of revolutionary upheaval; it discusses the functioning of the new administrative apparatus meant to contain the germ and examines the responses to the disease by local governmental and medical authorities in the age of bacteriology; it analyses the factors which enabled Saratov to exert better epidemic control between 1907 and 1910 than the neighbouring urban centres of Samara, Tsaritsyn and Astrakhan'; and finally, it asks why the city failed to eradicate cholera in the twentieth century. This section thus examines the changed nature of the relationship between local and national government initiatives, between the state and the medical profession, between administrative and medical officials and the population. In so doing, it places Saratov's sixth cholera epidemic within the context of the ongoing scientific and political revolution as it occurred within an autocratic state.

The government and cholera, 1904–1910

When cholera returned to Russia in 1904, the country already anticipated its outbreak. The bacterium had begun its sixth voyage to Europe in 1899. Travelling from Bengal northwards, the germ moved to the Punjab, Afghanistan and Persia, and reached the Caspian Sea in 1904. Alternatively, the epidemic took its traditional southern highway which led via Bombay and Madras to Ceylon and Jeddah; from here, pilgrims brought the contagion to Mecca, where it appeared in 1902, and thence dispersed it further across the Red Sea to Egypt, the Middle East and Africa. Russia, just as in the previous pandemic, was first afflicted at its eastern border. In late June 1902, cholera appeared among Korean sawmill workers at the river Ussura.[10] The unfortunate Koreans fled in panic and spread the *vibrio* to the surrounding villages. Soon the epidemic journeyed along the Ussuri railway (opened in 1899) to the urban centres of Vladivostok, Khabarovsk and Blagoveshchensk, which were most affected by the outbreak during the summer.[11] The *vibrio* then spread further through the provinces of Primor'e, Amur and Zabaikal'e, until it eventually reached Irkutsk.

As in 1892, the Russian government was fully aware of the threat. While Irkutsk was actually further away from central Russia than the Ganges delta, the disease could easily spread further by means of the Transsiberian railway.[12] The Ministry of Internal Affairs therefore immediately issued a new set of anti-cholera regulations in order to unify anti-epidemic measures and to place the fight against the disease on a new, stronger footing. In addition, the ministry took its first precautionary measures. Stringent health measures were implemented along the Chinese Eastern Railway and health staff and medical supplies were dispatched from St Petersburg to the afflicted region.[13] Fortunately, the onset of winter brought the *vibrio* to a halt in Irkutsk and in the following year the epidemic did not manifest itself on Russian soil at all.

Thus, the *vibrio* entered European Russia once again through its traditional gate of the Caspian Sea. During the summer of 1904 cholera had entered Persia from Baghdad and ferociously ravaged Herat.[14] Following its familiar route, the bacillus then moved through Meshed and Tauride towards Askhabad and from here journeyed westward to Baku and Erivan.[15] The two provinces suffered the heaviest losses, reporting a total of 7,144 cholera cases and 4,715 deaths at the end of the epidemic.[16] In comparison, cholera's northward movement along the Caspian Sea was much less vehement.[17] The lower Volga experienced only sporadic outbreaks, and in Samara province the cold weather eventually halted the germ before it could travel up the Volga. Altogether, the outbreak in 1904 caused 9,230 cholera cases, 6,700 of which proved fatal.[18]

Cholera's flare-up in 1904, brief yet virulent, signalled the epidemic's return for good. From this point on, the germ – with the exception of the year 1906 – never retreated from the country during the whole period from 1904 until 1911. 1905 witnessed a very limited epidemic confined to Russia's western border region.[19] From 1907, however, cholera spread widely across the whole country year after year. This progression overturned any established theories in the epidemiology of the disease. During the previous five pandemics, cholera followed clearly established and predictable patterns. Using Astrakhan' or Orenburg as its starting point, the germ systematically attacked place after place from south to north or from east to west. On the south–north axis, mortality was highest at the earliest affected places and descended in each succeeding province; on the east–west route, by contrast, cholera intensified as it moved westward. These patterns were usually reversed in the second year of the epidemic when the *vibrio* rolled back.[20]

From 1907, cholera deviated from its usual habit. To everybody's surprise, the disease flared up without any prior notice in the city of Samara on 3 July 1907.[21] It is impossible to know how the germ arrived in the city. Medical reports, both national and local, offer contradictory explanations. Some hold that the disease was imported by what medical experts by then called a 'Bazillusträger', i.e. people who carried the bacillus with them without being afflicted by the disease and who thus slipped unnoticed through the precautionary measures taken along the Persian border.[22] A second plausible, yet usually by most physicians discounted possibility, was the epidemic's arrival by means of the newly opened Orenburg–Tashkent railway (1906).[23] Most medical accounts surmise that the germ had probably lived on in the refuse of one of Samara's ravines throughout the years of 1905 and 1906.[24] From Samara, a migrant worker carried the infection by ship down to Astrakhan'. This great southern seaport, having lost its status as the germ's point of entry to Russia, was still a major centre for migrant workers from all over the country and thus continued to provide the crucial epidemiological link to Russia's heartland. Ship passengers, ship commanders and returning migrants first spread the disease across the Volga provinces and thence throughout the empire.[25] From now on, each outbreak established foci of contagion across the country, and in subsequent years the epidemic's emergence at many places was of local origin. 1908 witnessed cholera's first occurrence in Tsaritsyn, where the germ had lain dormant during the winter of 1907.[26] In 1909 the disease was first reported from St Petersburg where the bacillus had established a most enduring presence in 1908.[27] By 1910, it was already impossible for official authorities to identify the epidemic's beginning and to trace its journey through the country. Since January the disease had been reported from Moscow as well as from Baku, the Don Cossack Region and Ekaterinoslav.[28] Cholera became a fact of life. A medical journalist lamented in 1908:

> It seems already fully natural, that every year in July the information comes somewhere from the Volga that cholera cases were reported, then it is noted, that in other cities so and so many people got caught by the disease, and so and so many died. Every day the news is spread that cholera cases were reported in the south, and in the central provinces, and at the periphery [. . .] if on some wonderful day this information disappeared from the newspapers, the population would be irritated.[29]

The cholera outbreak in 1910 came to be the culmination of Russia's sixth pandemic. As Table 5.1 illustrates, the disease, much more extensive and intensive than in the previous three years, developed into a full-scale epidemic:

Yet the germ's new course notwithstanding, Russia's traditional epicentres maintained their national status as the most heavily stricken regions in the empire. Cholera's worst effects were felt in the Caucasus, which reported 45,923 cholera cases in the most virulent year of 1910.[30] Ferociously ravaged also were the Don Cossack Region, where cholera attacked 21,472 people in the same year, and Russia's southern provinces (Ekaterinoslav, Khar'kov, Tauride, Kherson), which counted 67,491 cholera cases.[31] The fourth hardest hit area was the provinces at the lower Volga (Simbirsk, Samara, Saratov, Astrakhan') with 34,000 cholera cases.[32] Finally, the outbreaks of cholera in St Petersburg marked particular high points of the sixth pandemic. Russia's capital was so violently attacked in 1908 and 1909 that the country's distinguished bacteriologist Nikolai Gamaleia compared the historical significance of the disease to that of the epidemic in Hamburg in 1892.[33]

Table 5.1 Cholera in Russia, 1907–1910

Year	Number of affected provinces	Cholera cases	Cholera deaths
1907	49	12,716	6,421
1908	68	20,623	10,294
1909	50	20,644	9,375
1910	72	208,707	98,050

Figures from V.I. Binshtok, "Kholernaia epidemiia 1910 goda v Rossii", p. 1353.

With cholera encroaching on European Russia in 1904, the government was occupied with international and domestic problems of the first magnitude. The war against Japan and the impending revolution presented more immediate concerns than cholera. Cholera's sixth pandemic came to crystallise the overlapping dramatic political and scientific events which shattered the empire. Prompted by the experience of 1892 and in particular the possible resurgence of plague in 1898, the government undertook significant changes in the management of epidemics. In 1899, on the occasion of an outbreak of plague in India, the Ministry of Internal Affairs established a Special Commission for Measures against Plague (soon called the Anti-Plague Commission).[34] Alongside medical considerations, in particular the need for unifying anti-epidemic policies, political considerations influenced the decision. In a time of heightened political activity on the part of local self-governing institutions, the Anti-Plague Commission was an ad hoc attempt to centralise Russia's disparate system of anti-epidemic management whilst leaving intact the authority of the many ministries responsible for public health and at the same time keeping local self-governing institutions under control.[35] In 1903, when cholera broke out in the Far East, the Ministry of Internal Affairs also charged the Anti-Plague Commission with protecting the country against the *vibrio cholerae*. One of the commission's first moves was the elaboration of a new set of anti-cholera regulations.[36]

As in the previous pandemic, the state (i.e. the Anti-Plague Commission) devised a cholera campaign which took full account of the latest scientific discoveries about cholera. Since 1892, medicine had come a long way. Koch's contagionist views on the disease had been validated during the course of the epidemic in Hamburg in 1892.[37] Further advances in bacteriology confirmed his approach. Scientific debates between contagionists and the proponents of miasmatism, to be sure, were still carried out for quite some time. As late as 1912, miasmatist theories of the transmission of cholera continued to circulate even in such a stronghold of bacteriology as Germany.[38] In Russia, where medical-scientific stances were used for political purposes, it was only in 1905 that the majority of the medical profession eventually recognised bacteriology as a medical specialty.[39] Yet despite these battles, the aetiology of cholera was fully explained by the early twentieth century. The bacteriological model of infectious disease had succeeded in establishing its pre-eminent position over miasmatist approaches. Koch's theory that cholera was caused by a microscopic bacillus, transmitted through infected water, food or clothing, was generally accepted; it was further acknowledged that the sources of infection – unfiltered water, poor housing, inadequate sanitation – were eradicable; and it was agreed that the disease was best contained by measures of quarantine, isolation and disinfection.

Once again, the international community responded to the latest scientific findings. In 1903, an International Sanitary Conference in Paris devised a new framework of defence measures against cholera that, above all, sought to forestall the economic damage cholera caused to international trade.[40] Up to that point, the sanitary conferences on cholera had expressed recommendations, which tried to limit the arbitrariness of coercive policies against the bacillus. The Paris

Convention of 1903, by contrast, established for the first time in the history of the disease an internationally unified set of anti-cholera measures.[41] On the basis of the bacteriological explanation for the epidemic, the treaty committed the signatory nations to rational public health policies. These involved the immediate notification of the international community about the appearance of the epidemic and continuous information about its course as well as the measures taken against it. They further comprised standardised precautionary measures and sanitary procedures to be taken by the afflicted states: land-based quarantine, sanitary cordons and military defence systems, the distinctive features of Russia's cholera combat in 1892, were explicitly forbidden. Maritime quarantine, by contrast, was preserved under the condition that it was conducted along rational principles based on the modern scientific understanding of the disease. The Russian delegation, which included among others Vasilii Anrep and Boris Shapirov, had signed the document.[42] It was ratified on 15 March 1904.[43]

As a signatory of the convention, Russia had to introduce fundamental changes in its anti-epidemic policies. St Petersburg had sounded the alarm when the disease ravaged Persia in 1904. As soon as the *vibrio* had reached the traditionally ominous centres of Tauride, Meshed and Herat, the government took its first steps to protect the Russian–Persian border. Unlike in 1892, however, the state abandoned its coercive strategy to contain the germ. Bound by international law, the government dismissed the deployment of soldiers and placed its principal emphasis on laboratory diagnostic techniques and on gaining public trust. The contrast was striking. Whereas in 1892 a few military physicians had been sent from the Caucasus to Persia in order to observe the epidemic's progress, in 1904, the state authorised Russia's top medical research institution, the Institute of Experimental Medicine, to prepare health staff, laboratories and medical supplies to actively support Persia's authorities in preventing the epidemic's spread. The Institute of Experimental Medicine dispatched some of the country's leading bacteriologists, including Semen Zlatogorov and V.A. Taranukhin, to Tauride.[44] During their time in Persia, the physicians built up contacts with local governing authorities, priests and Persian physicians who supported them in establishing laboratories, pharmacies and surgeries and provided them with information about both prevailing diseases and new cholera cases. To gain the trust of the local population, the doctors treated people suffering from all sorts of diseases for free. These efforts paid off. Returning in the summer of 1905, the physicians were able to rely on their experience with the population and make use of their increasing familiarity with local traditions.[45]

In pursuit of this policy, the government dropped its attempts at a military closure of the border and instead relied on a chain of medical observation points established in Ashkhabad, Kara-Kala, Kaachka, Chatlinsk and Chat.[46] As in 1892, national authorities aimed at identifying and isolating the *vibrio* as early as possible so as to prevent it from spreading further into the country. But to have expected these precautions to guard the border effectively was admittedly just as unrealistic as it had been in 1892. A medical report presented to the Pirogov Society in 1905 revealed that scientific medicine along the border, given local geographic, medical and economic conditions, still had to be replaced by improvisation. With local authorities uninformed and unprepared, the doctors from St Petersburg usually operated in no more than an ill-equipped tent.[47]

Yet medical defects notwithstanding, taking control of cholera along the border away from the military was a significant novelty. As the experience with the *vibrio* in 1892 had once again demonstrated, official policies, more than anything else, determined the popular response to cholera. The attempt to contain the disease by means of brutal force had not only caused physical suffering; it had also sent the message that the sick were like military enemies or at least dangerous criminals who had to be eliminated. At the same time, the arbitrariness of the cholera operation plainly exhibited the state's powerlessness to protect the population against the fatal disease. During the sixth pandemic, by contrast, the increased efforts to build up mutual confidence between medical authorities and the population clearly portrayed the disease as a medical affliction which could be avoided by following certain behavioural rules. From the very beginning, the state's anti-cholera policy spread the impression that the situation was under control and that there was no reason to panic.

In compliance with the new border policy, the state continued to conduct a more substantial campaign of preventive health inside the country. The Volga, in particular, was the greatest cause of concern for St Petersburg's officials. The cholera scare of 1892 had most clearly exposed the Volga's crucial strategic significance for maintaining the health of the nation. And the state's failure to arrange for any preparatory steps to rectify local medical inadequacies along the river had been a fatal flaw in the national cholera defence. By the early twentieth century, Russia's high-risk region had become even more of a threat. Since 1892, innumerable links by rail and road added to the diversified net of feeder streams and canals, linking the river with the whole of Russia's European heartland and with remote areas far away in central Asia and Siberia.[48] Moreover, the upturn in the river's economic activity had multiplied the number of seasonal migrant workers. Between 1891 and 1905, the turnover of goods on the river basin had more than doubled from 519 million pud to 1,300 million pud.[49] The Ministry of Ways and Communications recorded 73,823 ship workers on the Volga in 1900 versus approximately 100,000 in 1910.[50] Being the most susceptible victims to the disease, these people were the crucial carrier of the contagion as much as of the country's economy. The government's interest in preventing the spread of the bacillus along the river was therefore most acute. An epidemic on the river would halt trade, increase unemployment and raise the possibility of social tensions. Cholera threatened the nation's health and economy.

To avoid the spectre of economic disaster, the Russian government reinforced sanitary and medical observation along the river, in particular on its lower reaches, as soon as the germ showed itself in 1904. According to the principles agreed upon at the Paris Convention, the Anti-Plague Commission had regulated quarantine and isolation procedures on waterways on a strictly scientific basis. Existing legislation stipulated that every passenger ship had to be accompanied by physicians, medical students and feldshers.[51] Suspiciously ill passengers were to be isolated in specially prepared isolation cabins and their personal belongings disinfected. Every ship coming from a place affected by cholera had to undergo medical observation at its destination point and to be declared free of disease before the passengers could leave the ship. During all the measures taken, coercion was to be avoided. Instead of subjecting every person on a ship and the whole ship to a harassing process of cleansing and disinfection at its point of arrival, as was the rule in 1892, the Anti-Plague Commission decreed that every steamer had to undergo thorough disinfection procedures only at the end of the navigation period. Physicians, in addition to controlling the state of health on a ship, also made deliberate efforts to win the trust of the passengers by distributing pamphlets and brochures and by giving talks on individual measures of prevention.[52] As for the fleet of non-passenger ships, they were subjected to medical surveillance by special vessels (*kreisery*), which were brought into action at Astrakhan' and Saratov.[53] If a patient was found, he was immediately put under medical observation on the vessel and shipped to the nearest hospital. This way, sick passengers were spared the agonising journeys on barges without medically trained personnel. According to official reports, the use of vessels to transport the sick had a particularly positive impact in the Volga delta at Astrakhan' where the eight-hour journey from the observation point to the hospital had caused lots of suffering for the victims in the previous epidemic.[54]

In addition to strengthening medical observation on the Volga, the state recognised the need to support the organisation of sanitary surveillance and medical facilities at the banks. For the purpose of severing the link between the river and the banks, the Anti-Plague Commission had authorised the Ministry of Ways and Communications to cooperate with local self-governments in organising medical provision at the river's rural and urban settlements. Throughout the sixth pandemic, the Ministry built up cholera barracks on the banks;[55] it supplied them with health staff and laboratory equipment; it set up medical observation points; it enforced strict sanitary control at the landing docks, the most dangerous sources of contamination on the whole river; and, eventually, it sought to protect the ship workers by providing them with a healthy diet. With this aim in mind, the state also obliged ship owners to open soup kitchens for their workers or, alternatively, to give them 10 kopecks for the purchase of hot food.[56]

Historical scholarship has argued that Russia's new cholera plan produced dire results. Theodore Friedgut, for example, pointed to violent cholera riots in Iuzovka as late as 1910 as a response to the state's rigorous handling of the epidemic.[57] Likewise, in her analysis of the epidemic in 1904–05, Nancy Frieden argued that the measures taken evoked public fear and resistance towards medical authorities and thus undermined the physicians' attempts to gain popular trust.[58] Her interpretation also concurs with the grim reports presented by physicians to the Pirogov Society at the 'Cholera Congress' in 1905, on which, in fact, Frieden's study is based. However, a closer look at the course of the epidemic does not uphold such a verdict. Physicians at the 'Cholera Congress', as will be seen below, pursued both professional and political interests when they depicted the effects of the latest anti-epidemic policies in the darkest colours. It is necessary to disentangle their professional–political motives from medical events. In fact, due to the state's rejection of coercive measures and a more substantial policy of precautionary activity, the epidemic's impact in the early twentieth century differed considerably from that in 1892. In 1907 (and in subsequent years), as the disease was progressing towards Astrakhan' and up the Volga, it was no longer accompanied by major social disturbances. Admittedly, many doctors reported on the distrust of the population towards medical personnel and pointed to people's refusal to submit to treatment.[59] And at individual places in the empire, notably in the countryside, cholera could still create utter chaos.[60] Yet poisonous frenzy and public hysteria, which had played so prominent a role in 1892, did not overwhelm people's imagination any more. Even the big cities at the lower Volga, where once violent fracas in the streets and open revolt had paralysed official authorities, setting the tone for popular responses across the country, remained quiet. As some contemporaries noted, the moderate approach to quarantine itself had lowered the threat of rebellion: 'The previous panic, former anxiety we did not see any more, and, most of all, the awkward and, according to our contemporary view, pointless measures, with which some states still annoyed one another, are almost a thing of the past.'[61]

There were other calming factors. Most significantly, cholera mortality during the sixth pandemic was considerably lower than in 1892 when it seemed that the disease would sweep away all its victims. In European Russia, only the southern provinces of Voronezh, Khar'kov, Ekaterinoslav, Kherson and Tauride were as heavily hit by the disease in 1910 as they were in 1892.[62] Elsewhere, and even at the lower Volga, the bacillus did not launch the natural disaster which was the previous pandemic. Limited mortality, of course, does not necessarily prevent panic. Frank Snowden has shown how coercive sanitary policies inspired full-scale riots in Barletta, Trani and Molfana in 1910 despite the negligible demographic impact of the disease.[63] Yet in Russia, the lower level of mortality in many parts of the country nevertheless confirmed the impression that cholera was controllable and that human beings were not at the mercy of the *vibrio* any more.[64]

Another important element that reduced the social explosiveness of the disease was the strengthened position of Russia's medical profession at the beginning of the twentieth century. Since the previous epidemic, the achievements of zemstvo medicine, although more successful in some places than in others, had begun to accustom the population to medical care and physicians. Moreover, the deliberate efforts during the sixth pandemic to promote trust between the people and the medical profession yielded good results. Whilst the physicians at the 'Cholera Congress' reported about fearsome disinfection procedures in the Caucasus or at the Chinese border, many doctors from the lower Volga noted that the population related more calmly to the medical profession than in 1892. Even from Astrakhan', still the most vulnerable city at the river's lower reaches, physicians noted that:

> the population at the beginning was distrustful towards the medical personnel. Sometimes, distrust turned into hostility and there were threats to smash the hospitals following the example of previous epidemics, yet the calm and systematic activity of the municipal medical personnel – although quite few in number – ultimately enabled the elimination of this hostility.[65]

Yet despite these successes in combating cholera, Russia failed to eradicate the disease. Strictly speaking, the interventions undertaken by the government during the sixth pandemic were even less successful than the state's measures in 1892. At that time, the epidemic erupted with full fury in the year of its arrival yet receded in subsequent years – chiefly as an immediate result of emergency reforms in local medical administration. During the sixth pandemic, by contrast, cholera returned year after year with greater force, reaching its climax as late as 1910, the seventh year of the pandemic.

One major problem, which powerfully undermined the state's campaign, was environmental pollution. Russia's sixth cholera pandemic carried with it a heavy indictment of the country's sanitary conditions. Along the Volga, the disastrous conditions that had given rise to the epidemic of 1892 had not simply remained; the river was now even more at risk. Booming commercial activity in the 1890s and 1900s drove the Volga cities through two decades of rapid expansion. Existing sanitary and medical capacities could not keep up with growing population numbers, and new sources of pollution brought about by commercial and industrial growth further deteriorated the urban environment. Most alarming, cholera laid bare the cities' dangerous deficits in water supply and sewage disposal. At a regional cholera congress in Samara in 1908, physicians and public health experts from the river cities pointed out that not a single Volga city was provided with a canalisation system and proper sewage disposal.[66] Samara, Saratov, Tsaritsyn, Kazan', Nizhnii Novgorod and every urban centre at the river still emptied their urban refuse into the river, thus heavily contributing to its severe contamination. With increasing pollution of the Volga and ever-growing cities, the problems of supplying the urban inhabitants with adequate quantities of fresh water for drinking, cooking and washing became steadily more acute. The delegates at the Samara congress concluded that:

> sanitary conditions in the Volga cities need to be regarded as very bad and unfavourable: broad sections of the population, notably the poor, who live at the margins, are not provided with fundamental sanitary services such as water, housing, sufficient food; the soil of the cities is highly polluted, and medical-sanitary organisation in the Volga centres is either non-existent altogether or in its earliest infancy.[67]

By the turn of the century national and local public health experts unanimously regarded the Volga cities as the most dramatic health hazard to the whole nation. The damage that increasing commerce and urban growth were inflicting upon the river became the object of official attention. In 1899, the Medical Council dispatched a delegation of hygienists, chemists and physicians to the middle and lower Volga in order to examine the impact of fuel oil, the chief polluter of the Volga, on the water.[68] In the following year, prompted by the repeated occurrence of epidemics and diseases along the Volga and their spread all over Russia, the government established a sanitary inspectorate (*sanitarnyi nadzor*) along the river, covering the distance from Nizhnii Novgorod down to Astrakhan'.[69] Under the

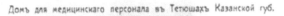

Домъ для медицинскаго персонала въ Тетюшахъ Казанской губ.

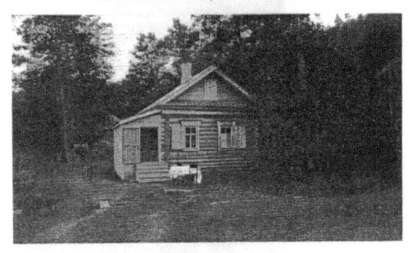

Плавучій окружной баракъ № 3, служившій въ навигацію 1910 г. врачебно-продовольственнымъ
пунктомъ въ г. Царицынѣ.

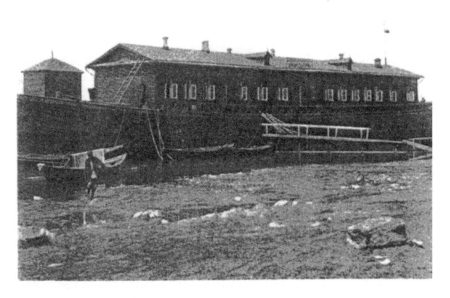

Figure 7 "Swimming cholera barrack" near Tsaritsyn and house for medical personnel
during the cholera, 1910, A.A. Desiatov, *Kholera 1907–1908–1909 i 1910 g.g.
na vodnykh putiakh Kazanskogo okruga putei soobshcheniia* (St Petersburg,
1911).

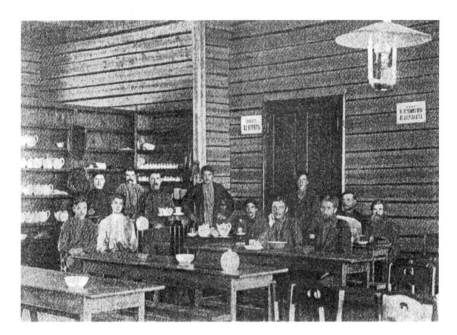

Figure 8 Medical observation point near Iurevets (Kostroma province), A.A. Desiatov, *Kholera 1907–1908–1909 i 1910 g.g. na vodnykh putiakh Kazanskogo okruga putei soobshcheniia* (St Petersburg, 1911).

auspices of the Ministry of Ways and Communications, the inspectorate employed nine physicians, based in Rybinsk, Nizhnii Novgorod, Kazan', Samara, Tsaritsyn and Astrakhan', who were charged with the task of carrying out investigations into the hygienic conditions of the ship workers and boatsmen, i.e. the poor who were most affected by the problem.[70] These physicians also assumed responsibility for controlling the implementation of sanitary measures on the Volga during times of epidemic crisis. Furthermore, the Anti-Plague Commission dispatched the country's best bacteriologists from St Petersburg to the Volga during the cholera epidemic in order to identify and investigate the chief sources of pollution in the cities.[71] All these initiatives sadly confirmed that the tasks confronted in the field of sanitation along the river were overwhelming. And, while the state had delegated public health and sanitation to the communes, municipalities along the river were both mis-administered and lacked financial means for their sanitary build-up. Given such conditions, Zlatogorov, one of the delegates of the Anti-Plague Commission to the lower Volga in 1907, returned to the capital with the unhappy premonition that 'the sanitary conditions of the cities will for a long time nourish various epidemics, and notably cholera'.[72]

Yet the cholera campaign was also impeded by other problems for which state authorities bore responsibility. Inefficient administration remained a fundamental defect in the country's cholera defence. The Anti-Plague Commission, after a century of creating non-governmental, autonomous agencies to fight against cholera, was as unsuited to combating the germ as Zakrevskii's cholera commission in 1830.[73] Its weakness began with its personnel composition. Comprising eight ministers from the Ministry of Finance, of Internal and Foreign Affairs, and of Ways and Communications (virtually the Committee of Ministers), Russia's new commission responsible for formulating and directing anti-epidemic policies lacked any medical expertise.[74] While this institution of high senior bureaucrats was of higher authority than the Medical Council, the state's highest advisory body for medical policies within the Ministry of Internal Affairs, the Medical Department, which had the administrative experience of the cholera campaign in 1892, was legislated out of existence in the course of Plehve's reform of the Ministry of Internal Affairs in 1904.[75]

Without any medical knowledge, the Anti-Plague Commission was charged with a multitude of difficult tasks. Above all, it had to govern the actions and movements of the many subsidiary governing institutions that were spread out across an immense territory. As such, the commission was an administrative body, which collected information from the infected areas; it published the received data in cholera bulletins; and it provided a channel of communication between local authorities and national ministries. In addition, the commission also served as the country's chief dispersal centre for medical personnel and supplies. Any requests for medical support had to be directed to the Anti-Plague Commission. This way, it was hoped, the supply of medical necessities would proceed with greater speed and efficiency than if they were distributed by several ministries.[76]

In order to streamline communication to the local level and to achieve some degree of coordination across the empire, control in the provinces was vested in newly created Sanitary Executive Commissions (SECs). In contrast to the Sanitary Executive Commissions from 1892/93, which placed the main responsibility for the combat against epidemics in the hands of physicians and local zemstvo and duma deputies, the new SECs were composed of non-medical administrators and governmental representatives of the central government.[77] Thus reconstituted, the commissions were charged with expanding and directing the whole arsenal of anti-cholera measures according to the instructions issued by the Anti-Plague Commission in 1903. All local officials were operating under the surveillance of the SECs and thus under the jurisdiction of the Anti-Plague Commission. The latter retained the highest authority over all decision-making. Any official acknowledgement of a particular locality as affected or threatened by the germ depended on its affirmation.[78] And any measures going beyond its instructions needed the approval of its central authority.[79]

In practice, the remodelled infrastructure complicated rather than rationalised governmental processes. The first shortcoming of St Petersburg's new defence scheme had to do with timing. Rapid decisions and their immediate execution, so crucial in particular during the early stages of the epidemic, were irreconcilable with the requirement that every move had to make its way via the capital. At the Volga River, the policy undermined the overriding concern for an early disclosure of cholera cases. Cholera barracks, medical personnel and supplies along the river needed to be provided before the epidemic occurred and not once the Anti-Plague Commission had acknowledged the cholera's presence. The impossibility of predicting when and where the disease would break out further complicated swift operation. As a result, the work of the sanitary inspectorate along the river usually began only after the germ had established its presence.[80]

Action was further delayed by the fact that most medical supplies were still in St Petersburg. Medical deficits in one area could not simply be remedied by reshuffling local resources. In 1907, Astrakhan's bacteriologist was sent up and down the lower Volga, which meant he was missing from Astrakhan', a city affected by the most virulent cholera attack.[81] On the Volga River, eight sanitary physicians could not provide more than a skeletal service for so large a territory extending from St Petersburg to Astrakhan', from Ufa and Perm in the east to Viatka in the west. Everywhere, as it turned out, medical supplies were impossible to obtain, and local authorities along the Volga chiefly criticised the Anti-Plague Commission for failing to prevent chronic medical shortages: 'the Anti-Plague Commission should pass its enormous means to the zemstva and dumas and not limit itself to the dispatchment of bacteriologists.'[82] Under these circumstances, the new anti-cholera policies were extremely difficult to enforce. A report about the measures taken on the Volga River summed up the living reality: 'Indeed, these requirements, of course, proved completely inapplicable, which is fully explainable to those who have an understanding about the traffic of the ships and the passengers on the Volga. [. . .] Willy-nilly,' the report concluded, 'the region had to ignore these requirements.'[83]

Even more fatally, as it turned out, the policies pursued by the Anti-Plague Commission alienated both local self-governing bodies and the medical profession. Given how much power had been granted to local institutions during the cholera in 1892, the new legislation, in fact, presented a major step backwards. Moreover, it rode roughshod over the achievements made by zemstvo and duma institutions notably in the field of public health and epidemic control after the cholera calamity of 1892. Throughout the sixth cholera pandemic a flood of petitions from zemstva and dumas across the country reached the Ministry of Internal Affairs demanding to review or, better still, abolish the new regulations.[84] First and foremost, the deputies regarded the reorganised SECs as an infringement on their local autonomy and authority. The regulations, they argued, violated the zemstvo statute from 1890 which had placed some public health jurisdiction, including that over the control of epidemics, into the hands of the zemstva.[85] Encroaching on zemstvo and medical prerogatives, they further held, these regulations only complicated epidemic control. In support of their claim local authorities pointed to the fact that some areas, for instance those under the jurisdiction of the Ministry of War or the Ministry of Ways and Communications, remained outside the legislation.[86] Moreover, zemstva and dumas were still entitled to enact their own measures which could contradict the initiatives taken by the SECs.[87] Local authorities were actually correct when they concluded that such 'amalgam of archaic decrees about institutions of public health' prevented what they were supposed to do, namely to unify and coordinate anti-epidemic measures at the local level.[88]

From the standpoint of the physicians, the new cholera regulations furthermore undermined the very structure that they considered vital for their work. After all, it was the physicians' alliance with the zemstva, albeit a tense one throughout the period under consideration, which had enabled them to strengthen their corporate consciousness and to gain some degree of professional autonomy. The infringement of zemstvo rights and privileges went right to the core of their professional ethos and work. Recent advances in medicine powerfully underlined the issue. In an era of revolutionary scientific breakthroughs, the Russian government placed the responsibility for critical medical questions into the hands of government officials without specialised knowledge. To the physicians, this dismissal of their professional authority, deriving from scientific knowledge and expertise, epitomised unacceptable medical policies: 'Being the result of bureaucratic-clerical creativity,' one physician remarked, 'they were recognised even before their implementation as incapable of surviving.'[89]

Faced with new scientific foundations and a completely reshuffled administrative framework, physicians from all over the country once again assembled in St Petersburg in order to discuss an appropriate set of anti-epidemic measures. Yet unlike 1892, when the central government had summoned the country's medical experts after the epidemic, it now was the Pirogov Society which initiated the famous 'Cholera Congress' in March 1905. Historical scholarship has correctly pointed out that the overriding concern of the Congress was professional-scientific.[90] Well-known scientists in the fields of bacteriology, epidemiology, hygiene and pathology summarised and discussed the recent scientific basis for methods of diagnosis, vaccination, disinfection and isolation procedures, and means of treatment.[91] At the same time, it was inevitable that the physicians took a stance on the new administrative rules affecting their ability to do their job. John Hutchinson claimed that the participants of the congress had dismissed the new official institutions from the very beginning. He concluded that 'Russian medical scientists and community physicians entirely bypassed the official anti-epidemic agencies of the government and created an alternative institutional network by which the scientific understanding of disease could be applied quickly and consistently at the local level.'[92]

Yet, as Russia's physicians were very aware, bypassing St Petersburg's authority was not so easy. It is true that the official resolution of the congress encouraged the country's physicians not to cooperate with the new SECs.[93] They were advised, primarily for medical reasons, to rely instead on local governing institutions which had, after all, proven their effectiveness in organising public health provision. In some places, like Saratov city for example, this strategy proved feasible and reasonably successful. Overall, however, the resolution created chaos and confusion. Not only did it increase the lack of clarity about current administrative mechanisms; it also carried with it a heavy indictment of the autocratic state. In the revolutionary situation of 1904/05, medical concerns turned into political demands.

It is important to recall the impact of the congress on the relationship between Russia's medical profession and the state with regard to the practical consequences for combating cholera.[94] During the 1890s and early 1900s, continuous confrontations with state authorities and local self-governing institutions had driven the physicians into the mainstream of the opposition movement. Until the 'Cholera Congress', however, the majority of the medical profession still advocated gradual political and social reform within an autocratic government. By issuing cholera regulations that completely dismissed cooperation with the medical profession at a time of great scientific discoveries, the central government had gone too far. Russia's physicians concluded that any improvement in the country's public health required first of all a change in the political system. Cholera, crystallising the problem of central and local governance since its first arrival in Russia, became the vehicle for the medical profession to openly express and mobilise opinion in favour of desired political reforms. At the 'Cholera Congress', both bacteriologists and community physicians spoke out for a constitutional assembly elected by equal, direct, secret and universal suffrage; for freedom of speech, press, assembly and for the inviolability of person; finally, they sought the release of political prisoners and the establishment of autonomous self-government.[95]

These events proved disastrous for the next few years. The Anti-Plague Commission could only perform its functions if it could rely on local authorities, whose autonomy it had abolished; meanwhile, physicians refused to acknowledge the authority of the new institutions and threatened a boycott of their services as cholera advanced in 1905. Local self-governing institutions, for their part, 'were suddenly caught between an obstinate Ministry of Internal Affairs and a determined group of physicians'.[96] Antagonisms between the three groups were exacerbated as the revolution got under way. Following the revolution, numerous zemstva destroyed their sanitary organisations. Physicians became much sought-after targets for recrimination in the wave of reprisals that swept the country.[97] Moreover, community medicine, and its political and social underlying assumptions, plunged into a deep crisis under the pressure of further innovations in bacteriology and sanitary science. At the same time, medical reform at the central level was hampered by the multiple jurisdictions over medical affairs and by the failure of St Petersburg's reformers to cooperate with the state-hostile physicians in the community medical institutions. A serious plan for the creation of a central ministry of public health was put forward only in 1910 by G.E. Rein, who had witnessed the cholera epidemic of the same year in the Donets Basin and Russia's southern provinces.[98] Yet his proposal was first blocked by Stolypin, Minister of Internal Affairs and head of the Medical Council, and eventually swept away by the beginning of the war in 1914.

As in 1892, in 1910 the Russian state was anxiously awaiting the renewed cholera threat to the country since the disease had broken out in the Far East. Owing to the disastrous experience with the bacillus during the previous epidemic, the government took two important decisions. The first was to centralise anti-epidemic management by assigning its direction to the newly created Anti-Plague Commission. The commission elaborated a new set of anti-cholera policies which, once again, took full account of the latest advances in preventive techniques following the cholera outbreak of 1892 in Hamburg. The main novelty of the remodelled scheme of defence, furthermore, was the decision to dismiss military force and coercion in order to contain the germ. In the era of bacteriology, and in agreement with international law, the government instead emphasised and conducted a strategy based on laboratory diagnostic techniques and medical precaution. As a result, the epidemic's social impact throughout the sixth pandemic was far removed from the tumultuous events of 1892.

Such an outcome notwithstanding, Russia's state authorities failed to eliminate the disease. In fact, one could even argue that the campaign in 1892 was more successful than the policies conducted as of 1904. Two major reasons account for the epidemic's return year after year until it reached its height in 1910. Firstly, rapid urban growth and booming commerce, at least at the Volga, had magnified the sanitary dangers along the river. Given the speed of urban development in light of a sanitary movement just at inception, the tasks confronted in the field of sanitation were overwhelming. Secondly, the Anti-Plague Commission was no solution whatsoever to the problem of how to unify and coordinate epidemic policies. Instead of rationalising anti-cholera management, the commission complicated swift operation and communication and created further confusion about current legislative responsibilities. Yet most fatally, it alienated local official and medical authorities. The new cholera regulations provoked not only medical boycotts; across the country, and with Saratov province in the lead, they also challenged the political authority of the regime. The revolution, eventually, changed the relationships between the state, local governing authorities and the physicians, and it left the medical profession fragmented and disorganised. Under these conditions, cholera flourished.

Local authority in crisis: cholera in Saratov, 1904–1910

Cholera's initial arrival in Saratov in 1904, just as in 1892, went unnoticed. Physicians were alerted to the threat when observing an increasing number of severe, often lethal cases of gastroenteritis during the summer.[99] According to official reports, however, the *vibrio cholerae* did not manifest itself until early September. The first acknowledged case was that of a railway worker who was diagnosed with the disease on 4 September through a bacteriological analysis in the municipal hospital.[100] On the same day, the zemstvo hospital reported the admission of two patients, a fruit seller from the *Beloglinskii* ravine and an oil worker from *Detiagin* Street, both of whom exhibited cholera-like symptoms. From then on, cholera spread as a succession of isolated cases through various streets affecting individual houses and household members. In total, 39 people, mostly local residents working as unskilled labourers at the landing docks, the railway or somewhere else in the city contracted the disease and 21 (51%) died of it.[101] The last officially recorded patient was the wife of a signalman who was struck by the *vibrio* on 2 November and discharged from the hospital on 18 November; her case marked the official end to the disease.

In contrast to 1892, local administrative and medical officials had already taken action against a possible outbreak when the epidemic was still advancing towards the city.[102] On 3 and 4 August, the provincial sanitary council (*sanitarnyi sovet*) elaborated a detailed plan with preparatory and therapeutic measures against the germ. The plan was approved at an emergency meeting of the provincial uprava on 26 August. Fortunately, so local physicians believed, the onset of autumn had ended the outbreak before it could develop into a full-scale epidemic. Low temperatures in September and October reduced the vitality of the *vibrio cholerae*, which thrives in warm and humid conditions. More importantly, in Saratov, cold weather also lowered the consumption of fruits, especially watermelons, and contaminated water, and it ended the bathing season in the Volga. Finally, the navigation period came to an end and tens of thousands of seasonal migrants, the most vulnerable recipients and effective transmitters of the bacillus, disappeared.

Nevertheless, Saratov's mild cholera flare-up still became an important event. During the autumn, the germ had managed to establish several foci of contagion across the province, which were expected to come to life the following spring. The neighbouring provinces of Astrakhan' and Samara, which had been much more affected by the disease than Saratov province, presented another serious threat for the coming year. Local physicians, moreover, knew that in 1904 plain good fortune had saved the city: 'without doubt, under different circumstances, with the occurrence of the disease in the spring or summer, we would have had to face a full-scale, dreadful epidemic.'[103] As elsewhere in Russia, Saratov's authorities therefore anxiously awaited a major cholera epidemic in 1905. The department of public health (*otdel narodnogo zdraviia*) was adamant: 'It is beyond doubt,' it argued, 'that Saratov province is required to prepare in the most serious way for the fight against cholera in the coming spring.'[104]

Times now were even more difficult than 12 years before. Cholera, to begin with, threatened to invade during a period of depression in the local economy. The all-important agricultural sector was already vulnerable because of low productivity, land shortages and a burgeoning rural population destined for unemployment and poverty.[105] Since Saratov province boasted areas of rich and fertile soil, peasants were also exposed to exorbitantly high rents, low wages and exploitative agricultural contracts.[106] Rural economic hardship was exacerbated still further in 1897, 1898, 1901 and 1905 when bad harvests befell the province. Throughout 1902–04 peasants across the province expressed their despair through various forms of collective violence, including arson strikes against the estates, plundering stores and attacks on local authorities.[107] The cities, too, got a taste of the tensions in the countryside: swamped with peasants, the provincial capital grew from 143,431 inhabitants in 1900 to 203,000 in 1906.[108]

The outbreak of the Russo–Japanese War in January 1904 aggravated the crisis.[109] War demands placed a heavy burden on Saratov's peasant society. The military call-up left many families without their main breadwinner. Industry also declined, making it even more difficult to find employment in the cities: in Saratov the number of factory workers decreased from 9,203 in 1903 to 6,906 in 1906.[110] Instead of providing relief measures, provincial and municipal budgets strained under the task of allocating mobilised troops and evacuating the wounded. In protest, postcards circulated in the capital showing a poorly built military barracks in the form of an enormous gravestone memorial with the inscription: 'Here are buried 80,000 rubles of the municipal reserve capital.'[111] In addition to causing economic hardship, the war profoundly restricted medical care throughout the province. Diseases in the Far East now took priority over epidemics at home. Saratov sent military hospitals, medications and medical staff to Manchuria and Kharbin.[112] When the provincial uprava tried to hire additional medical personnel in the autumn of 1904, only 40 of 100 physicians were able to take up employment due to military conscription.[113] Mobilised physicians included the most distinguished medical authorities in the capital, among them Nikolai Teziakov, head of the provincial medical board.[114] Local medical authorities grimly concluded: 'Obviously, the unfortunate war with its outrageous mass of victims is not confined to those who die in the fields of Manchuria; most likely, it also brings in its wake tens and hundreds of thousands of deaths here, in the heart of Russia, which is helpless to organise the fight against cholera.'[115]

In such an explosive context, 39 cholera cases had a major impact on the city, the province and the empire. Once again, the epidemic became a vehicle for the population to express its dissatisfaction and demands for change. It did so, however, without producing the hysteria and mass uprisings which had characterised the fifth pandemic. Reflecting the general picture at the lower Volga, Saratov city did not witness the tumults that had accompanied the epidemic in 1892. Nevertheless, cholera, which crystallised issues such as the relation between central and local governments, between science and the state, and between the population and its governors, was bound to serve as a catalyst as revolutionary events unfolded. A combination of factors and events involving the whole province combined to turn the medical challenge into a political sensation that resonated across the whole country.

As discussed above, the historiography of cholera epidemics to date has predominantly charted a rich and highly varied model of civil disorder as a social response to the epidemic. Richard Evans, most far-reaching, established a link between cholera epidemics and political upheaval, asking whether the germ might have played a decisive role in the coming of revolutions, for example in 1830 and 1848.[116] Indeed, in western Europe cholera classically manifested itself shortly after or during times of political upheaval: in 1830–1832, during the revolutionary wave in central and western Europe; in the revolutionary year 1848; in 1866 when the German Confederation was overthrown; and in 1871, which saw the end of the Second Empire in France.[117] Already Chevalier, therefore, has placed his work on the 1832 epidemic in the context of the history of the French Revolution in 1848.

The capacity of cholera to unleash social disorder notwithstanding, Evans's comparative analysis ultimately negates the germ's capacity to unleash a revolution: 'Cholera did not after all cause, or even precipitate, major social and political upheavals such as those which swept across Europe in the early 1830s and late 1840s.'[118] Moreover, Evans's study on the cholera in Hamburg in 1892 showed that the history of the epidemic is not as marked by social tumults as the existing studies on its earlier outbreaks might suggest. In striking contrast to other places in earlier times, Hamburg's experience of the epidemic lacked any rioting or public disturbances.[119] Paris, as well, kept calm during its final cholera outbreak in 1884.[120] The complexity of the history of cholera's social impact is further revealed in Frank Snowden's analysis of the epidemic in Naples. The return of the germ to Italy in 1910/11 led again to regional eruptions of social tumult and assaults on doctors, albeit on a much smaller scale than in 1884. The Neapolitan experience, however, provides a novel case in which the successful concealment of a major epidemic prevented public unrest – yet in the end undermined the moral authority of the Liberal regime, laying the political groundwork for its overthrow.[121]

Despite only minor occurrences, Saratov's cholera in 1904/05 continued to lay the ground for revolutionary upheaval. The new cholera regulations established the link between the disease and social discontent. The instructions, which provided the basis for the combat against cholera throughout the sixth epidemic, were for the first time put into effect by the Anti-Plague Commission in 1904. Since the germ did not travel beyond Samara that year, their implementation was confined to the Far East and the Volga River.

In Saratov, the fact that zemstva and dumas as executive organs were now required to pay for a plan devised by a provincial Sanitary Executive Commission heralded the breakdown of public order.[122] Whilst preparations were going on for the anticipated cholera outbreak in 1905, the new directives exacerbated prevailing tensions between the medical profession and governing officials, escalating into one of the most dramatic confrontations between the *intelligentsia* and the local administration in the whole country in the summer of 1905.

Trouble had begun the preceding winter. Physicians across the province, already in the 1890s well known for their active involvement in political agitation, were subjected to increasing harassment for their part in the growing opposition movement. Police and priests launched an anti-intellectual campaign spreading rumours about zemstvo employees having been bribed by the Japanese and the English to overthrow Russia's war effort.[123] In several villages, as a result, physicians were beaten up when lecturing about precautionary cholera measures. Additionally, public hygiene lectures across the province were sometimes violently disrupted by the police. In March 1905, police officials interrupted a lecture taking place in one of the capital's theatres, invading the building and leaving many people in the audience injured.[124] Outraged, physicians raised the spectre of cholera riots:

> Concerted action supported by the administration has been directed against the intelligentsia. Rumours, slanders, sermons from the clergy have disturbed and demoralised the countryside and have prepared the soil – so recently infertile – for cholera riots, which now seem to be unavoidable. To physicians, students, and other workers going to the villages, their lives in peril, the concern is not about how to control the epidemic or teach the population how to fight it, nor in using one or another measures, but to eliminate the artificially created distrust of medical workers. Whoever has worked in

the countryside knows the strength and tenacity of popular prejudices. Artificial barriers have been created consciously and have destroyed the possibility of fighting epidemics.[125]

The 'Cholera Congress' in March 1905 further inflamed the situation. Following the congress's resolutions, many physicians in the province refused to co-operate with the new SECs. Governing authorities responded promptly. In the district of Balashov, where one-third of the medical posts were vacant due to the military call-up, governor Stolypin fired six doctors and assistants;[126] likewise, Saratov's city duma unceremoniously dismissed its public health official I.S. Veger.[127] And, as a further response to the physicians' increasing political activity, Saratov's sanitary society, which had played such an important role in addressing the city's most urgent sanitary and medical issues, was closed.[128] The crisis gained momentum in early June, when Balashov's zemstvo physicians threatened to resign on 15 July if conditions were not improved.[129] While Stolypin forecast further arrests and repression, both district and provincial zemstvo failed to protect their employees. Finally, on 21 July, six days after the passing of the deadline, the situation exploded. Physicians were attacked by a crowd of peasants during negotiations with zemstvo deputies in Balashov over the prevention of the strike. Suspecting the worst, Stolypin joined the scene with a troop of cossacks. He promised to escort the doctors safely to the station under the soldiers' protection. Ignoring their duties, however, the cossacks instead assisted the mob and began beating up those whom they were meant to protect. Some doctors were stoned, others were brought to the Balashov jail and Stolypin, failing to control the situation, was wounded. To top it off, he displayed his total inability to maintain social order by sanctioning the peasants' attacks: on 25 August he ordered the arrest of 36 physicians – versus only 22 rioters. Since physicians across the province threatened a collective strike if the arrest warrant was implemented, provincial self-governing bodies (district zemstva, the provincial zemstvo and Saratov's duma) appealed to St Petersburg to annul Stolypin's order. Yet St Petersburg's police chief sent 35 army doctors as blacklegs instead, and the Balashov doctors' strike thus continued throughout the autumn.

Thomas Fallows has interpreted the disturbances in Balashov as an important step clearing the way for Stolypin to become prime minister. By September 1905, Stolypin had 'acquired a reputation as a strong governor who (as in the Balashov pogrom) could confront revolutionaries while preventing any deaths'.[130] According to this interpretation, Balashov demonstrated the governor's ability to cope with mounting discontent and actually displayed an instance of the regime's strength. Yet if contextualised within the broader picture of unfolding political, social and medical events, the clash between the medical profession and Saratov's local government indeed epitomised the collapse of the government's credibility.[131] The Ministry of Internal Affairs, by decreeing the subordination of local governing institutions and medical professionals under state direction, had grossly misjudged the political crisis that was brewing. The 'Cholera Congress' had created a forum for physicians to question the regime's right to rule. At Balashov, four months later, physicians felt openly betrayed by the exhibition of power and repression in the face of a coming cholera epidemic. For the medical profession, and the *intelligentsia* in general, the state lost whatever moral authority it had left. Balashov was a direct call to sweep the autocracy from power.

In 1905, then, cholera had once again demonstrated its capacity to unleash civil disorder. Yet it remains an open question how an epidemic outbreak might have affected Saratov's (and Russia's) revolutionary situation. For luckily, and in full defiance of the extensive predictions and preparations made by local and national authorities that year, Russia could declare itself cholera-free both in 1905 and 1906.[132]

Luck ran out in 1907. Within the next four years, cholera, once again, took thousands of lives at the lower Volga. Although mortality rates caused by the *vibrio* were significantly lower throughout the sixth pandemic as compared with 1892, Saratov province still recorded 3,838 cholera deaths between 1907 and 1910. In 1910, the province counted more than 7,000 cholera cases, of which about 2,000 were fatal.[133] As regards the river's urban centres, the four major cities at the lower Volga, Astrakhan', Tsaritsyn, Saratov and Samara, reported 4,807 cholera victims between 1908 and 1910, 2,710 in 1910 alone.[134] Strikingly, as Table 5.2 demonstrates, Saratov as the biggest city at the lower Volga displayed a limited vulnerability to the germ.

Judging from these figures, Saratov's fight against the epidemic during the sixth pandemic must have been more efficient and successful than elsewhere along the river, in particular if compared with its immediate neighbours Samara, Tsaritsyn and Astrakhan'. Indeed, a combination of factors aligned, which enabled Saratov to exert better epidemic control. Most importantly, by 1907 Saratov's medical profession – at both the municipal and the provincial level – was simply better organised. A brief comparison with the neighbouring cities and provinces of Astrakhan', Tsaritsyn and Samara, which were all much more heavily hit by cholera between 1907 and 1910, shows that medical improvements made in Saratov in the wake of 1892 were uniquely successful along the lower Volga.

During the sixth pandemic, owing to the impressive development of zemstvo medicine in the 1890s, the differences between the administrative set-ups

Table 5.2 Cholera at the lower and middle Volga, 1908–1910

City	Inhabitants	1908	1909	1910	Total
Astrakhan'	142,441	816	30	789	1,635
Tsaritsyn	102,452	645	23	377	1,045
Saratov	217,418	139	6	376	521
Samara	95,461	261	176	1,169	1,606
Simbirsk	52,378	34	3	290	327
Kazan'	179,201	109	6	239	354
Nizhnii-Novgorod	101,144	480	154	459	1,093

S.A. Novosel'skii, "Kholera i vodosnabzheniie v gorodakh Rossii", *Vrachebnaia Gazeta*, 1912, no. 8 (26.2.), pp. 21–23. Kazan' and Nizhnii-Novgorod have been included just for comparative reasons.

in various localities of the empire made themselves dramatically felt.[135] In Astrakhan', for example, as late as 1907, public health administration continued to be directed by far-away St Petersburg. Since medical affairs were still under the auspices of the outdated charitable board (*prikaz obshchestvennogo zreniia*), the province and the city did not benefit from the medical and sanitary progress accompanying the rise of zemstvo medicine in other provinces during the 1890s. The Ministry of Internal Affairs had equipped Astrakhan's capital with the only laboratory at the whole lower Volga that could meet modern standards. Yet it failed to address the fundamental structural deficits in the provincial and urban medical infrastructure – despite the seaport's important strategic significance for the spread of diseases. Hopelessly underfunded by the capital, the province suffered from a tremendous shortage of medical personnel, and during the whole of the epidemic in 1907 no bacteriologist was available to make use of the spectacular laboratory.[136] In addition, the dependency on St Petersburg relieved local officials of any sense of responsibility in medical matters. The municipal duma seems to have cared even less about the cholera bacillus than it had in 1892. In late August 1907, one month after the official beginning of the epidemic in the city, the provincial sanitary commission realised that the city administrators had not yet employed any extra sanitary physicians as they had been instructed; likewise, they had not begun medical night shifts; disinfection procedures were not organised; no carts had been purchased for the transport of the sick; out of seven surgeries only three surgeries were functioning; and the population was not provided with boiled water.[137] As ever, Astrakhan' remained one of Russia's most devastated places by cholera during the sixth pandemic.

Unlike Astrakhan', Tsaritsyn, the southern urban centre of Saratov province, could benefit from a comparably well-established provincial health organisation. Yet in contrast to the city of Saratov, Tsaritsyn had no medical-sanitary commission which would have directed long-term medical improvements and represented local doctors in the pursuits of the municipality. As late as 1908, when cholera attacked Tsaritsyn for the second time in a row, the city was therefore still medically completely unprepared for the epidemic. The report on the cholera outbreak in Tsaritsyn records that 'the first half of the epidemic, which requires considerable work, passed in the complete absence of epidemic personnel, and the second, less important, with a considerable surplus of physicians'.[138]

Compounding the lack of medical organisation, Tsaritsyn suffered from excessive urban growth. Although only half the size of Saratov, Tsaritsyn was the fastest growing city at the lower Volga, rising from 56,000 inhabitants in 1897 to 132,000 in 1913.[139] During the 1890s, the city's activities notably in the trade in naphtha, fish and salt, had begun to surpass turnovers in Saratov.[140] In 1895, an estimated 50,000 peasant migrants arrived in Tsaritsyn in search of work.[141] This figure was not far short of the 60,000 journeying through Saratov. By the beginning of the next century, however, Tsaritsyn had overtaken its northern rival and become the second biggest centre for migrant workers at the lower Volga after Astrakhan'.[142] Rapid urban growth, sanitary neglect and inadequate medical organisation provided the most favourable conditions for the cholera bacillus:

Tsaritsyn became the primary focus of contagion in the whole of Saratov province in 1907 and especially 1908.[143]

Finally, in the zemstvo province of Samara, since 1897 the junction of three major traffic routes, the Siberian and Tashkent railway lines and the Volga, public health organisation in 1907 was in a shambles. Across the province, for a start, the epidemic of 1892 had not inspired the efforts in medical-sanitary improvements that it had in its neighbouring province to the south. Despite Samara's high vulnerability to diseases, healthcare was badly funded throughout the 1890s;[144] as late as 1910, the zemstvo employed only three physicians for the sanitary build-up of the province as compared with eight who were responsible for Saratov province;[145] Samara's zemstvo also failed to elaborate permanent regulations to steer its involvement in the fight against epidemics on a long-term basis.[146] To top it off, just as cholera was approaching in 1907 and 1908, the two most important provincial health institutions were actually shut down.[147] When M.M. Gran', the sanitary physician, resigned from his post in 1907 in response to permanent constraints by the zemstvo administration, the zemstvo left the position vacant; one year later, it closed down the sanitary office (*sanitary biuro*), formerly headed by Gran', allegedly for financial reasons. The highest public health administrative organ in the province and chief executive institution in the fight against epidemics was thus demolished. Not surprisingly, the municipal duma in Samara's capital proved unable to implement any short-term emergency measures devised by a hastily improvised provincial Sanitary Executive Commission.[148] Medical and administrative reports from 1907–1910 overwhelmingly testify to the ineptness of local provincial and municipal authorities in coping with the crisis and to the continuously dramatic deficits in the provision of medical care.[149] Compared with its neighbour in the south, Samara's defence against cholera still was an anarchic battle.

In Saratov, the advances made in public health organisation since 1892 had paid off. Although medical authorities in Astrakhan' and Samara repeatedly stressed their complete lack of readiness for a cholera attack, Saratov's provincial sanitary physician Nikolai Teziakov could confidently declare in 1907 that 'the cholera epidemic, which unexpectedly erupted this year, at first at the Volga and then in other regions of Russia, did not completely take our medical-sanitary organisation by surprise'.[150] Indeed, due to the medical-administrative structures in both Saratov province and city, important regulations and administrative innovations introduced by the Anti-Plague Commission in 1903 were actually circumvented. The Anti-Plague Commission declared city and province at high risk of cholera on 24 July 1907, two days after the germ had manifested itself in Astrakhan', and demanded sanitary vigilance from provincial and municipal authorities for marketplaces, shops, riverbanks, cesspits and any possible sources of infection.[151] Yet Saratov's medical experts, much more alert to the epidemic than 15 years before, were no longer waiting for official confirmation of the medical threat. With cholera in Samara since the beginning of July, municipal physicians had already pointed to the need for reinforcing medical staff on 16 July. Three days later, the first team of epidemic personnel began to inspect courts, marketplaces and other high-risk localities. In order to break the potential link between infectious ship passengers and the city in due time, an observation point at the river went into operation on 20 July.[152] Moreover, the municipal Sanitary Executive Commission was quickly established, since it could basically rely on the representatives of the already existing *sanitarnoe biuro*; it promptly responded with further measures to the announcement by the Anti-Plague Commission.[153] On 26 July, it elaborated a detailed anti-cholera plan, which was officially approved by the provincial Sanitary Executive Commission on 3 August.[154]

The new scheme demonstrated that local authorities had learned their lessons. In 1892, when cholera's aetiology was not as yet fully known, Saratov's authorities had responded to the disease with an emergency attempt to enforce rigorously an all-encompassing medical surveillance of the city, its residents and their everyday life. A coercive policy of preventive health compounded illiteracy, lack of contact between the population and the medical profession, and bitterly resented social inequalities. These strategies exacerbated the profound distrust towards official authorities and generated conditions that exploded when confronted with a relentless killer. Just like the national authorities, however, Saratov's officials abandoned these coercive experiments in the twentieth century. The new era of bacteriology offered other means to prevent a medical catastrophe. Instead of resorting to the police and army, Saratov's new anti-cholera campaign envisaged the use of laboratory diagnostic techniques and, especially in 1908 and 1910, the cooperation of the population.

Laboratory medicine had reached the province in 1898 at the latest, when the zemstvo established a Pasteur institute in the capital. Local doctors began to take courses in microscopy and bacteriological analysis with the most distinguished authorities in the field. In 1902, the chief physician of the zemstvo hospital in Saratov city, S.L. Raskovich, was sent to the Robert Koch Institute in Berlin where he studied recent medical techniques with Robert Koch himself.[155] By 1907, Saratov's zemstvo and municipal hospitals were each provided with a small laboratory – although Zlatogorov, used to conditions and facilities at the Institute of Experimental Medicine in St Petersburg, thought them to be poorly equipped and far from satisfactory.[156]

In contrast to 1892, scientific advances now allowed authorities to address specific targets, which were directly involved in the spread of the *vibrio*. In accordance with bacteriological principles, Saratov's authorities began their offensive with energetic efforts to detect any sufferers as early as possible before they could contaminate water or food and pass the disease to others.[157] An important new element in the cholera plan was the aim to identify suspect cholera cases as quickly as possible and to ensure a rapid medical response. Such a practice was essential in view of the difficulties in diagnosis which numerous physicians and feldshers were nevertheless still facing. Even more significantly, and in a major difference to 1892, it meant that official and medical authorities were not going to wait to begin medical intervention until a full diagnosis was established and confirmed by the Anti-Plague Commission.

Initial measures were aimed at reducing likely niches of ferment for the *vibrio*. The marketplaces and riverbanks posed a particular health hazard. The Sanitary

Executive Commission therefore ordered the regular cleaning of the marketplaces (*bazary*) and enforced the relocation of the vegetable market; ship companies were ordered to establish public latrines at the landing docks; the police inspected waste removal practices by private and municipal companies and arranged the cleansing of particularly insanitary places. To reduce the possibilities of infection through food and water, the commission further tried to ensure a healthier diet for the population. People were warned about the risks of eating fruits and vegetables; a set of instructions on the sale of food products was distributed across the city. In order to guarantee the provision of boiled water during the crisis extra tearooms were opened at the banks and the inspection of *kvas* stalls arranged. Finally, the commission stationed physicians on 24-hour duty in each of the town boroughs and instructed them to bring faecal samples of suspected cholera victims to the municipal hospital as quickly as possible for bacteriological analysis. To speed up communication, the surgeries were equipped with telephones linking them to the hospitals. All these precautions were in place three weeks before the official outbreak of cholera in Saratov city on 21 August. They found full support from the provincial zemstvo which, according to the still valid anti-cholera plan from 1904, was involved in the city's fight against the epidemic in so far as it concerned 'measures significant to the entire province'.[158]

Once the epidemic had begun, medical vigilance was enforced. The control of new cholera cases, too, was carried out under a new premise. In 1892, as was seen, the arbitrary and coercive manoeuvres to locate and isolate the sick had caused even more suffering and evoked stormy resistance among the population. Since they were carried out by the police, the raids on the sick and healthy had eroded municipal and medical authority by linking their efforts with the work of repression. For the next pandemic, local authorities had learned their lesson. Already during the anxious years of 1904–05, city and zemstvo had set up sanitation teams of a very different ilk.[159] Their most important aim, apart from the traditional tasks of detecting new cholera cases and inspecting and cleansing particularly insalubrious places, was to break down the barriers of distrust between the population and official and medical authorities. To this end, the new network of medical guardians consisted not only of duma deputies but also of ordinary local residents who volunteered to aid in fighting the germ. In conducting the surveillance, these recruits were instructed to avoid any use of force or coercion. Instead, they were to operate by virtue of persuasion and reason, explaining their work and its protective significance to the population. Municipal and provincial medical authorities further supported this approach. Making use of the increasing familiarisation of the population with medical institutions and authorities over the previous 15 years, they held public lectures informing the population about the disease, showing the mechanisms of microscopes and discussing how individuals could protect themselves.

According to the delegate of the Anti-Plague Commission in 1910, N.Ia. Shmidt, it was precisely these aspects of medical precaution and provision, which distinguished Saratov from other urban centres at the Volga and placed it at an advantage when combating cholera. The facilities to localise and isolate new cholera cases at an early stage, Shmidt stated:

are built up well and gladden the heart at every step. Six surgeries with six physicians serve the timely disclosure of cholera cases. Twenty-four-hour duties are established; the municipal hospital maintains carriages with hospital orderlies.[160]

In addition to the timely discovery of cholera cases, medical provision of the sick, too, had considerably improved. Shmidt stressed the spacious, bright and clean rooms in the hospitals. Medical personnel in the hospitals were also sufficient. Disinfection procedures were carried out by three disinfection teams under the supervision of special physicians.[161] In addition, patients were no longer dragged into the hospital against their will. The disinfection of people's houses and belongings was only undertaken with the consent of the patient's relatives and conducted under the professional guidance of local doctors.

These principles presented a crucial qualitative novelty in the anti-cholera campaign as compared to that of 1892 and, indeed, in any previous epidemic. The ending of coercive policies ruled out the decisive factor that had fostered public anxiety and triggered the tumultuous violence in 1892. Reflecting the general picture in Russia between 1907 and 1910, the social impact of the epidemic in Saratov city and across the province was therefore far less disruptive than in 1892. Scattered incidents of poisoning phobia and assaults on doctors were still reported from the surrounding villages, but these compared neither in scale nor ferocity to the cataclysms of 1892 and did not resonate through the whole country. During the sixth pandemic, Saratov's doctors reported most often on the positive change in attitude of the population towards the medical profession.[162] Many people voluntarily called on medical help during the early stage of the disease; they were aware (not least because of the preceding epidemics) of potential means of infection and followed medical advice such as avoiding unboiled water or consuming raw vegetables; relatives of sufferers asked for disinfection and generally did not resist the isolation of the sick. As a result of both medical precautionary measures and better medical provision, Saratov reported a much lower level of mortality in the sixth pandemic as compared with the other cities at the lower Volga. As will be seen, the measures taken by local authorities were still far from being satisfactory. In marked contrast to 1892, however, the city had managed to keep the germ under control.

And yet, Saratov was still not free from cholera. Despite lowered mortality figures, the disease persisted throughout five years. Local and national medical and public health experts had no illusions about the circumstances that allowed the disease to prevail over the physicians' efforts. Medical provision notwithstanding, Saratov did not differ from any other Volga city in that serious sanitary deficiencies remained to be addressed. The delegates of the Anti-Plague Commission who visited Saratov in each epidemic year continually complained about the city's inadequate water supply, its defective sewer system, as well as the insufficiency of sanitary control at important public places such as markets, hotels, bath-houses or the banks. 'A city of 200,000 inhabitants has no sewage system,' Zlatogorov fiercely declared on returning from Saratov in 1907 and continued:

all refuse is released directly into the Volga and the water at the banks is decorated with blood. Public latrines are primitively built and in insufficient number. There is a disgusting lodging house for the migrant workers that is so overfilled with bedbugs that the migrants take refuge from it.[163]

Official reports and duma minutes lay bare an abundance of old perils and practices. Bathing and washing, unless it took place in the Volga, was a rare luxury; people continued to rid themselves of all kinds of waste, including their excrement, on the open streets and courtyards; sanitary regulations were comprehensively ignored and the vast majority of the population was living on a deficient diet, consuming 'foul products, which are not adequately controlled, which are contained in dirty stalls and the unboiled Volga water, which is seriously contaminated'.[164]

Saratov's municipal duma aggravated the sanitary mayhem. Unlike the provincial zemstvo administration, which conducted a comprehensive cholera campaign in good time, the duma followed old dilatory procedures and did little to support the physicians' medical efforts to protect Saratov's residents. The visiting bacteriologist S.I. Zlatogorov wondered at the mildness of Saratov's cholera outbreak in 1907 in view of the 'complete unpreparedness of the city for the fight against cholera and the obviously indifferent attitude of municipal organs towards a proper organisation of anti-cholera measures'.[165] In fact, the cholera announcement coming from the highest state authorities on 24 July in 1907 left Saratov's city fathers unaffected. For several weeks the city duma lapsed into inaction. Even when the germ had already invaded provincial territory at Dubovka on 6 August, and even when it was reported from Tsaritsyn four days later, the municipality did not show any sign of urgency. Municipal authorities postponed action until the *vibrio* had manifested itself in the city and the cholera threat was imminent. Only on 22 August did the duma discuss the full scheme devised by the municipal Sanitary Executive Commission a month before.[166] This was unfortunate, for the first measures taken by the Sanitary Executive Commission in July could not involve more than tentative preparations. While the timely organisation of preventive measures remained incomplete, therefore, and far from satisfactory, the preparation of therapeutic measures, which was the exclusive responsibility of the municipalities, began far too late.[167] In fact, the duma was only set in motion by the arrival of Zlatogorov, the delegate of the Anti-Plague Commission in early September 1907.

In addition to being late, Saratov's municipality sacrificed concerns about public health to worries about economic interests and public order. A constant theme throughout the decade, and the most urgent target of the municipal Sanitary Executive Commission and the physicians, was the water in the bay. Already in 1903, bacteriological investigations of the bay had revealed that the severely polluted Tarkhanka provided the most favourable environment for bacterial growth. It posed a particular threat to the whole city not only because local residents used the water in the boatyard for drinking, washing and other household necessities; more alarmingly, the municipal water pipe also began here. To prevent a major calamity, it was essential to eliminate the *vibrio* before it could enter the water pipe and perpetuate the disease throughout Saratov. The most effective solution to the problem, as official authorities openly acknowledged, would have been to relocate the pipes from the boatyard to the Volga itself.[168] However, such a possibility was generally regarded as unrealistic since the city would not be able to raise the colossal funds needed for the operation. Alternatively, the duma there-fore considered the removal of the boats and the closure of the boatyard – a measure which would have eradicated the major source of pollution. Yet even rumours about this idea caused some ship companies to avoid Saratov's port entirely and thus threatened the urban economy with considerable losses.[169] Moreover, an idle boatyard would have risked unemployment for many residents, who were living from all sorts of business brought about by the convoy. Anxiously recalling the events of 1892, the duma delegates reasoned that the closure of the boatyard might escalate into social unrest.[170] This idea, too, was therefore quickly dismissed. Eventually, the Sanitary Executive Commission issued a decree which arranged a compromise: it ordered the ships in the boatyard to be removed so that the opening of the water pipe was not blocked.[171] Within one week, bacteriological analyses revealed that the water of the Tarkhanka had become unrecognisable. Bacterial colonies were significantly reduced and the *vibrio cholerae* had disappeared completely. Still, Saratov's entrepreneurs expressed their indignation at the decision by submitting a complaint to the Minister of Ways and Communications, who was then travelling through the city.[172] It was the tardiness of Saratov's city duma to which Zlatogorov referred when criticising the city's unpreparedness for the epidemic. In his report to the Anti-Plague Commission, he was compelled to point out that 'if there had not been the zemstvo, then many cities would have had no tearooms, and insufficient medical help. [. . .] Concluding our observations, we have to say that the fight against the current epidemic in the cities of Saratov province was conducted completely without order and far from rationally.'[173]

Conclusion

Saratov encountered the sixth cholera pandemic under completely new scientific and administrative foundations. Following the revised national strategy to combat the disease, local authorities dismissed the deployment of military and police forces and instead conducted a campaign based on modern scientific principles. The more circumspect public health policy should be regarded as the fundamental change in the city's renewed anti-cholera scheme. It presented the chief factor preventing the disruptive societal turbulence which had accompanied Saratov's cholera epidemic in 1892 and which had resonated along the Volga up to St Petersburg.

Significant improvements in public health provision and medical care, follow-ing the epidemic of 1892, complemented the new approach. Among the lower Volga cities, Saratov was medically best prepared to cope with the disease. Above all, the medical profession in both city and province was much better organised and more alert to an outbreak of cholera than was the case in other urban centres along the river. Local physicians responded to the cholera threat before it was declared by the Anti-Plague Commission. In marked contrast to 1892, they followed a coherent strategy which placed emphasis on comprehensive preventive measures. Arrangements to inform the residents about the disease and to guarantee the immediate reporting of cholera cases were made weeks before the epidemic's arrival. In addition to greater medical vigilance and better diagnostic abilities, Saratov's physicians, moreover, benefited from people's increased familiarity with medical care.

Yet despite these achievements, cholera once again became a catalyst for political tensions. If in 1892 the physicians' activity had been obstructed by popular distrust and rebellion, in the early twentieth century, it was the official policies as conducted by state authorities in both St Petersburg and Saratov which ran counter to the physicians' efforts. The new administrative framework for anti-epidemic combat was nowhere more unacceptable than in Saratov, where the medical profession, when compared with other provinces, had gained a much higher professional and political standing during the 1890s. It was here, therefore, that medical experts clashed headfirst with official state authority and openly challenged the regime's legitimacy.

At the same time, the conflict at Balashov most clearly exposed the major obstacle preventing the elimination of cholera in Saratov during subsequent years: having been accustomed to more decision-making power after 1892, vested with scientific authority and confronted with a semi-centralised medical-administrative framework, the position of medical experts within duma, zemstvo, Anti-Plague Commission and state ministries in 1905 was, in fact, more complex and tense than it had been in 1892.

Conclusion: Saratov, cholera and the empire

Russia's cholera history had no counterpart in the European history of the disease. The *vibrio cholerae* mercilessly blanketed the tsarist empire alone at a time when the authorities in every nation on the European continent had long since triumphed over the disease. In western Europe, only Hamburg and Naples still suffered major cholera outbreaks as late as 1892 and 1910–11. Autocratic Russia therefore presents a new perspective on the comparative history of Asiatic cholera. Saratov's story of the epidemic in the period 1892–1910 makes a novel study in exploring the link between the history of cholera and the broader concerns of its political, social, cultural and urban history in an autocratic state.

The *vibrio*'s fifth visitation to Russia, which forms the centre-piece of this study, was more virulent than any previous outbreak in the century. Although the dramatic course of the outbreak in 1892 evoked the history of the cholera in 1830–31 among contemporaries, the significance of Russia's fifth and sixth pandemics differed considerably from the country's first encounter with the disease. The impact of cholera on Saratov between 1892 and 1910 was more severe than when cholera had first arrived in the city in 1831. The medical challenge of 1892 was an important transformative event and, moreover, became and enduring concern for the city, its administrators and its residents in the early twentieth century. A crucial factor which explains both the shock of the disease in 1892 and the consequences was the timing of the onslaught. Until mid-century, Russia's dramatic cholera experiences had very much conformed to the general European pattern. Yet in contrast to most parts of western Europe, which had been particularly vulnerable to the epidemic when it was still little known, Russia was ravaged by the most virulent cholera attack of the nineteenth century when the disease had become preventable. Although the disease was not yet fully under-stood, the link between poor sanitation, overcrowded living conditions, poverty and the *vibrio* was well established in western European countries, especially Britain.

Yet timing involved more than a medical dimension. The tsarist authorities, after all, had been fully aware of foreign experiences with the disease and the medical debates surrounding it since cholera's first arrival on European soil. By 1892, however, the epidemic arrived at a crucial point in Russian history. By the early 1890s, the process of political, social, economic and cultural modernisation, triggered by the Crimean War, was well under way. The transformation of the economic and social order was irreversible. In large parts of European Russia, local institutions of self-government, which were supposed to take over the responsibility for public health, had been in place for 20 years. And, continued state oppression notwithstanding, the institutional innovations made at Russian universities during the Reform Era, most importantly the introduction of laboratory science, provided fertile ground for appropriating and developing modern scientific medicine. True, Russia had been affected by cholera in 1871–72. At that time, however, the reforms were too recent to be challenged by the disease. In 1892, by contrast, cholera presented a crucial test to the new order established with the Great Reforms. The official newspaper in the capital city, *Sankt-Peterburgskie Vedomosti*, established the link when it reported the cholera riots that year:

> Neither the Great Reforms of the last tsar, nor the increasing schools have achieved their civilising mission. There is no enlightenment. Cultural foundations are still not deeply embedded. This 'symptom of the time' commands attention, whether you want it or not, and indicates into which direction state and public concerns have to be persistently steered.[1]

This complaint touched upon some much larger issues. By the early 1890s, medical opinion agreed that cholera was a social disease caused by economic hardship and social inequality. The fact that the epidemic could claim more than 200,000 victims at such a late date blatantly revealed that the promises of progress and social improvement had not been fulfilled. On the contrary, the cholera riots that overwhelmed Saratov and the lower Volga showed that social conflict and economic misery had reached an explosive stage. By exacerbating their despair at social injustice and economic misery, cholera became a tool for Saratov's residents to express their discontent and dissatisfaction with the governing authorities. The violence that erupted in the streets of Saratov, Astrakhan' and Tsaritsyn demonstrated the alienation of large parts of the population from governmental institutions, which had not only created the conditions for the epidemic's spread, but also demonstrated little respect for civil liberties in handling the cholera. Ultimately, the brutal repression of the riots by means of military force suggested that the general breakdown of public order in the lower Volga region posed a serious threat to local and national statecraft while at the same time eroding governmental authority even further.

It is these multiple aspects to the political challenge presented by the medical tragedy that explain the significance of Saratov's cholera outbreak in 1892, and the tremendous response it evoked among national and local governing officials, medical experts and the educated public. Accordingly, cholera's most important legacy was political. As has been seen, the efforts to improve Saratov's sanitary conditions, such as improvements to the sewage system and water supply, were short lived or, in the case of housing reform, never even begun. A major reason for the city's continuous sanitary disrepair was the administrative and legislative framework within which municipal policies were conducted. By delegating responsibility and financial expenses for the nation's health to local authorities, the autocratic government ensured that the civilian population was medically neglected. Throughout the period under consideration, Saratov, like most other Russian cities, was too much in debt and badly administered to assume the task. Given these conditions, as Saratov's physicians recognised very well, the application of modern laboratory medicine as embraced in St Petersburg made little sense. The introduction of bacteriology could not effectively alleviate the city's health problems. They required instead a fundamental renewal of the social and urban infrastructure.

Politically, however, the epidemic did mark a turning point and effected an important transformation. In conjunction with the famine, the cholera in 1892 activated the radical *intelligentsia*, the liberal opposition movement and the zemstvo employees. New legislation encouraged individual initiative in the field of philanthropic work and thus opened new spheres of social commitment in the autocratic state. Similarly, the reforms in public health administration in the immediate aftermath of the epidemic endowed the medical profession with hitherto unknown authority. Although its new influence was constantly under threat, physicians nevertheless now had an active voice in public policy. While economic and social transformations took place in the 1890s, Saratov's doctors enhanced their professional status and social prestige. By the time of the social unrest brewing at the beginning of the twentieth century, they were fully prepared to defend their interests and positions. Within a decade, and in crucial difference from 1892, Saratov's doctors would not only demand more professional rights but join the call for a change in the constitution itself.

It was only fitting that cholera, which crystallised the ongoing conflicts between central and local governments, between the state and medical science, between the population and official authorities, once again posed a political challenge upon its return in 1904. Strikingly, the scientific advances that mitigated the former tensions between the physicians and the population now shifted the main source of conflict to the physicians and the state. In a complete reversal of its 1892 strategies, the government modernised its anti-epidemic policies in 1903, but at the same time it excluded medical experts from any decision-making processes. To Saratov's medical professionals, as to the country's physicians at large, these new policies signified a betrayal and eroded the legitimacy of the tsarist regime. The interweaving of medical interests with political pursuits destroyed their professional cooperation during the revolution of 1905–06. However, Saratov's medical infrastructure was still better organised than in most other cities in the country. Even so, medical achievements had limited success when political influence and rights were granted only to a minority and burning social issues remained unaddressed. In early-twentieth-century Saratov, cholera returned year after year. The First World War, eventually, brought the disease back under incomparably more difficult and chaotic conditions.

The history of cholera in Saratov between 1892 and 1910 demonstrates not only the strains inherent in Russia's process of modernisation. It also illuminates the complexity of converting to the modern cause. As AIDS and SARS have reminded us, the powers of modern science are limited and depend on the social and political context in which they occur. In late-imperial Russia, the achievements of bacteriology could not eradicate cholera. The control of the disease required a profound change of the country's social and political network. As it turned out, it was only the political, social, administrative and intellectual upheaval of 1917 which opened the doors to eliminating the disease once and for all.

Notes

Introduction

1 Thus the fall of the Duvalier regime in Haiti in 1986 has been claimed to be caused by AIDS. Richard J. Evans, "Epidemics and Revolutions: Cholera in Nineteenth-Century Europe", *Past and Present*, no. 120 (August 1988), pp. 123–146, here: p. 123. For the role of epidemics and diseases in the history of civilisations, see William H. McNeill, *Plagues and Peoples* (Oxford, 1977).

2 For a general introduction see Sheldon Watts, *Epidemics and History: Disease, Power and Imperialism* (New Haven, 1997).

3 Paul Slack, *The Impact of Plague in Tudor and Stuart England* (London, 1985); John T. Alexander, *Bubonic Plague in Early Modern Russia: Public Health and Urban Disaster* (Baltimore, 1980); Hans Heilbronner, "The Russian Plague of 1878–79", *Slavic Review*, 1963, pp. 89–112; Arcadius Kahan, "Social Aspects of the Plague Epidemics in 18th-century Russia", *Economic Development and Cultural Change* 27 (1979), pp. 255–266.

4 Cholera's first arrival in Astrakhan' is analysed in detail by Roderick E. McGrew, *Russia and the Cholera, 1823–1832* (Madison, 1965), esp. chap. 1.

5 R. Pollitzer, *Cholera* (Geneva, 1959); Richard J. Evans, "Epidemics and Revolutions", p. 124.

6 Ibid., p. 125.

7 Asa Briggs, "Cholera and Society in the Nineteenth Century", *Past and Present*, 19 (August 1961), pp. 76–96, here: p. 96.

8 Louis Chevalier (ed.), *Le Choléra: la première épidémie du xixe siècle* (Paris, 1958), p. xv.

9 McGrew, *Russia and the Cholera*, p. 3.

10 Charles Rosenberg, *The Cholera Years: The United States in 1832, 1849 and 1866* (Chicago, 1962; 2nd edn., with new afterword, 1987); Charles Rosenberg, "Cholera in Nineteenth Century Europe: A Tool for Social and Economic Analysis", *Comparative Studies in Sociology and History*, vol. 8 (1956–6), pp. 452–463.

11 Margaret Pelling, *Cholera, Fever and English Medicine, 1825–1865* (Oxford, 1978), p. 5.

12 Richard J. Evans, *Death in Hamburg. Society and Politics in the Cholera Years, 1830–1910* (Oxford, 1987); Frank M. Snowden, *Naples in the Time of Cholera, 1884–1911* (Cambridge, 1995).

13 See, for instance, the interpretation by Orlando Figes, *A People's Tragedy. The Russian Revolution 1891–1924* (London, 1996), esp. pp. 157–164; Geoffrey Hosking, *Russia. People and Empire* (Cambridge, MA., 1997), esp. pp. 398–399; Nancy M. Frieden, *Russian Physicians in an Era of Reform and Revolution, 1856–1905* (Princeton, 1981), esp. p. 161; see also the catalyst role ascribed to the famine and the cholera by Adele Lindenmeyr, *Poverty is not a Vice. Charity, Society, and the State in Imperial Russia* (Princeton, 1996).

14 Lindenmeyr, *Poverty is not a Vice*; Frieden, *Russian Physicians*.
15 Frieden, *Russian Physicians*, esp. pp. 158–160; also her "Physicians in Pre-Revolutionary Russia: Professionals or Servants of the State", *BHM*, vol. 49 (1975), pp. 20–29; John F. Hutchinson, "Society, Corporation or Union? Russian Physicians and the Struggle for Professional Unity (1890–1913)", *JfGO*, vol. 30 (1982), pp. 37–53.
16 The major Soviet works on late imperial Russian medicine are Ivan D. Strashun, *Russkaia obshchestvennaia meditsina v period mezhdu dvumia revoliutsiami 1907–1917 gg.* (Moscow, 1964); Petr E. Zabliudovskii, *Istoriia otechestvennoi meditsiny, chast' 1, period do 1917 goda* (Moscow, 1960); M.M. Levit, *Stanovleniie obshchestvennoi meditsiny v Rossii* (Moscow, 1974); E.I. Lotova, *Russkaia intelligentsiia i voprosy obshchestvennoi gigieny: Pervoe gigienicheskoe obshchestvo v Rossii* (Moscow, 1970).
17 See, for instance, Henry E. Sigerist, *Socialized Medicine in Soviet Russia* (New York, 1928); idem, *Medicine and Health in the Soviet Union* (Cambridge, Mass., 1957); Susan Gross Solomon, John F. Hutchinson (eds), *Health and Society in Revolutionary Russia* (Bloomington, 1990); and in particular Paula Michaels, *Curative Powers: Medicine and Empire in Stalin's Central Asia* (London, 2003).
18 A few years earlier, the first outbreak had also received attention in an article by M.V. Netchkina, K.V. Sivkov, Al. Sidorov, "La Russie", Louis Chevalier (ed.), *Le Choléra. La première épidémie du XIXe siècle* (La Roche-sur-Yon, 1958), pp. 143–155.
19 Nancy M. Frieden, "The Russian Cholera Epidemic, 1892–93, and Medical Professionalisation", *Journal of Social History*, 10 (1977), pp. 538–559; John F. Hutchinson, "Tsarist Russia and the Bacteriological Revolution", *Journal of the History of Medicine and Allied Sciences*, vol. 40 (1985), pp. 420–439.
20 Richard G. Robbins, *Famine in Russia, 1891–1892* (New York, 1975).
21 As Frank Snowden has pointed out, the history of cholera in the countryside still needs to be written. Russia would certainly provide a valuable case study for such claim.
22 See, for example, S. Frederick Starr, *Decentralization and Self-Government in Russia, 1830–1870* (Princeton, 1972); George L. Yaney, *The Systematization of Russian Government: Social Evolution in the Domestic Administration of Imperial Russia, 1711–1905* (Urbana, 1973); Terence Emmons, Wayne S. Vucinich (eds), *The Zemstvo in Russia. An Experiment in Local Self-Government* (Cambridge, 1982); Ben Eklof, *Russian Peasant Schools: Officialdom, Village Culture, and Popular Pedagogy* (Berkeley, 1986); Richard Robbins, *The Tsar's Viceroys. Russian Provincial Governors in the Last Years of the Empire* (Ithaca, 1987); Lindenmeyr, *Poverty is not a Vice*. Frieden, *Russian Physicians*.
23 Frieden, *Russian Physicians*, esp. chap. 12; John F. Hutchinson, *Politics and Public Health in Revolutionary Russia, 1890–1918* (Baltimore, 1990); see also Samuel C. Ramer, "The Zemstvo and Public Health", Emmons, Vucinich (eds), *The Zemstvo in Russia*, chap. 8.
24 An exception is Theodore H. Friedgut, "Labor Violence and Regime Brutality in Tsarist Russia: The Iuzovka Cholera Riots of 1892", *Slavic Review* (1988), pp. 245–265. However, Friedgut's article focuses mainly on the city's labour movement and not on its cholera history.
25 Louise McReynolds, "Urbanism as a Way of Russian Life", *Journal of Urban History*, vol. 20, no. 2 (February 1994), pp. 240–251.
26 Michael J. Hittle, *The Service City: State and Townsmen in Russia, 1600–1800* (Cambridge, MA, 1979). For the administrative status of Russia's cities see also V.A. Nardova, *Samoderzhavie i gorodskie dumy v Rossii v kontse XIX-nachale XX veka* (St Petersburg, 1994) and Boris Mironov, "Bureaucratic- or Self-Government: The Early Nineteenth Century Russian City", *Slavic Review*, 52, no. 2 (summer 1983), pp. 233–255. See also the case studies by Michael F. Hamm, "Khar'kov's Progressive Duma, 1910–1914: A Study in Russian Municipal Reform", *Slavic Review*, 40, no. 1 (March 1981), pp. 17–36 and James Bater, "Some Dimensions of Urbanization and the Response of Municipal Government: Moscow and St Petersburg", *Russian History*, 5, pt. 2 (1978), pp. 46–63.

27 William Blackwell, "Modernization and Urbanization in Russia: A Comparative View", in Michael F. Hamm (ed.), *The City in Russian History* (Lexington, 1976), pp. 291–330, here: p. 303.
28 For instances see Daniel Brower, *The Russian City between Tradition and Modernity, 1850–1900* (Berkeley, 1990); Louise McReynolds, *The News under Russia's Old Regime: The Development of a Mass Circulation Press* (Princeton, 1991); Alexander J. Rieber, *Merchants and Entrepreneurs in Imperial Russia* (Chapel Hill, 1982); Laura Engelstein, *The Keys to Happiness. Sex and the Search for Modernity in Fin-de-Siècle Russia* (Ithaca, 1992). For further studies see the reference material in the bibliography.
29 In two essay collections Michael Hamm has begun to redress the imbalance: Michael F. Hamm (ed.), *The City in Russian History* (Lexington, 1976) and his *The City in Late Imperial Russia* (Bloomington, 1986).
30 See in particular the works by Donald Raleigh, *Revolution on the Volga: 1917 in Saratov* (Ithaca, 1976); idem, *Experiencing Russia's Civil War: Politics, Society and Revolutionary Culture in Saratov, 1917–1922* (Princeton, 2002) and *A Russian Civil War Diary: Alexis Babine in Saratov, 1917–1922* (Durham, 1988); also Jonathan Sanders, "Lessons from the Periphery: Saratov, January 1905", *Slavic Review*, no. 2 (1987), pp. 229–244, Rex A. Wade, Scott J. Seregny (eds), *Politics and Society in Provincial Russia: Saratov, 1590–1917* (Ohio, 1989).
31 In particular historical scholarship of the Cold War era highlighted the differences. The classic work is Alexander Gerschenkron's, *Economic Backwardness in Historical Perspective* (Cambridge, MA, 1962); also Theodor von Laue, *Why Lenin? Why Stalin?* (Philadelpia, 1964); see also, more recently, Daniel Chirot (ed.), *The Origins of Backwardness in Eastern Europe* (Berkeley, 1989). In Chirot's volume, the spread of modernity stopped around the Elbe, Oder, or Vistula.
32 This view was also the starting point of the essay collection edited by Edith W. Clowes, Samuel D. Kassow, and James L. West, *Between Tsar and People*; see also Harley D. Balzer (ed.), *Russia's Missing Middle Class* (New York, 1996).
33 David L. Hoffmann, Yanni Kotsonis, *Russian Modernity. Politics, Knowledge, Practices* (New York, 2000); also Jane Burbank, David L. Ransel, *Imperial Russia. New Histories for the Empire* (Bloomington, 1998).
34 For examples from other non-European countries see John Z. Browers, *When the Twain Meet: The Rise of Western Medicine in Japan* (Baltimore, 1980); Ming-chang Lo, *Doctors within Borders: Professions, Ethnicity and Modernity in Colonial Taiwan* (Berkeley, 2003); Annette H.K. Son, "Modernization of Medical Care in Korea (1876–1990)", *Social Science and Medicine*, vol. 49, no. 4 (1999), pp. 543–550; see also Paula Michaels, *Curative Powers: Medicine and Empire in Stalin's Central Asia* (London, 2003).
35 Before the 1870s, the province constituted the basic unit of statistical investigations. For basic information on the development of statistics in Russia see I. Miklashevskii, "Statistika", Brokgauz-Efron, pp. 497–98; also S. Frederick Starr, *Decentralization and Self-Government in Russia, 1830–1870* (Princeton, 1972), p. 98. For local medical statistics, see the article by G. Khlopin and F. Erisman, "Meditsina i narodnoe zdravie", Brokgauz-Efron, vol. 27 (1899), pp. 214–227. The history of Saratov's provincial statistics is brilliantly analysed in Martine Mespoulet, "Statisticiens des *Zemstva*. Formation d'une nouvelle profession intellectuelle en Russie dans la période prérévolutionnaire (1880–1917). Le cas de Saratov", *Cahiers du Monde Russe*, vol. 40, no. 4, (Oct.–Dec. 1999), pp. 573–623.

1 Cholera in Russia

1 Numbers can only be an estimate at best and were probably higher. My figures are from Reiner Olzscha, "Die Epidemiologie und Epidemiographie der Cholera in Russland. Ein Beitrag zur Geomedizin", *Zeitschrift fuer Hygiene und Infektionskrankheiten*,

vol. 121, no. 1 (Berlin, 1939), pp. 1–26, esp. p. 10. According to Olzscha the exact number of deaths from cholera for the period from 1823 to 1914 was 2,145,838.

2 See introduction pp. 6–7.

3 For descriptions of the cholera routes in the various pandemics see R. Pollitzer, *Cholera* (Geneva, 1959). The most thorough and detailed description of the cholera germ along traditional camel caravans through Persia during the first pandemic can be found in the first Russian medical report on the disease by Dr. J. Reman, "Poiavleniie vostochnoi kholery na Sredizemnom i Kaspiiskom More", *Voenno-Meditsinskii Zhurnal*, chast' III, no. 1 (1824), pp. 3–14; chast' III, no. 2 (1824), pp. 159–195. See also McGrew, *Russia and the Cholera*, pp. 18–25. A comprehensive historical analysis of the first cholera outbreak in Astrakhan' is offered by Barbara Dettke, *Die asiatische Hydra. Die Cholera von 1830/31 in Berlin und den preussischen Provinzen Posen, Preussen und Schlesien* (Berlin, New York 1995), pp. 26–35.

4 "Nastavlenie o lechenii bolezni, nazyvaemoi kholera (Cholera morbus), sostavlennoe Meditsinskim Sovetom", *Voenno-meditsinskii zhurnal*, vol. III, no. 2 (1824), pp. 177–193.

5 For a thorough account of Russia's first anti-cholera institution see McGrew, *Russia and the Cholera*, pp. 23–25.

6 Reman, "Poiavlenie vostochnoi kholery", *Voenno-meditsinskii zhurnal*, vol. III, no. 2 (1824), pp. 169–177. Also M.K. Shchepot'ev, *Chumnye i kholernye epidemii v Astrakhan'skoi gubernii* (Kazan', 1884), p. 4.

7 Reman, "Poiavlenie vostochnoi kholery", *Voenno-meditsinskii zhurnal*, in particular vol. III, no. 2 (1824), pp. 159–193. A brief summary of Reman's article in English is provided in the *Edinburgh Medical and Surgical Journal*, XXIII, (1825), Jan.–April, pp. 432–435; also Dettke, *Die Asiatische Hydra*, p. 31. Local efforts to protect Astrakhan's residents also played an eminent role in the outbreak in 1830; see McGrew, *Russia and the Cholera*, p. 53.

8 Dettke, *Die asiatische Hydra*, p. 3.

9 Shchepot'ev, *Chumnye i kholernye epidemii*, p. 3; Arkhangel'skii, *Kholernye epidemii v Evropeiskoi Rossii*, p. 104.

10 For medical debates and discussions raised by Orenburg's first cholera outbreak see further down, p. 29–30. A thorough analysis of the medical dimensions of the outburst is offered by McGrew, *Russia and the Cholera*, pp. 43–49.

11 For Orenburg's cholera outbreak in 1829 see McGrew, *Russia and the Cholera*, pp. 41–49 and also Dettke, *Die asiatische Hydra*, pp. 35–38; the standard first-hand account is Jeremias Lichtenstaedt, *Cholera in Russland, 1829–1830*, pp. 110–117. Lichtenstaedt's work is translated into English in the *Supplement to the Edinburgh Medical and Surgical Review* (Edinburgh, 1832), pp. x–xiii.

12 Numbers from Pavlovskii, *Kholernye gody v Rossii*, p. 33. Figures for Orenburg's first cholera outbreak vary considerably. In the city of Orenburg, according to Dettke, 1,135 people were infected and 208 died. Dettke, *Die asiatische Hydra*, p. 37.

13 That figures of cholera cases and deaths do not sufficiently explain the social impact and historical significance of an epidemic is thoroughly discussed by Snowden, *Naples in the Time of Cholera*, p. 178. For the course of the cholera in Orenburg see McGrew, *Russia and the Cholera*, pp. 41–49.

14 Theodor Schiemann, *Geschichte Russlands unter Kaiser Nikolaus I.*, Bd. 3: *Kaiser Nikolaus im Kampf mit Polen und im Gegensatz zu England und Frankreich. 1830–1840* (Berlin 1913), p. 1–31. Chapter II gives a good overview of the significance of the cholera and the Polish Revolution for Russian political decision-making in 1830. Dettke, *Die asiatische Hydra*, pp. 39–42.

15 Numbers for the first cholera epidemic in the Caucasus are difficult to come by. According to Pavlovskii, the disease afflicted 21,000 people in the whole of the Caucasus, of whom 11,000 died. Dettke mentions the eyewitness account of the French Consul Gamba, who estimates the number of cholera victims in Tiflis to be up to 5,000. However, according to

Dettke it is more likely that 2,222 people fell ill and 1,575 died in the city. Pavlovskii, *Kholernye gody v Rossii*, p. 2.; Dettke, *Die asiatische Hydra*, pp. 42–43. For the cholera outbreak in Tiflis see also McGrew, *Russia and the Cholera*, p. 53–54.

16 Cholera was reported from Gurev on 26 July. A small village of 1,124 residents Gurev, reported 120 cholera cases, 42 of which were fatal. Arkhangel'skii, *Kholernye epidemii v Evropeiskoi Rossii*, p. 104.

17 Ibid., pp. 103–104.

18 Pavlovskii, *Kholernye gody v Rossii*, p. 33. According to McGrew, 3,633 cholera cases and 2,935 deaths were reported from Astrakhan', see McGrew, *Russia and the Cholera*, p. 52.

19 For the symptoms of cholera see the description by Snowden, *Naples in the Time of Cholera*, pp. 112–121; also Evans, *Death in Hamburg*, p. 227; McGrew, *Russia in the Time of Cholera*, pp. 21–22.

20 For the collapse of local administration in Astrakhan', see McGrew, *Russia and the Cholera*, pp. 52–53. See also H. Haurowiz, *Topographisch-medicinische Beobachtungen über den südlichen Theil des Saratowschen Gouvernements* (St Petersburg, 1836), p. 204.

21 McGrew, *Russia and the Cholera*, p. 55. According to Haurowiz the first cholera case had been reported in Tsaritsyn already on 1 August. Haurowiz, *Topographisch-medicinische Beobachtungen*, p. 205.

22 Haurowiz, *Topographisch-medicinische Beobachtungen*, p. 208.

23 Based on English reports on the epidemic in India, contagiousness had originally been denied in 1819 in the first documents on cholera. See McGrew, *Russia and the Cholera*, p. 22.

24 For the Council's first instructions see Reman, "Poiavlenie vostochnoi kholery", *Voenno-meditsinskii zhurnal*, vol. III, no. 2 (1824), esp. pp. 138–193.

25 Ibid., pp. 189–190.

26 McGrew, *Russia and the Cholera*, p. 43–45. For contemporary western European concepts of the disease see R.J. Morris, *Cholera, 1832: The Social Response to an Epidemic*, (London, 1976), pp. 28–29. Excellent discussions about early western European explanations of cause, contagiousness and cure of cholera in relation to later cholera theories are offered by Evans, *Death in Hamburg*, pp. 336–341 and by Snowden, *Naples in the Time of Cholera*, especially pp. 121–129.

27 McGrew, *Russia and the Cholera*, p. 44. See also from the first pandemic the classic report by Dr. Lichtenstädt, "Fragmente aus einer ausführlichen zur Fortsetzung meiner Schriften über die asiatische cholera in Russland bestimmten Abhandlung von Prof. Dr. Lichtenstädt", *Mittheilungen über die Cholera-Epidemic zu St. Petersburg im Sommer 1831, von praktischen Aerzten daselbst*, unter Redaktion der Herren Doktoren Lichtenstädt und Seidlitz, 2 vols, vol. 1, (St Petersburg, 1831), pp. 67–94; also for the second pandemic the extensive report by G.I. Blosfel'd, "Zamechaniia o vostochnoi kholere, svirepstvovavshei v gorode Kazani v 1847 godu, sobrannye is nabliudenii professorov meditsinskago fakul'teta imperatorskago Kazanskago Universiteta", *Uchenye Zapiski*, izdavaemye Imperatorskim Kazanskim Universitetom 1848, kn. 1 (Kazan', 1848), pp. 1–102, in part. pp. 1–21.

28 Lichtenstädt, *Fragmente*, pp. 80–91; Blosfel'd, *Zamechaniia o vostochnoi kholere*, pp. 37–39, 68–73, and in particular 47–102.

29 Spanish pepper (another word for cayenne pepper), which contains capsaicin, had been used for centuries as a remedy against both gastrointestinal and circulatory diseases. Remedies such as calomel and opium were common throughout Europe during the first pandemic and were taken from the English reports on cholera in India.

30 Snowden, *Naples in the Time of Cholera*, pp. 124–125.

31 McGrew, *Russia and the Cholera*, pp. 41–51.

32 Violent plague riots, brought about by strict sanitary regulations, had indeed exploded in Sevastopol' in May 1830. See McGrew, *Russia and the Cholera*, pp. 50–51.

33 Quarantine against cholera was first introduced during the Orenburg outbreak in 1829. Two laws, from 8 July and 12 August 1830, issued the general regulations concerning quarantine for cholera. In the second law, the government lay all responsibility for anti-cholera quarantine on the central government. McGrew, *Russia and the Cholera*, p. 48. The government only put the rules against plague into force on 12 September, see Pavlovskii, *Kholernye gody v Rossii*, p. 55.

34 The cholera riots in Russia during the first pandemic have been in detail described by McGrew, *Russia and the Cholera 1823–1832*, esp. pp. 67–74.

35 Ibid., esp. chap. 3. See also Netchkina, Sivkov, Sidorov, "La Russie", p. 143–155.

36 Evans, *Death in Hamburg*, p. 245.

37 Chevalier, "Le Choléra a Paris", Louis Chevalier (ed.), *Le Choléra*, pp. 21–24. See also Catherine J. Kudlick, *Cholera in Post-Revolutionary Paris. A Cultural History* (Berkeley, 1996).

38 Durey, *The Return of the Plague*, chap. 7.

39 Evans, *Death in Hamburg*, p. 243–251.

40 McGrew, *Russia and the Cholera*, pp. 41–51.

41 Pavlovskii, *Kholernye gody v Rossii*, esp. pp. 52–53.

42 McGrew, *Russia and the Cholera*, chap. 4.

43 Ibid., esp. chap. 3 and pp. 153–158. Also Pavlovskii, *Kholernye gody v Rossii*, p. 53.

44 McGrew, *Russia and the Cholera*, p. 54–55; Arkhangel'skii, *Kholernye epidemii*, pp. 110–112; Pavlovskii, *Kholernye gody v Rossii*, pp. 8–51.

45 Since population figures of the Caucasus did not exist for those years it was impossible for Archangel'skii, the most authoritative analyst of the epidemic, to give precise figures for the cholera's intensity in that region. Archangel'skii had to base his estimates on a census conducted in the Caucasus in 1851 when the Caucasus numbered 700,000 people. With 11,795 cholera victims in 1830 the intensity was 16.8 victims per thousand inhabitants. Population figures in 1830, however, were presumably much lower than in 1851. Arkhangel'skii, *Kholernye epidemii*, p. 111–112.

46 Ibid., p. 113–115.

47 Absolute numbers of cholera victims in these provinces were: Chernigov 14,698; Poltava 14,552; Ekaterinoslav 7,340; Khar'kov 10,276; Tauride 2,960; Don Cossack Region 5,703. Arkhangel'skii, *Kholernye gody*, pp. 116–117.

48 In 1830, cholera claimed an approximate 68,000 cholera cases and 37,600 victims. Numbers from Pavlovskii, *Kholernye gody v Rossii*, p. 4. Also Arkhangel'skii, *Kholernye epidemii*, p. 31.

49 McGrew, *Russia and the Cholera*, chap. 5.

50 For an overview of the historiography see the introduction and also the references in the bibliography.

51 Evans, *Death in Hamburg*, pp. 470–478; Snowden, *Cholera in Naples*, in particular pp. 152–154.

52 McGrew, *Russia and the Cholera*, pp. 153–158. Russia was not the exception. As in most other European countries, the first pandemic did not lead to any major reform efforts.

53 Ibid., p. 128.

54 Ibid., p. 128.

55 Europe's post-1832 cholera outbreaks are generally neglected in the historiography on cholera. Given the present inadequate state of research and the scarcity of sources, especially statistics, on Russia's third cholera pandemic in particular, my account is mainly based on the most authoritative description of the course of the cholera in 1847–48 by Arkhangel'skii, *Kholernye epidemii*, pp. 136–143 and on the work by Pavlovskii, *Kholernye gody v Rossii*, pp. 5–6. See also Patterson, "Cholera Diffusion in Russia", esp. pp. 1177–1179.

56 The most devastating mortality of the country was, once again, recorded in Stavropol (26.8 per thousand). In general, however, the Caucasus was unevenly affected by the

outbreak in 1847. In European Russia, the disease reached its highest intensity in the Don Cossack region (13.3 per thousand), followed by Astrakhan' (12.1 per thousand) and, again, Saratov (9.3 per thousand). Less severely affected were other traditional epicentres such as Ekaterinoslav with a mortality rate of 4.1 per thousand, Khar'kov (2.7 per thousand), and Voronezh (3.4 per thousand). For figures see Arkhangel'skii, *Kholernye epidemii*, pp. 144–146. Real figures were probably higher. According to McGrew more than a million people died in the period 1847–1851, see *Russia and the Cholera*, p. 5.

57 The first occurrence of cholera in Siberia is mentioned in the *Otechestvennye zapiski*, 1848, no. 9–10, t. 60, vnutrennye izvestiia, Otd. VIII, S. 49–50.

58 For a good overview of the year 1848 in Russia see David Saunders, "A Pyrrhic Victory: The Russian Empire in 1848", R.J.W. Evans; Hartmut Pogge von Strandmann (eds.), *The Revolutions in Europe 1848–1849* (Oxford, 2000), pp. 135–154. Saunder's' article considers mainly the political situation in 1848 and mentions the internal crises caused by cholera and the famine only marginally. For more on the cholera of that year see W. Bruce Lincoln, *Nicholas I. Emperor and Autocrat of All the Russians* (London, 1978), pp. 269–290.

59 Figures from Arkhangel'skii, *Kholernye epidemii v Evropeiskoi Rossii*, pp. 158–159. Contemporary statistics provide much lower numbers. According to official reports of the epidemic as published in the *Otechestvennye Zapiski* 290,318 people fell ill and 116,658 perished during the period from 16 October 1846 until 23 June 1848. See *Otechestvennye Zapiski*, 1849, no. 1–2, t. 62, vnutrennye izvestiia, Otd. VIII, pp. 1–36; for cholera see in particular pp. 22–23.

60 Podolsk recorded 92,933 cases and 32,977 deaths (mortality rate of 21.4 per thousand), Kiev 97,682 cases and 36,865 deaths (21.3 per thousand) and Chernigov 77,752 cases and 31,521 deaths (22.4 per thousand). Voronezh and Khar'kov suffered a mortality of 25.6 per thousand and 20.9 per thousand respectively. Figures from Arkhangel'skii, *Kholernye epidemii*, pp. 158–159. In general, the 1848 epidemic is by far less documented than the second pandemic, including the compilation of statistical material. For contemporary accounts of the third pandemic see in particular the "Obozrenie khoda i deistvii kholernoi epidemii v Rossii v 1847 godu", *Zhurnal Ministerstva Vnutrennikh Del*, vol. 23, no. 9 (1848), pp. 472–485; also "Istoricheskoe obozrenie sobytii v Rossii za 1848 god", *Otechestvennye zapiski*, 1849, t. LXII, pp. 1–36, esp. p. 22.

61 For the European context of Russian quarantine policy in the wake of the first cholera epidemic see Evans, *Death in Hamburg*, pp. 243–247; Snowden, *Naples in the Time of Cholera*, pp. 78–85.

62 For the history of Russia's quarantine legislation see John T. Alexander, *Bubonic Plague in Early Modern Russia. Public Health and Urban Disaster* (Baltimore, 1980), esp. pp. 31–35.

63 Nikolai Gogol' was detained for 14 days at Odessa in 1848 on his return from his journey to Syria. The detail is mentioned in Pavlovskii, *Kholernye gody v Rossii*, p. 55.

64 Unfortunately, sources about the 1848 outbreak are much more difficult to come by than for the first pandemic. The available material contains mostly mortality figures, yet one hardly finds reports about local measures in combating the epidemic or about local rioting in 1848. It is highly likely that local quarantine precautions were conducted just as rigorously as in 1830–31. That the state itself did not pursue a national quarantine campaign as during the second pandemic is explicitly laid out in the work by Arkhangel'skii, *Kholernye epidemii*, p. 142.

65 The epidemic caused an estimated 249,788 cholera cases and 100,083 deaths in 1853 and 331,025 cases and 131,327 deaths in 1855. Figures from Olzscha, "Die Epidemiologie und Epidemiographie der Cholera in Russland", esp. p. 10.

66 The classic works are Max von Pettenkofer, *Untersuchung und Beobachtung über Verbreitung der Cholera, nebst Betrachtungen über Massregeln derselben Einhalt zu thun* (Munich, 1855) and John Snow, *On the Mode of Communication of Cholera*,

reprinted in *Snow on Cholera* (New York, 1936), pp. 1–139. For a concise account of Pettenkofer's work on cholera and its implications for urban sanitation see Evans, *Death in Hamburg*, pp. 237–243.

67   Beginning in 1851 anti-cholera measures came to be discussed at seven international sanitary conferences: 1851–1852 (Paris), 1866 (Constantinople), 1874 (Vienna), 1885 (Rome), 1893 (Dresden), 1897 (Venice), 1903 (Paris). For the history of quarantine in the nineteenth century see in particular the article by J.C. McDonald, "The History of Quarantine in Britain during the Nineteenth Century", *Bulletin of the History of Medicine*, no. 25, 1951, pp. 22–44. For the sanitary conferences on cholera see Valeska Huber, "Unification of the Globe by Disease? The International Sanitary Conferences on Cholera, 1851–1894", *Historical Journal*, vol. 49, no. 2 (2006), pp. 453–467; see also Daniel Panzac, *Quarantaines et Lazarets. L'Europe et la Peste d'Orient (xvii-xx siecles)*, (Aix-en-Provence, 1986), pp. 120–125. A Russian view on the quarantine conference in Paris in 1851 is provided in an account which the Ministry of Internal Affairs added to the new legislation of 1866: *PSZ*, II, vol. 16, no. 43061 (1 March 1866), pp. 209–218.

68   By the end of July, the first cholera cases were reported from Podolia and Kherson; in August the epidemic appeared in Volhynia and on the Crimean, in September in Kiev, and in October in Ekaterinoslav. For an overview of the course of the fourth pandemic in Russia see Arkhangel'skii, *Kholernye epidemii*, p. 209. Unlike Russia, western Europe was severely affected in the 1860s. Austria, Hungary, Turkey and Prussia, too, were severely struck.

69   E.A. Ames, "A century of Russian railroad construction: 1837–1936", *American Slavic East European Review*, vol. 6, 1947, pp. 57–74.

70   The epidemic caused an estimated 322,711 cholera cases and 124,831 deaths in 1871 and 312,607 cases and 113,196 deaths in 1872. Figures from Olzscha, "Die Epidemiologie und Epidemiographie der Cholera in Russland", esp. p. 10.

71   *PSZ*, II, vol. 16, no. 43061 (1 March 1866), pp. 209–218. For a valuable analysis of the new quarantine legislation and it shortcomings with regard to the cholera outbreak in 1892 see N. Druzhinin, "Bor'ba s kholeroiu", *Nabliudatel'*, 1893, pp. 232–319.

72   The continuity between strategies against plague and cholera is well analysed by Frank Snowden, *Naples in the Time of Cholera*, pp. 78–81. For Russia's anti-plague policies during the seventeenth and eighteenth centuries see Alexander, *Bubonic Plague in Early Modern Russia*, pp. 29–35.

73   *PSZ*, II, vol. 16, no. 14614 (4 June 1841), pp. 435–497. The more than 60-page-long document was cut down to merely 9 pages in 1866.

74   Pettenkofer's cholera model is explained by Evans, *Death in Hamburg*, pp. 237–243. For Pettenkofer's influence in France in the early 1880s see Snowden, *Naples in the Time of Cholera*, p. 68.

75   Reman, "Poiavlenie vostochnoi Kholery", *Voenno-meditsinskii zhurnal*, vol. III, no. 2, 1824, pp. 159–193, p. 164. The influence of foreign, in particular British, medical theories on early Russian thinking about cholera during the 1820s is described by McGrew, *Russia and the Cholera*, pp. 18–25.

76   F.C.M. Markus, *Rapport sur le choléra-morbus de Moscow* (Moscow, 1832). Markus's account is evaluated by McGrew, *Russia and the Cholera*, pp. 84–97.

77   For examples see G.G. Blosfel'd, "Zamechaniia o vostochnoi kholere svirepstvovavshei v gorode Kazani v 1847 godu", *Uchenye Zapiski izdannye Imperatorskim Kazanskim Universitetom* (Kazan', 1848), pp. 1–102; "Obozreniie khoda i deistvii kholernoi epidemii v Rossii v techeniie 1848 goda", *JMVD*, chast' 27, kniga 9 (1849), pp. 315–36, in particular p. 328. These early cholera studies anticipated the analysis of the standard Russian work on the epidemic by Arkhangel'skii, *Kholernye epidemii*, which is an entirely localist document. The significance of the first and second cholera pandemics on the development of preventive medicine in Russia is also discussed by Frieden, *Russian Physicians*, pp. 78–81. With regard to the lower Volga an early general

topographic-medical study on Saratov province was conducted by H. Haurowiz, *Topographisch-medicinische Beobachtungen über den südlichen Theil des Saratowschen Gouvernements* (St Petersburg, 1836).

78 For the social history and scientific profile of Russia's most renowned medical scientists of the nineteenth century see the encompassing study by Frieden, *Russian physicians*, pp. 78–96.

79 For a short account on F.F. Erismann and his formidable work in Russia see Frieden, *Russian Physicians*, pp. 99–104. So far, an encompassing study on Russia's Pettenkofer still needs to be written.

80 See the classic article by Erwin Ackerknecht, "Anticontagionism between 1821 and 1867", *Bulletin of the History of Medicine*, 22 (1948), pp. 562–593.

81 Evans, *Death in Hamburg*, pp. 237–264. See also on pp. 264–275 Evans's analysis of the political, social and economic context explaining the triumph of contagionism in the 1880s and 1890s.

82 Snowden, *Naples in the Time of Cholera*, pp. 225–230. For reasons of clarity, the two positions, miasmatist and contagionist, are juxtaposed in the text. Yet neither of the two theories presented a coherent system of medical and political concepts. Lines between them were fluid, leaving much room for intermediate opinions. Pettenkofer himself presents more of a contingent-contagionist than an anti-contagionist position. The classic article on the two medical concepts on cholera is Ackerknecht, "Anticontagionism between 1821–1867", pp. 526–293. For the relativisation of the strict opposition of the two theories see Pelling, *Cholera, Fever and English Medicine*. A concrete example of the complex interweaving of medical and political arguments in the two approaches towards cholera is thoroughly discussed by Evans, *Death in Hamburg*, pp. 226–284.

83 McGrew, *Russia and the Cholera*, pp. 49–50.

84 Frieden, *Russian Physicians*, p. 37.

85 S. Frederick Starr, *Decentralization and Self-Government in Russia, 1830–1870* (Princeton, 1972).

86 Frieden, *Russian Physicians*, pp. 77–104.

87 For an analysis of the relation between Pettenkofer's medical thinking and decentralised politics see Evans, *Death in Hamburg*, pp. 237–243 and Snowden, *Naples in the Time of Cholera*, p. 195 and 436.

88 Sanitary surveillance on railways had been regulated through a series of circulars since 1881. However, these orders were not usually distributed widely enough, which created general uncertainty as to their validity.

89 Hans Heilbronner, "The Russian Plague of 1878–1879", *Slavic Review*, vol. 21 (March 1962), pp. 89–112.

2 Saratov on the eve of the epidemic

1 Figures are from the standard work by Arkhangel'skii, *Kholernye epidemii*, p. 31. To compare, in Astrakhan', a city of 30,770 inhabitants in 1830, the disease counted 2,935 deaths and mortality stood at 90%%.

2 Ibid., p. 154.

3 Ibid., p. 221.

4 The history of the cholera commission during the first pandemic is described by McGrew, *Russia and the Cholera*, pp. 41–74.

5 S. Gusev', A. Khovanskii, *Saratovets. Ukazatel' i putevoditel' po Saratovu* (Saratov, 1881), p. 27–29.

6 See the evaluation by F.V. Dukhovnikov, "Pamiati M.I.Semevskogo: Referat, chitannyi v saratovskoi uchenoi arkhivnoi komissii", *Russkaia Starina*, 1892 (December), pp. 685–689. See also the report by P.P. fon'-Gets', "Dnevnik pastora Ioanna Gubera: kholera v Saratove, v iune i iule 1830 g.", *Russkaia Starina*, 1878 (August), pp. 581–190. The preceding cholera epidemics also became a popular subject in

Saratov's feuilletonistic literature. For examples see Gusev, Khovanskii, *Saratovets*, p. 27–29 and the feuilletonistic articles in the local newspapers. For the significance of the plague in Vetlianka see the article by Hans Heilbronner, "The Russian Plague of 1878–79", *Slavic Review*, 1963, pp. 89–112.

7 These figures were established by the Medical Department in St Petersburg and published in B.V. Vladykin, *Materialy k istorii kholernoi epidemii 1892–95 v predelakh evropeiskoi Rossii* (St Petersburg, 1899), pp. 16–23. In contrast to western Europe Russian investigations of the 1892 epidemic for the country as a whole are rare. Vladykin's work, a dissertation written at the Imperial Military Medical Academy under the guidance of L.F. Ragozin, Director of the Medical Department of the Ministry of Internal Affairs, provides the best and most detailed account for European Russia. It was also the first to use the abundant statistical material of the Medical Department of the Ministry of Internal Affairs. Slightly bigger numbers (161,957) are given by L.A. Kharitonov, whose work is based on English reports of the fifth pandemic. L.A. Kharitonov, "Kholernaia epidemiia v Rossii v 1892–95 godakh", *VOGSPM*, 1902 (April), pp. 1–16; (November), pp. 16–23.

8 Figures, again, refer to European Russia. Vladykin, *Materialy k istoii kholernoi epidemii*, p. 8.

9 The death rate in 1831 stood at 42.4%% and in 1848 at 39.5%%. See Arkhangel'skii, *Kholernye epidemii*, p. 115.

10 A.V. Amsterdamskii, "Kholernaia epidemiia 1892 goda v Saratove i ee sviaz' s sanitarnymi usloviiami goroda", *SSO*, 1895, no. 1–4, pp. 89–120, here: p. 90. For reasons discussed below, real figures were almost certainly higher.

11 The discovery of the cholera bacillus by Robert Koch is discussed in the context of the 1892 epidemic in Hamburg by Evans, *Death in Hamburg*, pp. 264–284.

12 A thorough analysis of Saratov's early history is James G. Hart, "From Frontier Outpost to Provincial Capital: Saratov, 1590–1860", Rex A. Wade, Scott J. Seregny (eds), *Politics and Society in Provincial Russia: Saratov, 1590–1917* (Columbus, 1989), pp. 10–27; also S. Kedrov, "Kratkii obzor istorii Saratovskogo kraia", *Saratovskii Krai. Istoricheskie ocherki, vospominaniia, materialy* (Saratov, 1893), pp. 3–18.

13 Hart, "From Frontier Outpost to Provincial Capital", pp. 15–21; it is striking that almost all of the millers who made Saratov city the major centre of grain production and grain trade in Russia at the end of the nineteenth century were descendants of German colonists. See V.N. Semenov, N.N. Semenov, *Saratov Kupecheskii* (Saratov, 1995).

14 For the Volga region's tradition of peasant rebellion see Orlando Figes, *Peasant Russia, Civil War. The Volga Countryside in Revolution (1917–1921)* (Oxford, 1989), esp. pp. 19–27.

15 See in the following the analysis in I.V. Porokha (ed.), *Ocherki istorii Saratovskogo Povolzh'ia* (Saratov, 1995), vol. 2, part 1 (1855–1894), chap. 5; also Orlando Figes, *Peasant Russia, Civil War*, esp. pp. 17–27.

16 The first proposals to link the eastern end of the St Petersburg–Moscow Railway line with the rich agricultural lands of the south-east of the empire reached back to 1846. In 1859 the Moscow–Saratov railway line was officially authorised. The section from Moscow to Riazan was completed in 1864 and the final link from Tambov to Saratov in 1871. See Richard Mowbray Haywood, *Russia Enters the Railway Age, 1842–1855* (New York, 1998) pp. 558–559.

17 These numbers are from V.P. Semenov T'ian-Shanskii (ed.), *Rossiia. Polnoe geograficheskoe opisanie nashego otechestva* (St Petersburg, 1901), vol. 6, p. 478. Generally, figures are difficult to determine and differ considerably from reality. The officials at the port who were responsible for reporting the arriving cargo significantly reduced the freight for the reports so as to evade paying taxes. For the same reason, a good part of the freight was unloaded at other places than the official jetties. Therefore, a special Duma commission was authorised to collect data about the freight. These are

reported in the work by S. Gusev', A. Khovanskii, *Saratovets*, pp. 52–55. Semenov's figures, however, are probably more reliable and authoritative.

18 "Krupchatoe mukomol'noe delo v volzhskom raione", *Vestnik finansov, promyshlennosti i torgovli*, 19.9. 1893, pp. 640–643.

19 See G. Saar, *Saratovskaia promyshlennost' v nachale 90-kh g.g.* (Saratov, 1928). Information on Saratov's labour population can also be found in Michael Melancon, "Athens or Babylon? The Birth of the Socialist Revolutionary and Social Democratic Parties in Saratov, 1890–1905", Rex A. Wade and Scott J. Seregny (eds), *Politics and Society in Provincial Russia: Saratov, 1590–1917*, pp. 73–112, here pp. 74–75.

20 Saar, *Saratovskaia promyshlennost'*, p. 27. Figures, again, need to be handled with care as the lines between workers and artisans were constantly blurred.

21 According to a local census in 1917 Saratov counted 24,242 workers, 50% of whom were engaged in the 150 factories. The remainder worked as artisan workers, in domestics or on the docks. To compare, Kiev, twice as large as Saratov and the fifth largest city of the empire in 1910, counted 15,000 industrial workers in 1912. The city's largest six enterprises occupied approximately 500 employees. By contrast, in Moscow and Petersburg one-third of the factory labour force worked in factories with more than 1,000 employees. See Michael Hamm, "Continuity and Change in Late Imperial Kiev," in Michael Hamm (ed.), *The City in Late Imperial Russia* (Bloomington, 1986), pp. 79–121.

22 This was the official view: see, for instance, the evaluation in Brokgauz-Efron, 1900, vol. 28, p. 417; also V.P. Semenov T'ian Shanskii (ed.), *Rossiia*, vol. 6, p. 474.

23 Most valuable information on Saratov's topographic history can be found in I.N. Kokshaiskii, *Gorod Saratov v zhilishchnom otnoshenii* (Saratov, 1922), esp. chap. 1.

24 A physician at the Military-Medical Academy, Ekk was the Russian delegate to the International Sanitary Conference in Rome in 1885. The mentioned paper is published in *Mezhdunarodnaia Klinika* 1888, no. 5, pp. 1–15.

25 The official name of the commission was the 'commission for the improvement of sanitary conditions and the decline of mortality in Russia' (*kommisiia ob uluchshenii sanitarnykh uslovii i umen'shenii smertnosti v Rossii*). The earliest beginnings of the Botkin Commission are described in D.A. Sokolov, V.I. Grebenshchikov, *Smertnost' v Rossii i bor'ba s neiu* (St Petersburg, 1901). See also Frieden, *Russian Physicians*, pp. 137–138. The commission's work ended with Botkin's death in 1889.

26 For this evaluation see also G. Khlopin's and F. Erisman's article "Meditsina i narodnoe zdravie v Rossii", *Brokgauz-Efron*, 1899, vol. 27, p. 214–227, here: p. 226.

27 For the development of Russia's programme of "healthification" at the beginning of the twentieth century see in particular the work by John F. Hutchinson, *Politics and Public Health in Revolutionary Russia, 1890–1918* (Baltimore, 1990).

28 The first attempt to assess the sanitary conditions in Russia's cities, a volume compiled by the *Imperatorskoe Russkoe Geograficheskoe Obshchestvo* and entitled *Sanitarnoe sostoianie gorodov Rossiiskoi Imperii v 1895 godu*, begins with analysing the cities in those provinces which boasted the highest mortality rates during the preceding 10 years and also the highest mortality figures caused by the cholera in 1892: Nizhnii Novgorod, Kazan', Simbirsk, Saratov, Penza, and Ufa.

29 P.N. Sokolov, "Sanitarnyi ocherk g. Saratova", *SZN*, 1904, no. 5, pp. 51–69 and 1904, no. 6–7, pp. 116–123 offers the best discussion of Saratov's morbidity and mortality between 1894 and 1904; see also N.I. Matveev, *Gorod Saratov v sanitarnom otnoshenii v 1906 godu. Otchet sanitarnogo vracha* (Saratov, 1908), esp. pp. 72–96.

30 In Britain, mortality rates stood at 19 per thousand, in France at 22, in Germany at 24. See the article on "smertnost'", Brokgauz-Efron, 1901, vol. 27, p. 99.

31 This point was stressed by Sokolov, "Sanitarnyi ocherk g. Saratova", pp. 51–69.

32 Ibid., p. 67. Sokolov used the official figures of the Medical Department.

33 To compare, life expectancy in Switzerland and Germany was 70 years. Matveev, *Gorod Saratov v sanitarnom otnoshenii*, p. 85.

34 Sokolov, "Sanitarnyi ocherk goroda Saratova", *SZN*, 1904, no. 6–7, p. 117. National registration recorded a male infant mortality of 300 per 1,000 live births and a female infant mortality of 265 per 1,000 live births for the orthodox Russian population. See *Brokgauz-Efron*, 1890, vol. 27, p. 100.

35 Matveev, *Gorod Saratov v sanitarnom otnoshenii*, p. 86. It can be assumed that under the term gastro-intestinal disorders, many deaths from other diseases were classified as well.

36 Ibid., p. 87. The province's high infant mortality became a widely discussed issue at the beginning of the twentieth century. Teziakov, N.I., *Materialy po izucheniiu detskoi smertnosti v Saratovskoi gubernii s 1899 po 1901 g.* (Saratov, 1904); For infant mortality at the end of the nineteenth century see also David Ransel, *Mothers of Misery. Child Abandonment in Russia* (Princeton, 1988).

37 Although typhus epidemics erupted in Saratov every year, it is impossible to assess the extent of these epidemics. The diagnosis of the disease was so unclear to the local physicians that, Saratov's medical statisticians classified the disease under four categories: Sypnyi tif (typhus), briushnoi tif (typhoid), vozvratnyi tif (recurrent typhus), and neopredeliennyi tif (indeterminate typhus). The last category registered almost twice as many typhus-like cases between 1895 and 1896 as typhus itself.

38 "Malen'kaia Stolitsa", *Nedelia*, 1891, no. 20, p. 630.

39 The link between water-supply and cholera had been established by John Snow, *On the Mode of Communication of Cholera* (London, 1849), repr. in *Snow on Cholera* (New York, 1936).

40 By 1914, only 17 cities in the Russian Empire had centralised sewage systems while the rest resorted to private contractors, wells – and rivers. William Gleason, "Public Health, Politics, and Cities in Late Imperial Russia", *Journal of Urban History*, vol. 16, no. 4 (August 1990), pp. 341–365, here p. 353.

41 This system of garbage disposal had existed in Saratov since 1880. Before then, rubbish and waste were brought out of the city during the summer (11.4.–11.11.) whereas during the winter it was, with the approval of the municipality, simply discharged onto the ice of the Volga. For a description of the development and the practices of Saratov's sewage disposal see M.I. Krotkov, *Doklad o neobkhodmoi i vozmozhnoi zamene nyne praktikuemykh sposobov udaleniia iz goroda Saratova nechistot i otbrosov gorodskoi zhizni i uborki ikh na svalochnom uchastke gorodskoi zemli luchshimi sposobami ikh udaleniia i uborki* (Saratov, 1899) and in particular the supplement to the article by the same author, *Neobkhodimost' zameny sposoba uborki vyvozimykh iz goroda Saratova nechistot svalkoiu ikh v iamy sposobom udobreniia imi khleborodnykh i vygonnykh polei, prinadlezhashchikh gorodu.*

42 Already in 1888 the situation at the dumping site was condemned at a meeting of the municipal duma. See Krotkov, *Doklad*, p. 72.

43 Ibid., p. 29. The same percentage is given by Matveev. He gives concrete numbers for the year 1896: from the 180,000 pud of daily refuse 18,000 pud were carried out of the city. See Matveev, "Sanitarnye ocherki berega Volgi u Saratova," *VOGSPM*, 1906 (November).

44 Ibid., p. 41.

45 Krotkov, *Doklad*, p. 40.

46 Khlopin, *Materialy po ozdorovleniiu Rossii*, p. 211; Saratov's housing problems and attempts to reallocate the ravine inhabitants are discussed in Chapter 3.

47 Because of their hazardous sanitary conditions, both ravines, and the *Glebuchev* ravine in particular became a place of more or less regular investigation by local as well as national medical authorities, usually during or after times of epidemic crises. Due to these investigations the following sources are available: Matveev, *Glebuchev ovrag, 1871–1906* (Saratov, 1907); P.N. Sokolov, "O sanitarnom sostoianii ovragov Beloglinskogo i Glebucheva", *SZN*, 1905, no. 3, pp. 29–46; 1905, no. 4, pp. 14–30; V.I. Al'mazov, "K voprosu ob uporiadochenii Glebucheva ovraga", *Izvestiia Saratovskoi Gorodskoi*

Dumy, no. 4 (1907), pp. 487–496; B.I. Likhachev, *Sanitarnoe opisanie Povolzh'ia* (St Petersburg, 1898); G.V. Khlopin, *Materialy po ozdorovelniiu Rossii. Sanitarnoe opisanie g.g. Astrakhana, Samary, Saratova i Tsaritsyna s ukazaniem mer, neobkhodimykh dlia ikh ozdorovleniia* (St Petersburg, 1911), pp. 191–246.

48 Sokolov, "O sanitarnom sostoianii ovragov Beloglinskogo i Glebucheva", *SZN*, no. 4, 1905, pp. 14–30, here: p. 23.

49 Khlopin, *Materialy po ozdorovleniiu Rossii*, p. 211.

50 Matveev, *Glebuchev Ovrag*, pp. 6–12; N.P. Sokolov, "O sanitarnom sostoianii," *SZN*, 1905, no.4, pp. 14–30.

51 Khlopin, *Materialy po ozdorovleniiu Rossii*, pp. 210–219.

52 Matveev, "Sanitarnye ocherki berega Volgi u Saratova", *VOGSPM*, 1906 (November), pp. 41.

53 Ibid., p. 44. Matveev adds that the actual number was much higher due to the masses of unemployed people roaming the banks.

54 V.I. Almazov, "O kanalizatsii v Saratove. Doklad gorodskoi dume", *ISGD*, 1907, no. 1, pp. 114–136.

55 The water pipes only covered one fifth of the urban territory, which meant they could have supplied 56,269 inhabitants with water. Since not all houses were connected to the water pipes, however, only 32,030 people received water from the water-supply system in the 1890s. Krotkov, Doklad, p. 33.

56 Khlopin, *Materialy po ozdorovleniiu Rossii*, pp. 224–229.

57 Ibid., p. 227.

58 Ibid., pp. 227–228.

59 Sokolov, "O sanitarnom sostoianii", pp. 40–46. The generally accepted norm was 150–300 colonies. Khlopin, *Materialy po ozdorovleniiu Rossii*, p. 228.

60 V.I. Likhachev, *Sanitarnoe opisanie Povol'zhia* (St Petersburg, 1898).

61 Matveev, "Sanitarnye ocherki berega Volgi ", p. 45.

62 Sokolov, "O sanitarnom sostoianii"; p. 39; see also G.V. Khlopin, "Vlianie neftianykh produktov na rybnoe naselenie rek i na kachestvo ikh vody", *Vrach*, no. 51 (1898), pp. 232.

63 Matveev, "Sanitarnye ocherki berega Volgi", p. 39.

64 J.N. Westwood, *A History of Russian Railways* (London, 1964).

65 For the effect of new modes of transportation on the course of the cholera in 1892 see Frank Clemow, M.D. Edin, *The Cholera Epidemic of 1892 in the Russian Empire* (London, 1893), p. 3 and 34–35.

66 Migration in late-nineteenth-century Russia has been investigated in a wide array of studies. See for instance Barbara Anderson, *Internal Migration during Modernization in Late Nineteenth Century Russia* (Princeton, 1980); Barbara Alpern Engel, *Between the Fields and the City. Women, Work, and Family in Russia, 1861–1914* (Cambridge, 1995); Joseph Bradley, *Muzhik and Muscovite. Urbanization in Late Imperial Russia* (Berkeley, Los Angeles, London, 1985); a unique biographical account of a peasant migrant's experience in Saratov is left by Semen Kanatchikov. See the edition by Reginald E. Zelnik, *A Radical Worker in Tsarist Russia. The Autobiography of Semen Ivanovich Kanatchikov* (Stanford, 1986).

67 According to the census in 1897, population numbers of the biggest cities on the middle and lower Volga were as follows: Kazan' 130,000; Simbirsk 41,700; Samara 90,000; Saratov 137,000; Tsaritsyn 55,200; Astrakhan' 112,800. See I.N. Kokshaiskii, *Gorod Saratov v zhilishnom otnoshenii (po dannym perepisi 1916 g.)* (Saratov, 1922), p. 21.

68 In 1910, Oslo had 243,000 inhabitants, Prague 224,000, Bordeaux 266,000, and Genoa 272,000. See B.R. Mitchell, *European Historical Statistics 1750–1970* (London, 1978), pp. 12–14.

69 Kokshaiskii, *Gorod Saratov*, p. 20.

70 N.I. Teziakov, "Otkhozhie promysly i rynki naima sel'sko-khoziaistvennykh rabochikh v Saratovskoi gubernii", *SZN*, 1903, no. 1, 1–39, p. 15.

71 A. Ershov, *Ocherk chernorabochego dvizheniia v Saratovskom krae* (Saratov, 1909), pp. 4–8.

72 Labour migration certainly was at its most intense in the Central Industrial Region (including the provinces of Iaroslavl', Tver', Kostroma, Kaluga, Moscow, Vladimir and Nizhnii Novgorod). Historiographical scholarship on the migration movement has therefore concentrated on this area. The migration movement from the Central Black Earth Zone to the steppe region has received less attention. However, a thorough analysis of seasonal work in the steppe region is offered by Timothy Mixter, "The Hiring Market as Workers' Turf: Migrant Agricultural Laborers and the Mobilization of Collective Action in the Steppe Grainbelt of European Russia, 1853–1913", Esther Kingston-Mann and Timothy Mixter (eds), *Peasant Economy, Culture, and Politics of European Russia, 1800–1921* (Princeton, 1991), pp. 294–340. According to Mixter, the annual number of peasants migrating to the steppe for the harvest season had reached between 1 and 1.5 million people by the mid-1880s (p. 294). The Central Black Earth Zone includes the provinces of Orel, Kursk, Tambov, Voronezh, Tula and Riazan. Some definitions also include Saratov, Penza, Simbirsk and Samara provinces. In Saratov province, only its northern districts were black earth soil regions.

73 There has been much debate over taxes and peasant living standards. For a summary see David Moon, *The Abolition of Serfdom in Russia* (Harlow, 2001), pp. 114–115. For the Central Black Earth and the Volga regions, however, Stephen Wheatcroft has identified an agrarian crisis in "Crises and the Condition of the Peasantry in Late Imperial Russia", Esther Kingston-Mann, Timothy Mixter (eds), *Peasant Economy, Culture, and Politics of European Russia*, pp. 128–172. In Saratov, a household was charged 11,435 rubles in taxes as compared, for instance, to 50 rubles in Kursk. Theodore H. von Laue, "Russian Labor between Field and Factory", p. 35–36.

74 A.P. Engel'gardt, *Chernozemnaia Rossiia. Ocherk ekonomicheskogo polozheniia kraia* (Saratov, 1902).

75 See Richard G. Robbins, *Famine in Russia 1891–92. The Russian Government Responds to a Crisis* (New York, 1975), p. 185–189.

76 I.V. Parokh, *Ocherki istorii Saratovskogo Povolzh'ia (1855–1894)* (Saratov, 1995), vol. 2, p. 136.

77 On weekdays numbers ran up to only between 50 and 150 people. N. Ponomarev, "O peredvizhenii sel'sko-khoziastvennykh rabochikh, napravliaiushchikhsia v iugo-ostochnye mestnosti Rossii", *Sel'skoe khoziaistvo i lesovodstvo*, 1896, no. 2, p. 13.

78 N.I. Teziakov, "Otkhozhie promysly i rynki naima sel'sko-khoziaistvennykh rabochikh v Saratovskoi gubernii", *SZN*, 1903, no. 1, 1–39.

79 For the functioning of the passport system see the article by Jeffrey Burds, "The Social Control of Peasant Labor in Russia: The Response of Village Communities to Labor Migration in the Central Industrial Region, 1861–1905", Esther Kingston-Mann, Timothy Mixter (eds), *Peasant Economy, Culture, and Politics of European Russia*; also David Moon, "Peasant Migration, the Abolition of Serfdom and the Internal Passport System in the Russian Empire, c. 1800–1914", D. Eltis (ed.), *Free and Coerced Migration: Global Perspectives* (Stanford, 2002), pp. 324–57.

80 N.I. Teziakov, "Otkhozhie promysli", p. 34; also A. Ershov, *Ocherk chernorabochego dvizheniia*, pp.4–8.

81 Cited from Ershov, *Ocherk chernorabochego dvizheniia*, p. 12.

82 See, for instance, Barbara Alpern-Engel, *Between the Fields and the City. Women, Work, and Family in Russia, 1861–1914* (Cambridge, 1996).

83 For an analysis of the sanitary conditions of the boatsmen on the ships see A. Desiatov, "Ocherk sanitarno-ekonomicheskogo polozheniia rabochikh na parokhodakh basseina reki Volgi", *Materialy dlia izucheniia sanitarnogo sostoianiia vnutrennykh vodnykh putei. VIII sbornik otchetov i dokladov vrachei sanitarnogo nadzora na r.r. Volge i Kame i na Mariinskom sisteme za 1903 g.* (St Petersburg, 1904), pp. 119–135.

84 Matveev, "Sanitarnye ocherki berega Volgi", p. 15.

85 Teziakov, "Otkhozhie promysly", pp. 6–8.

86 Ibid., pp. 7–8.

87 Ibid., p. 8. On malaria in Russia see Mary Schaeffer Conroy, "Malaria in Late Tsarist Russia", *BHM*, vol. 56, no. 1, (1982), pp. 41–55.

88 N.I. Teziakov, *Materialy dlia kharakteristiki Saratovskoi Aleksandrovskoi gubernskoi zemskoi bol'nitsy, kak obshche-gubernskogo lechebnogo uchrezhdeniia. Doklad VIII gubernskomu s"ezdu vrachei i predsedatelei zemskikh uprav Saratovskoi gubernii* (Saratov, 1907), p. 12.

89 Ibid., p. 13.

90 S.I. Kuz'min, A.I. Ershov, *Kratkii ocherk sostoianiia Saratovskoi Aleksandrovskoi gubernskoi zemskoi bol'nitsy v 1906, 1907 i otchasti v 1905 godu. Doklad IX gubernskomu s"ezdu vrachei i predsedatelei zemskikh uprav Saratovskoi gubernii,* (Saratov, 1908), p. 8.

91 Saar, *Saratovskaia promyshlennost'*, p. 10–11.

92 Numbers of workers at the mills increased from 468 in 1891 to 1,239 in 1904. Saar, *Saratovskaia promyshlennost'*, p. 13.

93 Workers at the railway workshops numbered 320 in 1891 and 1,582 in 1904. Saar, *Saratovskaia promyshlennost'*, p. 22.

94 In 1895 Saratov counted 2,431 artisans in the manufacturing of clothes and shoes, an additional 759 shoemakers, 751 tailors, 529 millers, 598 bricklayers, 580 joiners, and 436 blacksmiths. See the article "Saratov", Brokgauz-Efron, 1900, vol. 28, pp. 417–419.

95 Saar, *Saratovskaia promyshlennost'*, p. 27.

96 A rich description of the lives of migrants in British cities earlier in the century is presented by Raphael Samuel, "Comers and Goers", Dyos, H.J. and Wolff, Michael (eds), *The Victorian City. Images and Realities*, 2 vols. (London, 1973), vol. 1, pp. 123–153. See also the literature cited above, note 67.

97 Matveev, "Sanitarnye ocherki berega Volgi", p. 44.

98 Ibid., p. 42; Ershov, *Ocherk chernorabochego dvizheniia*, p. 9.

99 Ibid., p. 9–11.

100 Ibid., p. 10.

101 Matveev, "Nochlezhie doma, artel'nye kvartiry i postoialye dvory goroda Saratova", *SZN*, 1896, no. 39, pp. 502–511, p. 507.

102 Matveev, "Sanitarnye ocherki berega Volgi", p. 16.

103 Ibid., p. 46.

104 See, for instance, the interpretation of the basic study on public health in revolutionary Russia by John F. Hutchinson, *Politics and Public Health in Revolutionary Russia, 1890–1918* (Baltimore, London, 1990), p. 4–7.

105 Frieden, *Russian Physicians*, p. 136.

106 Frank Clemow, *The Cholera Epidemic of 1892 in the Russian Empire* (London, 1893).

107 Ibid., p. 79. Clemow's evaluation corresponds to Richard Robbins's conclusion on the role of the central government during the famine of 1891. See Richard G. Robbins, *Famine in Russia,* esp. chap. 11.

108 Tiflis reported 570 cases, 261 of which proved fatal. Clemow, *The Cholera Epidemic,* p. 27.

109 Detailed and informative analyses of the development of Russian medical organisation and administration during the seventeenth and eighteenth centuries are provided by John T. Alexander, *Bubonic Plague in Early Modern Russia* (Baltimore, 1980), esp. chap. 1, pp. 36–61; see also his "Medical Developments in Petrine Russia", *Canadian-American Slavic Studies* 7 (summer 1974), pp. 198–221; also McGrew, *Russia and the Cholera*, pp. 17–41. For the particular focus on medical education see Mirko Grmek, "The History of Medical Education in Russia", in C.D. O'Malley (ed.), *The History of Medical Education*, UCLA Forum in Medical Sciences, no. 12 (Berkeley, 1970), p. 303–325.

110 The history of the *aptekarskii prikaz* and the pharmaceutical profession in late-nineteenth-century Russia is investigated by Mary Schaeffer Conroy, *In Health and in Sickness. Pharmacy, Pharmacists, and the Pharmaceutical Industry in Late Imperial, Early Soviet Russia* (New York, 1994). See esp. chap. 1.

111 A parallel process occurred in the management of famine relief. See the analysis by Robbins, *Famine in Russia 1891–92*, chap. 2.

112 For the history of the Great Plague see Alexander, *Bubonic Plague in Early Modern Russia*.

113 For the development of Cameralism and the idea of the medical police, which played an important role in Russia until 1917, see the comprehensive article by George Rosen, "Cameralism and the Concept of Medical Police", *Bulletin of the History of Medicine*, 27 (1953), pp. 21–42. Johann Peter Frank, the main theoretical advocate of the concept of medical police, worked as first physician of Alexander I at the beginning of the nineteenth century. He accepted the chair of practical medicine at the Medical-Surgical Academy in Petersburg and later became rector of the institution. See Mirko Grmek, "The History of Medical Education in Russia", p. 313.

114 For Catherine's administrative reforms see George L. Yaney, *The Systematization of Russian Government. Social Evolution in the Domestic Administration of Imperial Russia, 1711–1905* (Urbana, 1973), chap. 2, pp. 67–76. The European context of the reforms is provided by Marc Raeff, *The Well-Ordered Police State: Social and Institutional Change through Law in the Germanies and Russia, 1600–1800* (New Haven, 1983).

115 The functions of local public health authorities before the Great Reforms are described by Frieden, *Russian Physicians*, pp. 63–65. In expectation of another cholera outbreak Committees on Public Health were introduced in the provinces in 1852. They operated alongside the medical boards and were responsible for the implementation of epidemic measures as well as for hygiene education. See Frieden, *Russian Physicians*, p. 64.

116 The first retired military practitioners had already been dispatched to the provinces since 1737. In the cities, medical control came into the hands of city-physicians. City-physicians appeared for the first time in Moscow and Petersburg in 1733. See Alexander, *Bubonic Plague*, p. 51.

117 The laws for the medical police were incorporated into volume 13 of the *Collection of Laws: The Statutes on Food Supply, Social Welfare, Medical Practice and the Medical Police*, which provides the basic source for all questions concerning medical administration.

118 For the ministerial reforms in 1803 see Daniel T. Orlovskii, *The Limits of Reform: The Ministry of Internal Affairs in Imperial Russia, 1802–1881* (Cambridge, Mass., 1981).

119 Similarly, in eighteenth-century Germany, the concept of the medical police could not be fully realised in practice. On its functioning see Evans, *Death in Hamburg*, p. 206.

120 For the reform in medical administration see also Chapter 1, pp. 41–42.

121 Exceptions are the works by William Gleason, "Public Health, Politics, and Cities in Late Imperial Russia", *Journal of Urban History*, vol. 16 (August 1990), pp. 341–365 and Joseph Bradley, *Muzhik and Muscovite. Urbanization in Late Imperial Russia* (Berkeley, 1985). However, they study the functioning of municipal health, sanitation and public welfare in the two capitals, which traditionally were equipped with excellent medical institutions and personnel and therefore are not representative of the majority of Russian cities.

122 For the municipal reform in particular see V.A. Nardova, "Municipal Self-Government after the 1870 Reform", Ben Eklof, John Bushnell, and Larissa Zakharova (eds), *Russia's Great Reforms, 1855–1881* (Bloomington, 1994), pp. 181–196; also Walter Hanchett, "Tsarist Statutory Regulation of Municipal Government in the Nineteenth Century", Michael Hamm (ed.), *The City in Russian History* (Lexington, 1976).

123 Nardova, "Municipal Self-Government", p. 184.

124 *PSZ*, II, vol. 54, no. 59399 (9 March 1879). The measures which could be taken included the cleanliness and order of streets, squares, wells; the construction and cleanliness of cesspits; the maintenance of slaughterhouses and factories; and also the possibility to prohibit the carrying of dead bodies through the streets in open coffins.

125 See Frieden, *Russian Physicians*, pp. 63–75.

126 V.Ia. Kanel', "Obshchestvennaia meditsina v sviazi s usloviiami zhizni naroda", *Istoriia Rossii v xix veke*. 9 vols. (St Petersburg, 1909–1911), vol. 8, pp. 156–262, here: p. 229.

127 The institution of a municipal hospital was the exception even at the beginning of the twentieth century. Only 12.4% of Russian cities financed a municipal hospital. See Kanel', "Obshchestvennaia meditsina", p. 231.

128 See generally for the public image of physicians Frieden, *Russian Physicians*, pp. 110–113.

129 Hutchinson, *Politics and Public Health in Revolutionary Russia*, p. 17.

130 Cit. in Kanel', "Obshchestvennaia meditsina", p. 230.

131 *Svod zakonov Rossiiskoi Imperii*, vol. 13 (1906), *Ustav vrachebnyi*, art. 48.

132 For the salary of zemstvo physicians see Frieden, *Russian Physicians*, p. 336.

133 *PSZ*, II, vol. 54, no. 59399 (9 March 1879).

134 *PSZ*, II, vol. 54, no. 59399 (9 March 1879).

135 For the tasks and composition of the *Meditsinskii Sovet* see N.B. Frejberg, *Vrachebno-sanitarnoe zakonodatel'stvo v Rossii*, (St Petersburg, 1908), chap. 1.

136 D-r Ukke, "Epidemii i nashi meditsinskie poriadki", *Vestnik Evropy*, 1882, vol. 6, pp. 827–852.

137 Freiberg, *Vrachebno-sanitarnoe zakonodatel'stvo v Rossii*, chap. 1.

138 Ukke, "Epidemii i nashi meditsinskie poriadki", p. 852.

139 There were many other institutions and authorities responsible for medical jurisdiction. I have mentioned those which were particularly important during epidemics. See *Svod zakonov Rossiiskoi Imperii*, vol. 13 (1906), *Ustav vrachebnyi*, art. 1.

140 G.E. Rein, *Iz perezhitogo 1907–1918*, 2 vols (Berlin, 1935), vol. 1, chap. 2, pp. 23–26.

141 Heilbronner, "The Russian Plague of 1878–79", p. 99.

142 For the activity of the commission see Frieden, *Russian Physicians*, pp. 291–292.

143 E. Nikolaev, "Saratovskoe sanitarnoe obshchestvo," *CZN*, 1905, no. 6–7, pp. 59–65, pp. 59–65; V.I. Miropol'skii, *Obshchii ocherk deiatel'nosti "Obshchestva Saratovskikh Sanitarnykh Vrachei", s maia 1886 t. po ianvar' 1893 goda* (Saratov, 1893).

3 Cholera in Saratov, 1892

1 These figures were established by the medical department in St Petersburg and published in B.V. Vladykin, *Materialy k istorii kholernoi epidemii 1892–95 v predelakh Evropeiskoi Rossii* (St Petersburg, 1899), pp. 16–23. In contrast to western Europe, Russian investigations into the 1892 epidemic for the country as a whole are rare. Vladykin's work, a dissertation written at the Imperial Military Medical Academy under the guidance of L.F. Ragozin, director of the medical department of the Ministry of Internal Affairs, provides the best and most detailed account for European Russia. It was also the first to use the abundant statistical material of the Medical Department of the Ministry of Internal Affairs. Slightly higher numbers (161,957) are given by L.A. Kharitonov, whose work is based on English reports of the fifth pandemic. L.A. Kharitonov, "Kholernaia Epidemiia v Rossii v 1892–95 godakh", *VOGSPM* (April, 1902) pp. 1–16; (November, 1902), pp. 16–23.

2 The severe cholera year in 1831 recorded 466,457 cholera cases and 197,069 deaths. All figures refer to European Russia. They are taken from the standard work by Arkhangel'skii, *Kholernye epidemii*, pp. 2–4.

3 The death rate in 1831 stood at 42.4 and in 1848 at 39.5 per thousand population. Again, figures refer to European Russia. Arkhangel'skii, *Kholernye epidemii*, pp. 2–4. Real figures, again, were probably higher. See the discussion of misdiagnosis in the appendix of Richard Evans's *Death in Hamburg*, pp. 567–592.

4 Articles in the national public and medical press on this issue are abundant. For examples see "Iz zhizni i pechati", *Russkii Vestnik*, vol. 221 (July 1892), pp. 262–269; "Iz provintsial'noi pechati", *Severnyi Vestnik*, 1892, no. 8, pp. 45–57; L.G. Karchagin, "Po povodu kholernoi epidemii v Rossi v 1892", *Vrach*, 1892, no. 32, pp. 79– 81; Physicians in particular complained about their dependency on local and national governmental agencies. Frieden, *Russian Physicians*, pp. 154–160, also pp. 135–138; Hutchinson, *Politics and Public Health in Revolutionary Russia*, pp. 6–7.

5 V. Kolpenskii, "Kholernyi bunt v 1892 godu!", *Arkhiv istorii truda v Rossii*, 1922, no. 3, p. 111. See also Frieden, *Russian Phyisicians*, pp. 147–148.

6 A highly instructive source which demonstrates the variety of the cholera experience in Russia on all levels (medical, administrative, social) are the *Trudy s"ezda vrachei prinimavshikh neposredstvennoe uchastie v bor'be s kholernoi epidemiei 1892 g. v Rossii s 13. po 20 dekabria 1892* (St Petersburg, 1893).

7 Frieden, *Russian Physicians*, pp. 143–148; also "Iz zhizni i pechati", *Russkii Vestnik*, vol. 221 (July 1892), pp. 262–269, esp. p. 268; on the difficulties physicians encountered in the countryside of Saratov province see the *Sbornik otchetov vrachei i studentov rabotavshikh po kholernoi epidemii 1892 goda v Saratovskoi gubernii* (Saratov, 1893) edited by the provincial zemstvo.

8 An abundance of reports from various regions and cities can be found in the abovementioned *Trudy s"ezda vrachei*. Frank Clemow stresses the importance of the living habits of the Karakalpaks and Uzbeks whose partly nomadic lifestyle at rivers and in tents heavily affected the severity of the epidemic in central Asia. Equally, the population in the Caucasus (Armenians, Georgians, Ossetians, Kurds, Turks, Kalmyks, Tatars and Cossacks) led a half-settled, half-nomadic life, which made them particularly vulnerable to the disease. Clemow, *The Cholera Epidemic of 1892*, pp. 10–25. Theodore Friedgut points to the fact that the English and Jewish population at Iuzovka did not even fall ill whereas the Russians died. Theodore H. Friedgut, "Labor Violence and Regime Brutality in Tsarist Russia: The Iuzovka Cholera Riots of 1892", *Slavic Review*, 1988, pp. 24–265, p. 255.

9 Samara and Iaroslavl', to name just two examples from the Volga, survived the epidemic without further social disarray. This was mainly because quarantine measures were carried out on a voluntary basis. *Trudy s"ezda vrachei*, p. 246.

10 An analogous thought is elaborated already for the first pandemic by McGrew, who stressed the necessity to pay attention to the geographical, ethnic, social and cultural diversity of the empire and thus to go beyond the all-explaining notion of the 'crisis of the feudal order' offered by M.V. Nechkina, K.V. Sivkov and A.L. Sidorov in their examination of the epidemic in 1830/31. In McGrew's words 'The "crisis of the feudal order", if such it actually was, was so diverse in its individual aspects as to cast doubt on the meaning of the phrase.' McGrew, *Russia and the Cholera*, p. 12. M.V. Nechkina, K.V. Sivkov, A.L. Sidorov, "La Russie", Louis Chevalier (ed.), *Le Choléra*, pp. 143–155, esp. p. 154.

11 Briggs, "Cholera and Society in the Nineteenth Century", p. 76.

12 Ibid., p. 76.

13 This argument is elaborated in the two classic articles by Briggs, "Cholera and Society in the Nineteenth Century", p. 76 and 89, and Evans, "Epidemics and Revolutions", esp. pp. 123–127.

14 These are the official figures provided by medical authorities. A.V. Amsterdamskii, "Protokol 87-go zasedaniia obshchestva saratovskikh sanitarnykh vrachei, 30 oktiabria 1892 goda", *Protokoly zasedanii obshchestva za 1890, 91, 92*, p. 197. The number of cholera cases in the city equalled 27.2 per thousand population. To compare, the highest figures were recorded in Astrakhan' (50.8 per thousand), Petrovsk (60.4 per thousand), Samara (35.5 per thousand) and Tsaritsyn (32.4 per thousand). From then on, figures of

cholera cases declined to Simbirsk (23.8 per thousand), Kazan' (21.2 per thousand), Kursk (19.7 per thousand), Voronezh (17.1 per thousand). See the tables in Vladykin, *Materialy k istorii kholernoi epidemii*, pp. 34–77.

15 A description of the course of the epidemic can be found in R. Pollitzer, *Cholera Studies: History of the Disease, Bulletin of the World Health Organization* (Geneva, 1959). The standard contemporary works on cholera in Russia are Arkhangel'skii, *Kholernye epidemii*; N. Pavlovskaia, *Kholernye gody v Rossii* (St Petersburg, 1892); Vladykin, *Materialy k istorii kholernoi epidemii*; L.A. Kharitonov, "Kholernaia epidemiia v Rossii v 1892–95 godakh", *VOGSPM*, April 1902, pp. 1–160; November 1901, p. 16–23. A very informative account of the epidemic of 1892 is also written by Frank Clemow, member of the Epidemiological Society in London, who worked at the English Hospital in Kronstadt in 1892–93. Frank Clemow, *The Cholera Epidemic of 1892*.

16 RGIA, f. 565, op. 7, 1886, d. 19907. Also Kharitonov, "Kholernaia epidemiia v Rossii v 1892–95 godakh", *VOGSPM* (April 1902), pp.1–160, p. 3; and Vladykin, *Materialy k istorii kholernoi epidemii*, p. 7. The outbreak which claimed 258 cases and 152 deaths was quickly and efficiently brought under control by local authorities.

17 RGIA, f. 565, op. 5, 1886, d. 19907.

18 A.A. Lipskii, "Mery bor'by s kholeroiu, proektirovannye v Rossi v 1883–1885 godakh", *VOGSPM*, vol. 9 (January–March 1890), pp. 36–46. The government's instructions of 1892 are published in M.I. Galanin, *Meropriiatiia protiv kholery russkogo i inostrannykh pravitel'stv i ikh nauchnye osnovy dlia vrachei i adminis-tratorov* (St Petersburg, 1892). Local governments, as well, had prepared cholera instructions in accordance to their local conditions. Some of these are also published in Galanin's work.

19 For the following see especially N. Danilov, "Obzor epidemii asiatskoi kholery v Mesopotamii i Persii v 1889 g.; mery, priniatye protiv zanosa ee v predely Rossii", *Meditsinskaia beseda*, vol. 4 (April 1890), pp. 145–147.

20 Ibid., p. 146. Also P.A. Glavatskii, "Meropriiatiia po bor'be s kholeroiu na Kavkaze", *Trudy s"ezda vrachei*, pp. 31–35.

21 *Pravitel'stvennyi Vestnik*, no. 128, 14.6.1892.

22 The available sources do not allow one to trace the detailed motivation of the ministry to take action. However, it suggests itself that the ministry was eager to prevent any crisis which might have destroyed its economic pursuit of establishing a stable currency. See the discussion by Richard G. Robbins, *Famine in Russia 1891–92: The Imperial Government Responds to a Crisis* (New York, 1975), chap. 3.

23 Kharitonov, "Kholernaia epidemiia v Rossii v 1892–95 godakh", p. 16.

24 For the early development of bacteriology in Russia see the article by John F. Hutchinson, "Tsarist Russia and the Bacteriological Revolution", *Journal of the History of Medicine*, vol. 40 (October 1985), pp. 420–439.

25 Sergei S. Botkin was the son of the famous internist and court physician S.P. Botkin (1832–1889), founder of the Pirogov Society and head of the Botkin Commission mentioned in Chapter 1. Nikolai Gamaleia (1859–1949) had been a student of Il'ia Mechnikov at Odessa. Mechnikov was also head of the Pasteur Institute in the city.

26 For personnel policies in the Russian medical establishment in the 1890s see Hutchinson, "Tsarist Russia and the Bacteriological Revolution", p. 422–429.

27 The Russian titles were: *Vestnik obshchestvennoi gigieny, sudebnoi i prakticheskoi meditsiny, Voenno-meditsinskii zhurnal*, and *Zhurnal obshchestva okhraneniia narodnogo zdraviia*.

28 Short instructions on the investigation of the dejecta of suspicious cases for the presence of the *comma bacillus* of Koch (Army Medical Scientific Committee, 8 May 1892), printed in Clemow, *The Cholera Epidemic of 1892*.

29 *Pravitel'stvennyi Vestnik*, no. 128, 14.6. 1892; also Kharitonov, "Kholernaia epidemiia v Rossii v 1892–1895 godakh", p. 16–20; and Clemow, *The Cholera Epidemic of 1892*, esp. pp. 64–79.

30 S.M. Ershov, "Epidemiia asiatskoi kholery v 1889 godu i mery bor'by s neiu", *Mezhdunarodnaia klinika*, no. 3 (1890), pp. 1–20, here: pp. 11–12.

31 The detail is mentioned by Kharitonov, "Kholernaia epidemiia v Rossii v 1892–1895 godakh", p. 16.

32 Ibid., p. 16; *Pravitel'stvennyi Vestnik*, no. 128, 14.6.1892.

33 P.A. Poliakov, "Kholernaia epidemiia 1892 goda v g. Askhabade", *Voenno-meditsinskii zhurnal*, vol. 177 (May 1893), p. 43–102, here: p. 44; Kharitonov, "Kholernaia epidemiia v Rossii", p. 16; Vladykin, *Materialy k istorii kholernoi epidemii*, p. 13–14; P.A. Glavatskii, "Meropriiatiia po bor'be s kholeroiu na Kavkaze", *Trudy s"ezda vrachei*, pp. 32–35.

34 Poliakov, "Kholernaia epidemiia 1892 goda v g. Askhabade", p. 44.

35 Glavatskii, "Meropriiatiia po bor'be s kholeroiu", p. 32.

36 C.A. Mark, "Kholera v selenii Kaachka Zakaspiiskoi oblasti", *Voenno-meditsinskii zhurnal*, vol. 179 (January 1894), pp. 1–47, here: p. 7. Frank Clemow, *The Cholera Epidemic of 1892 in the Russian Empire*, p. 2; Vladykin, *Materialy k istorii kholernoi epidemii 1892–95 gg.*, p. 13.

37 Kharitonov, "Kholernaia epidemiia v Rossii", p. 17. Mark, "Kholera v selenii Kaachka Zakaspiiskoi oblasti", p. 7.

38 Vladykin, *Materialy k istorii kholernoi epidemii 1892–95*, p. 13.

39 Mark, "Kholera v selenii Kaachka Zakaspiiskoi oblasti", pp. 1–47; see also Kharitonov, "Kholernaia epidemiia v Rossii", p. 17.

40 For an exhaustive report on the epidemic in Transcaspia and the measures taken against it see the *Otchet o kholernoi epidemii 1892 goda v voiskakh i naselenii oblastei podvedomstvennykh voennomu ministerstvu po rasporiazheniiu glavnovo voenno-meditsinskogo inspektora. Sostavlen sanitarno-statisticheskoii chastiiu Glavnogo Voenno-Meditsinskogo Upravleniia* (St Petersburg, 1893), pp. 5–59; on the events in Kaachka in particular see Mark, "Kholera v selenii Kaachka Zakaspiiskoi oblasti"; also Kharitonov, "Kholernaia epidemiia v Rossii", p. 17.

41 Kharitonov, "Kholernaia epidemiia v Rossii", pp. 17–18. Kharitonov's report concurs with the report of the director of the medical department of the civil administration in the Caucasus, Glavatskii, which he delivered at the cholera conference held in St Petersburg in December 1892. Glavatskii, "Meropriiatiia po bor'be s kholeroiu na Kavkaze", p. 33.

42 Cited in *Otchet o kholernoi epidemii 1892 v voiskakh i naselenii oblastei podvedomstvennykh voennomu ministerstvu*, p. 6; also Kharitonov, "Kholernaia epidemiia v Rossii", p. 18; Glavatskii, "Meropriiatiia po bor'be s kholeroiu na Kavkaze", p. 33.

43 Kharitonov, "Kholernaia epidemiia v Rossii", p. 18; Mark, "Kholera v selenii Kaachka Zakaspiiskoi oblasti", p. 20; see also the report by Lunkevich, "Obshchii otchet po komandirovkam v Zakaspiiskuiu oblast', po sluchaiu poiavleniia asiatskoi kholery, i v Persiiu, po povodu rassledovaniia slukhov o liudskoi chume", *Voenno-meditsinskii zhurnal*, vol. 176 (January 1893), pp. 49–72.

44 *Otchet o kholernoi epidemii 1892 v voiskakh i naselenii oblastei*, p. 6; Kharitonov, "Kholernaia epidemiia v Rossii", p. 18.

45 As already mentioned, for the large majority of provinces and cities the first cholera cases are impossible to identify. The dates given in the text follow the *Otchet o kholernoi epidemii 1892 v voiskakh i naselenii oblastei podvedomstvennykh voennomu ministerstvu*, pp. 16–32.

46 Kharitonov, "Kholernaia epidemiia v Rossii", p. 18; according to Poliakov the *vibrio* reached Uzun-Ada even earlier, on 22.5.1892. Poliakov, "Kholernaia epidemiia 1892 goda v g. Askhabade", p. 44.

47 This is the officially acknowledged date for the arrival of cholera in the city. As will be seen in the second part of this chapter, local physicians surmised the first cases occurred already on 1 June 1892.

48 Mery po ograzhdeniiu Imperii ot zanosa kholery s poberezh'iakh Kaspiiskogo moria, *Pravitel'stvennyi Vestnik*, no. 115, 30.5.1892.

49 "Nastavlenie dlia proizvodstva dezinfektsii tovarov, provozimykh cherez karantinno-nabliudatel'nye stantsii", Galanin, *Meropriiatiia protiv kholery*, pp. 56–57.

50 These regulations confirmed regulations which had already been issued in 1890: "Pravila snabzheniia sudov i pristanei trebuemymi, vysochaishe utverzhdennymi, 13-go iiulia 1890 g., pravilami sanitarnogo nadzora za rechnym sudokhodstvom v neblagopoluchnoe po kholere vremia, prinadlezhnostiami i osmotra takovykh sudov", Galanin, *Meropriiatiia protiv kholery*, pp. 66–67.

51 For the following see also Chapter 1.

52 Anti-plague measures certainly varied from country to country, but they generally included the closing of borders, the sealing off of infected places and areas, isolation of patients, and disinfection as well as fumigation of their belongings. Frequently, these measures were accompanied by the prohibition of public assemblies, burial regulations, orders concerning the cleanliness of streets and houses. John T. Alexander, *Bubonic Plague in Early Modern Russia: Public Health and Urban Disaster* (Baltimore, 1980); F.A. Derbek, *Istoriia chumnykh epidemii v Rossii s osnovaniia gosudarstva do nastoiashchego vremeni* (St Petersburg, 1905); See also with reference to Britain the articles by J.C. McDonald, "The History of Quarantine in Britain during the 19th Century", *BHM*, 25 (1951), pp. 22–44 and by Charles F. Mullett, "A Century of English Quarantine (1709–1825)", *BHM*, 23 (1949), pp. 527–545. For the significance of anti-plague measures for cholera epidemics see the analysis by Snowden, *Naples in the Time of Cholera*, pp. 78–90.

53 The swing of opinion on quarantine policy in medical and official circles is analysed by Evans, *Death in Hamburg*, pp. 243–251; see also Snowden, *Naples in the Time of Cholera*, pp. 78–84.

54 Snowden, *Naples in the Time of Cholera*, p. 84.

55 Ibid., esp. part II, chap. 2–4.

56 See also Chapter 1, pp. 21–23.

57 Evans, *Death in Hamburg*, esp. pp. 264–268.

58 Ibid., p. 275.

59 Pavlovskii, "Ob organisatsii i primenenii mediko-sanitarnykh mer, priniatykh protiv kholery v Povolzh'e, mezhdu Nizhnim Novgorodom i Astrakhan'iu i v Kamskom krae, po rekam Kame, Viatke i Beloi, v epidemiiu 1892 goda", *Trudy s"ezda vrachei*, pp. 368–382, here p. 377.

60 *Saratovskii Dnevnik*, no. 131, 23.6.1892.

61 At the above-mentioned conference in St Petersburg in December 1892 a whole session was dedicated to quarantine policies during the epidemic. The discussions and reports from the conference outline the various loopholes of the regulations. See esp. "Doklad redaktsionnoi kommissii o predupreditel'nykh protiv zanosa kholery merakh", *Trudy s"ezda vrachei*, pp. 206–251.

62 Ibid., p. 208.

63 P.N. Alianchikov, "Otchet o deiatel'nosti vo vremia prikomandirovaniia k Bakinskomu karantinu", *Trudy s"ezda vrachei*, pp. 320–336, here p. 326; also I.Z. Loris-Melikov, "Iz otcheta o poezdke v Persiiu", *VOGSPM*, vol. 27 (July 1895), pp. 1–38, here: p. 37.

64 Ibid., p. 37.

65 Alianchikov, "Otchet o deiatel'nosti", pp. 318–319. The regulation that passengers from Persia were not allowed to enter Russia existed until mid-September.

66 *Ustav Vrachebnyi*, art. 1082.

67 This critique was articulated by all the physicians coming from the various ends of the Caspian Sea. See, for instance, Alianchikov, "Otchet o deiatel'nosti", p. 320.

68 Ibid., p. 318.

69 Ibid., p. 329.

70 "Mediko-sanitarnyi nadzor vo vremia plavaniia i stoianki sudna" (MVD, 27.5.1892, §7), Galanin, *Meropriiatiia protiv kholery*, pp. 78.

71 Alianchikov, "Otchet o deiatel'nosti", p. 328. See also the reports of the physicians in the "Doklad redaktsionnoi kommissii o predupreditel'nykh protiv zanosa kholery merakh", *Trudy s"ezda vrachei*, pp. 206–251.

72 Alianchikov, "Otchet o deiatel'nosti", p. 329.

73 See the reports by the physicians Vorob'ev, Erem'ev and Proskuriakov (Astrakhan') as well as Alianchikov (Baku) in the "Doklad redaktsionnoi kommissii o predupreditel'nykh protiv zanosa kholery merakh", *Trudy s"ezda vrachei*, pp. 206–251.

74 Ibid., p. 220.

75 Ibid., p. 220.

76 Ibid., p. 214.

77 *Saratovskii Dnevnik*, no. 131, 23.6.1892; no. 134, 26.6.1892; the episode is also mentioned in Clemow, *The Cholera Epidemic of 1892*, p. 70; see also Frieden, *Russian Physicians*, p. 147.

78 R.V. Popov, "Kratkii obzor meropriiatii, vypolnennykh zemstvami Moskovskoi gubernii v vidu ugrozhaiushchei kholery", *Trudy s"ezda vrachei*, pp. 35–43, here: p. 35.

79 *Pravitel'stvennyi Vestnik*, no. 128, 14.6.1892. For the official acknowledgement of the cholera threat see Kharitonov, "Kholernaia epidemiia v Rossii", p. 17.

80 *Saratovskii Listok*, no.131, 23.6.1892.

81 On Baku during this period see the article by Audrey Altstadt-Mirhadi, "Baku. Transformation of a Muslim Town," Michael F. Hamm (ed.), *The City in Late Imperial Russia* (Indiana, 1986), pp. 283–318.

82 Ibid., p. 289.

83 Cited in Clemow, *The Cholera Epidemic of 1892*, p. 25.

84 Ibid., p. 26.

85 Estimates of this figure vary considerably. The administration of the Transcaucasian railway counted 44,000 fugitives. The newspaper *Kaspii* came to 100,000 as it counted another 30,000 fleeing by ship and the remainder fleeing by road. The *Saratovskii Dnevnik* came to 50,000 fugitives. See *Saratovskii Dnevnik*, no. 145, 9.7.1892. Clemow refers to official estimates giving the number of 75,000. Although he does not cite his source, this figure is probably more realistic. See Clemow, *The Cholera Epidemic of 1892 in the Russian Empire*, p. 71.

86 *Saratovskii Dnevnik*, no. 145, 9.7.1892.

87 *Saratovskii Dnevnik*, no. 139, 3.7.1892; also *St Peterburgskie Vedomosti*, no. 178, 16.7.1892; Clemow, *The Cholera Epidemic of 1892*, pp. 70–71.

88 Again, my dates follow the dates given by Clemow, *The Cholera Epidemic of 1892*, pp. 26–28.

89 Clemow, *The Cholera Epidemic of 1892*, p. 28.

90 For the course of the epidemic in Astrakhan' see N.I. Grigor'ev, "Kholera v Astrakhani v 1892 godu", *Zhurnal russkogo obshchestva okhraneniia narodnogo zdraviia*, 1892, no. 5, pp. 348–413.

91 The events circulated through the country's newspapers. My depiction is based on the article in the *Saratovskii Listok*, no. 134, 26.6.1892.

92 To compare, the epidemic needed 60 days to travel the 600 miles from Ekaterinoslav to Smolensk along the Dnepr.

93 Frank Clemow, *The Cholera Epidemic of 1892*, p. 34.

94 Amsterdamskii's examination of the epidemic is reported in "Protokol 87-go zasedaniia obshchestva saratovskikh sanitarnykh vrachei, 30.10.1892", *Protokoly zasedanii obshchestva Saratovskikh sanitarnykh vrachei za 1890,91,92 gg.* (Saratov, 1894), pp. 168–199, here p. 194. Official and medical documents demonstrate, however, that the first cholera case simply escaped any attention. According to I.I. Molleson, for instance, the epidemic began in the city on 19 June. Following Vladykin, it started on 22 June (when the epidemic's presence in the city was officially declared by St Petersburg). I.I. Molleson, "Organisatsiia dela bor'by s kholeroiu v Saratovskoi gubernii", *Trudy s"ezda vrachei*, pp. 27– 30, p. 27. Vladykin, *Materialy k istorii kholernoi epidemii*, p. 14.

95 For the following see the article by A.V. Amsterdamskii, "Kholernaia epidemiia 1892 goda v Saratove i ee sviaz' s sanitarnymi usloviiami goroda", *SSO*, 1895, no. 1–4, pp. 89–120; no. 5, pp. 180–189; no. 6, pp. 219–235; also his report in "Protokol 87-go zasedaniia obshchestva saratovskikh sanitarnykh vrachei, 30.10.1892", *Protokoly zasedanii obshchestva Saratovskikh sanitarnykh vrachei za 1890,91,92 gg.*, p. 195.

96 Amsterdamskii, "Kholernaia epidemiia 1892 goda v Saratove", pp. 90–91.

97 Ibid., p. 90; "Protokol 87-go zasedaniia obshchestva saratovskikh sanitarnykh vrachei, 30.10.1892", *Protokoly*, p. 199.

98 Rosental' was the head physician (*starshii vrach*) of Saratov's zemstvo hospital. "Doklad readaktsionnoi kommissii po voprosam ob organizatsii vrachebnoi pomoshchi naseleniiu, o sposobe obnaruzheniia pervogo sluchaia kholery i o registratsii zabolevaiushchikh i umiraiushchikh", *Trudy s"ezda vrachei*, pp. 142–194, p. 154.

99 See the report on the epidemic by the municipal physician I.V. Aleksandrovskii, which he gave to Saratov's sanitary society in December 1892. "Protokol 88-go zasedaniia obshchestva Saratovskikh sanitarnykh vrachei, 22.12.1892", *Protokoly*, p. 207.

100 Thus the conclusion by Amsterdamskii, "Protokol 87-go zasedaniia obshchestva saratovskikh sanitarnykh vrachei, 30.10.1892", *Protokoly*, p. 195.

101 "Ekstrennyi s"ezd vrachei i predstavitelei zemstv saratovskoi gubernii 25 iiunia 1892 goda", supplement to the *SSO* (July 1892), pp. 1–13.

102 *Saratovskii Listok*, no. 118, 7.6.1892; *Saratovskii Dnevnik*, no. 118, 7.6.1892.

103 *Saratovskii Dnevnik*, no. 118, 7.6.1892.

104 *Saratovskii Listok*, no. 120, 10.6.1892.

105 "Pervye meropriiatiia administratsii v vidu kholery", *Saratovskii Vestnik*, no. 133, 25.6.1892.

106 Frieden, *Russian Physicians*, p. 153.

107 Ibid., p. 153.

108 These extended rights were formalised in the zemstvo statute of 1890. See Frieden, *Russian Physicians*, pp. 286–287.

109 Witte held the ministry until August 1892 when he took over the Ministry of Finance.

110 This last point was articulated at the special provincial zemstvo meeting which only took place on 3.7. 1892. See *Saratovskii Dnevnik*, no. 140, 4.7.1892. Zemstvo institutions were established at both the provincial and the district levels. Most important for Saratov city, of course, was the collaboration with the provincial zemstvo. Yet the double institution of the zemstvo in the province and in the districts (uezdy) added another 10 institutions in Saratov province with which the provincial zemstvo had to coordinate its work.

111 The decree was published in the *Pravitel'stvennyi Vestnik*, no. 123, 13.6.1892.

112 According to Nancy Frieden the Sanitary Executive Commissions, institutionalised in 1893 as a result of the epidemic, were the decisive moment which changed the power relationships in the local administration of public health. Yet the commissions were for the first time established in 1892 to combat the cholera during the first year of the epidemic. As it turned out, in many places the Sanitary Executive Commissions faced the same problems as all the other local cholera committees: their responsibilities overlapped with many other institutions, financial resources were not clear, and, in the end, they could not act independently as neither their relation to the state nor to public institutions was clarified. In most places, the commissions therefore created more confusion instead of clarifying power relationships. For this reason their role and function were intensely discussed at the conference in St Petersburg. See "Doklad redaktsionnoi kommissii po voprosu ob organisatsii sanitarno-ispolnitel'nykh kommissii i sanitarnogo nadzora", *Trudy s"ezda vrachei*, pp. 1–58.

113 Leonid Dashkevich, *Nashe Ministerstvo Vnutrennykh Del* (Berlin, 1895), p. 69. On cholera see pp. 68–72.

114 The Russian terms of the provincial institutions were: *vrachebnaia uprava, gubernskii komitet obshchestvennogo zdraviia, gubernskoe zemskoe sobranie, gubernskaia*

zemskaia uprava. The function of the medical board (*vrachebnaia uprava*) was to assist the provincial governor. It mainly supervised medical personnel and institutions and supported the medical police; the *gubernskii komitet obshchestvennogo zdraviia* (provincial committee on public health) had the task to coordinate emergency measures and to distribute hygiene information. Both institutions worked under the auspices of the provincial governor. The Russian terms for the district institutions were *uezdnoe zemskoe sobranie, uezdnaia zemskaia uprava*. See Frieden, *Russian Physicians*, p. 64. For a concise analysis of provincial medical administration see in particular Samuel C. Ramer, "The Zemstvo and Public Health", Terence Emmons, Wayne S. Vucinich (eds), *The Zemstvo in Russia. An Experiment in Local Self-Government* (Cambridge, 1982), pp. 279–314.

115 Reports on the meetings can be found in *Saratovskii Listok*, no. 123, 13.6.1892; *Saratovskii Listok*, no. 124, 14.6.1892; *Saratovskii Dnevnik*, no. 125, 15.6.1892.

116 *Saratovskii Dnevnik*, no. 125, 15.6.1892.

117 Extensive reports on the duma meeting in *Saratovskii Dnevnik*, no. 127, 17.6.1892; *Saratovskii Listok*, no. 129, 20.6.1892.

118 The statute dated back to 14.12.1884. Unfortunately, it is not included in Galanin's work; yet its main points are set out in the *Saratovskii Dnevnik*, no. 140, 4.7.1892.

119 The official date of the epidemic's beginning in Astrakhan' was 18 June.

120 The report on the meeting in *Saratovskii Listok*, no. 130, 21.6.1892.

121 *Saratovskii Listok*, no. 130, 21.6.1892.

122 The dispute about the criteria for an official diagnosis of cholera was not confined to Russia. In Hamburg during the same summer, the Chief Medical Officer also followed the old method of diagnosis according to the symptoms of the disease, and thus decisively contributed to the series of delays which made the Hamburg epidemic so devastating. Evans, *Death in Hamburg*, pp. 285–290. For diagnosis as practised during the 1873 epidemic (the last epidemic in Hamburg before the bacteriological revolution), see pp. 251–256. Hamburg, however, presented an exceptional case in Germany.

123 "Doklad redaktsionnoi kommissii po voprosam ob organisatsii vrachebnoi pomoshchi naseleniiu, o sposobe obnaruzheniia pervogo sluchaia kholery i o registratsii zabolevaiushchikh i umiraiushchikh", *Trudy s"ezda vrachei*, pp. 141–193.

124 For this problem see the contribution by the physician from Iaroslavl' during the conference in St Petersburg. "Doklad redaktsinonnoi kommissii", pp. 144–145.

125 According to Amsterdamskii a number of cholera cases during the first week was diagnosed as *disenteria, gastro-enteritis*, or *cholera nostras* instead of *cholera asiatica*. Amsterdamskii, "Kholernaia epidemiia 1892 goda v Saratove", p. 90. The results of the laboratory analysis were revealed only on 24.6.1892. See A. Briusgin, "Epidemiia asiatskoi kholery v g. Saratove v 1892 g.", *Zhurnal russkogo obshchestva okhraneniia narodnogo zdraviia*, 1896, no. 6, pp. 537–549; also *Saratovskii Dnevnik*, no. 130, 22.6.1892.

126 Briusgin, "Epidemiia asiatskoi kholery v g. Saratove v 1892 g.", p. 541; *Saratovskii Listok*, no. 133, 25.6.1892.

127 The report of the meeting of the provincial health board in *Saratovskii Listok*, no. 130, 21.6.1892.

128 According to the plan from 1884 the uprava had to take the initial preparatory measures against the epidemic on its own, including the provision of disinfection means, accommodation and linens for the sick. As soon as the *vibrio* entered European Russia, however, the uprava had to convene a special zemstvo meeting to devise the full cholera plan. *Saratovskii Dnevnik*, no. 140, 4.7.1892; also *Saratovskii Listok*, no. 128, 19.6.1892.

129 Reports on the meeting of the zemstvo assembly (*zemskoe sobranie*) in *Saratovskii Dnevnik*, no. 140, 4.7.1892; *Saratovskii Dnevnik*, no. 142, 6.7.1892.

130 "Ekstrennyi s"ezd vrachei i predstavitelei zemstv Saratovskoi gubernii po voprosu o bor'be s kholeroiu, 25-go iiunia 1892", supplement to the *SSO*, June 1892, pp. 3–13.

There is also an extensive report on the meeting in *Saratovskii Dnevnik*, no. 137, 1.7.1892.
131 The measures elaborated by the provincial physicians essentially addressed the same problems as those suggested by the municipal sanitary commission and included a general clean-up of the city, the provision of healthy food, and the establishment of temporary cholera barracks at the banks. "Ekstrennyi s"ezd vrachei i predstavitelei zemstv", June 1892, p. 4.
132 I.I. Molleson, "Organisatsiia dela bor'by s kholeroiu v Saratovskoi gubernii", *Trudy s"ezda vrachei*, pp. 27–30; *Saratovskii Dnevnik*, no. 143, 4.7.1892.
133 *Saratovskii Dnevnik*, no. 136, 26.6.1892; *Saratovskii Listok*, no. 133, 25.6.1892.
134 *Saratovskii Dnevnik*, no. 127, 17.6.1892.
135 *Saratovskii Listok*, no. 129, 20.6.1892; *Saratovskii Listok*, no. 130, 21.6.1892; *Saratovskii Dnevnik*, no. 127, 17.6.1892.
136 *Saratovskii Dnevnik*, no. 138, 2.7.1892; *Saratovskii Listok*, no. 134, 26.6.1892; "Protokol soedinennogo zasedaniia obshchestva saratovskikh sanitarnykh vrachei s chlenami fiziko-meditsinskogo obshchestva, 24.6.1892," *Protokoly*, pp. 175–179.
137 *Saratovskii Listok*, no. 130, 21.6.1892.
138 I.I. Molleson, *Derevenskie besedy po kholere* (Saratov, 1893). These recommendations were also widely circulated in the newspapers. See, for instance, *Saratovskii Vestnik*, no. 133, 25.6.1892; *Saratovskii Dnevnik*, no. 140, 4.7.1892.
139 For the debates on the Demidov house and its opening see *Saratovskii Listok*, no. 124, 14.6.1892; *Saratovskii Dnevnik*, no. 131, 23.6.1892.
140 Apart from the Demidov house the city established another cholera hospital for 50 patients on 24 June; three more barracks were established by the municipality on 5 July with 54 beds each. *Saratovskii Listok*, no. 134, 26.6.1892; *Saratovskii Listok*, no. 136, 28.6.1892. *Saratovskii Dnevnik*, no. 143, 6.7.1892. The zemstvo cholera hospital was opened on 8 July, *Saratovskii Dnevnik*, no. 145, 9.7.1892.
141 *Saratovskii Listok*, no. 132, 24.6.1892; also *Saratovskii Listok*, no. 136, 28.6.1892.
142 The Demidov house provided another 75 beds, but the building was burned down during the riots, shortly before the epidemic reached its peak.
143 *Saratovskii Dnevnik*, no. 127, 17.6.1892. *Saratovskii Listok*, no. 134, 26.6.1892.
144 *Saratovskii Dnevnik*, no. 140, 4.7.1892; the original plan of the duma calculated 400 vigilants, *Saratovskii Dnevnik*, no. 130, 22.6.1892.
145 *Saratovskii Listok*, no. 133, 25.6.1892.
146 *Saratovskii Dnevnik*, no. 130, 22.6.1892.
147 The municipality rejected this idea on the grounds that it would provide a 'dangerous precedent'. *Saratovskii Listok*, no. 129, 20.6.1892; also *Saratovskii Dnevnik*, no. 140, 4.7.1892.
148 *Saratovskii Dnevnik*, no. 128, 20.6.1892.
149 *Saratovskii Dnevnik*, no. 143, 7.7.1892. Numerous other examples were reported in the newspapers. The physicians, too, complained about the unthorough and incompetent conduct of the police during disinfection procedures not only at private homes but also at the railway station and at the river. See the report on Saratov by Dr. Parfenovskii in "Doklad subkommissii po ustanovleniiu nadzora za peredvizheniem naseleniia po razlichnym putiam coobshcheniia", *Trudy s"ezda vrachei*, pp. 283–301, esp. p. 288.
150 These are the figures provided by medical officials. Amsterdamskii, "Protokol 87-go zasedaniia obshchestva saratovskikh sanitarnykh vrachei, 30 oktiabria 1892 goda", *Protokoly*, p. 197.
151 Evans, *Death in Hamburg*, pp. 292–298. To compare, in Glasgow in 1832 cholera mortality stood at 15 per thousand and in Paris in 1832 at 21.8 per thousand. In St Petersburg in 1832 it ran to 40 per thousand. The highest cholera mortality rates were recorded in Montreal in 1832 (74 per thousand) and in Hungary as late as 1873 (65 per thousand), see ibid., p. 294.

152 Again, this is only an approximate figure. It is calculated from the absolute numbers of deaths provided by N. Matveev for the time between 1895 and 1906. N. Matveev, *Gorod Saratov v sanitarnom otnoshenii v 1906 godu* (Saratov, 1908), p. 88.

153 Ibid., p. 87.

154 P.N. Sokolov, "Sanitarnyi ocherk goroda Saratova", *SZN*, 1904, no. 5, p. 54. The figures given by the police can only be used as an indicator here. It is impossible to check how these numbers were calculated and what the exact reasons were for such a difference.

155 "Protokol 87 ocherednogo zasedaniia Obshchestva Saratovskikh sanitarnyk vrachei, 14 oktiabria 1892 goda," *Protokoly*, p. 197; Amsterdamskii, "Kholernaia epidemiia 1892 goda v Saratove", p. 97.

156 These and the following figures were provided by Amsterdamskii, "Kholernaia epidemiia 1892 goda v Saratove", p. 92–93. Unfortunately, the city issued no health bulletin which would allow one to trace the number of cholera cases and deaths on a daily basis.

157 *Saratovskii Dnevnik*, no. 140, 4.7.1892. The cemetery recorded 249 adults and 613 children in one month in 1892 as opposed to 135 adults and 569 children in the whole year of 1891.

158 This was, in particular, Louis Chevalier's approach to study the epidemic. Chevalier, *Le Choléra*, esp. pp. 13–24.

159 Evans, *Death in Hamburg*, chap. 5, pp. 403–469.

160 *Sbornik otchetov vrachei i studentov*, pp. 317–342; Amsterdamskii, "Kholernaia epidemia 1892 goda v Saratove", pp. 94–95; A. Briusgin, "Epidemiia asiatskoi kholery v g. Saratove v 1892 g.", *Zhurnal russkogo obshchestva okhraneniia narodnogo zdravia*, 1896, no. 6, pp. 537–459.

161 See the report by Amsterdamskii in "Protokol 87-go ocherednogo zasedaniia obshchestva Saratovskikh sanitarnyk vrachei, 30 oktiabria 1892 goda", *Protokoly*, pp. 194–198.

162 Amsterdamskii, "Kholernaia epidemiia 1892 goda v Saratove", p. 96.

163 Ibid., pp. 98–114.

164 The map is reprinted in Matveev, *Gorod Saratov v sanitarnom otnoshenii*.

165 These included among others the clergy (4), honorary citizens (2), military (5), merchants (1), nobility (1), students (1), feldsher (1), Austrian citizens (2), officials (*chinovniki*) (2). *Sbornik otchetov vrachei i studentov*, p. 333.

166 Briusgin, "Epidemiia asiatskoi kholery v gorode Saratove v 1892 g.", p. 544.

167 *Sbornik otchetov vrachei i studentov*, p. 333.

168 Ibid., pp. 333–334. The high percentage of migrant workers in the hospital is also confirmed by Briusgin, "Epidemiia asiatskoi kholery v gorode Saratove v 1892 g.", p. 544.

169 *Saratovskii Dnevnik*, no. 128, 18.6.1892. Clemow, in his account on the cholera, refers to the legend as well. In Clemow's version 'God ordered the cholera to carry off five hundred victims: in the end 3000 died. Five-sixths died from fear.' See Clemow, *The Cholera Epidemic of 1892*, p. 62. The journalist revived a widespread view which explained the epidemic in terms of moral reasons or psychological disturbances. First and foremost, however, the legend stands in a religious context which ascribed the outbreak of epidemic diseases to the wrath of God. For the moral and psychological explanatory model of the disease see Evans, *Death in Hamburg*, pp. 235–236. The theology of cholera is discussed by Snowden, *Naples in the Time of Cholera*, pp. 71–74.

170 *Saratovskii Dnevnik*, no. 128, 18.6.1892.

171 Louis Chevalier, *Le Choléra*, p. 23.

172 Briggs, "Cholera and Society in the Nineteenth Century", p. 76.

173 The Haymarket riot is analysed by McGrew, *Russia and the Cholera*, pp. 111–114; see also Hubertus Jahn, "Der St. Petersburger Heumarkt im 19. Jahrhundert.

Metamorphosen eines Stadtviertels", *JfGO*, vol. 44 (1996), pp. 162–177, esp. pp. 167–168.

174 David Steel, "Plague Writing: From Boccaccio to Camus", *Journal of European Studies*, xi (1981), pp. 88–110. Alexander Pushkin, "Pir vo vremia chumy", A.S. Pushkin *Sobranie sochinenii v desiati tomakh*, vol. 4 (Moscow, 1960), pp. 371–381.

175 The riots at the lower Volga during the first pandemic happened in 1830, the year before the Haymarket riots. In 1831, the regions worst affected were Volhynia and Podolia. McGrew, *Russia and the Cholera*, esp. pp. 67–74; for the course of the epidemic in 1831 see pp. 98–100.

176 See Snowden, *Naples in the Time of Cholera*, esp. chap. 2, pp. 138–154; also Snowden, "Cholera in Barletta 1910".

177 For the discussion of the social response in Hamburg see Evans, *Death in Hamburg*, pp. 346–372.

178 Frequent articles in the newspapers reported on the refugees. The first comments appeared around mid-June. See, for instance, *Saratovskii Listok*, no. 127, 18.6.1892.

179 V. Kolpenskii, "Kholernyi bunt v 1892 godu", *Arkhiv istorii truda v Rossii*, vol. III (Petrograd, 1922), pp. 104–113, see pp. 107–108.

180 *Saratovskii Listok*, no. 120, 10.6.1892; no. 129, 20.6.1892.

181 *Saratovskii Dnevnik*, no. 128, 18.6.1892.

182 I.I. Molleson, "V ozhidanie kholery", *SZN*, 1892, no. 2, pp. 425–434. See also the comment in *Saratovskii Listok*, no. 130, 21.6.1892.

183 According to Russian quarantine law the minimum punishment for the violation of quarantine regulations was eight years of hard labour. For the significance of the plague at Vertlianka for the people's perception of the cholera epidemic see the report by Dr Shiklarskii, a district physician in Saratov province, at the conference in St Petersburg in December 1892. "Doklad redaktsionnoi kommissii o predupreditel'nykh protiv zanosa kholery merakh", *Trudy s"ezda vrachei*, pp. 206–208.

184 Kharitonov, "Kholernaia Epidemiia v Rossii v 1892–1895 godakh", pp. 8–15. Matveev, "Kholera v Saratove", *Saratovskii Dnevnik*, no. 127, 17.6.1892.

185 Gusev, Khovanskii, *Saratovets*, pp. 27–29.

186 Ibid., p. 27.

187 For a series of reasons cholera never produced such extreme social reactions as did the bubonic plague. In part, the explanation for the lower level of violence caused by cholera lies in the fact that the epidemic never claimed as many victims as the plague. See the discussion by Snowden, *Naples in the Time of Cholera*, pp. 151–153.

188 Clemow, *The Cholera Epidemic of 1892*, p. 44.

189 *Saratovskii Listok*, no. 131, 23.6.1892. Reports in the local newspapers about overcrowded ships are abundant. See also *Saratovskii Dnevnik*, no. 140, 4.7.1892; *Saratovskii Dnevnik*, no. 139, 3.7.1892.

190 *Saratovskii Listok*, no. 196, 18.7.1892; see also *Saratovskii Dnevnik*, no. 129, 19.6.1892.

191 This belief was maintained in the local newspapers: *Saratovskii Listok*, no. 196, 18.7.1892; *Saratovskii Dnevnik*, no. 129, 19.6.1892.

192 *Saratovskii Listok*, no. 196, 18.7.1892.

193 *Saratovskii Dnevnik*, no. 143, 7.7.1892.

194 McGrew, *Russia and the Cholera*, p. 109.

195 Ibid., p. 109.

196 *Saratovskii Listok*, no. 129, 20.6.1892.

197 *Saratovskii Dnevnik*, no. 134, 26.6.1892; *Saratovskii Listok*, no. 133, 25.6.1892.

198 *Saratovskii Dnevnik*, no. 134, 26.6.1892.

199 Galanin, *Meropriiatiia protiv kholery russkogo i inostrannykh pravitel'stv*, p. 59.

200 Daniel Defoe, *A Journal of the Plague Year* (London, 1722); Alessandro Manzoni, *The Betrothed* (Milan, 1827).

201 See the complaint by the physician A.M. Sal'ko on a meeting of the municipal duma on 26 June. The report on the duma meeting in *Saratovskii Listok*, no. 136, 28.6.1892.

202 Cited in Kolpenskii, "Kholernyi bunt v 1892 godu", p. 108. The document was sent to the newspaper *Novoe Vremia* on 28 June but was intercepted by the police in the printing-house.

203 This is pointed out by Evans, *Death in Hamburg*, p. 228–320.

204 Evans, *Death in Hamburg*, p. 227; Snowden, *Naples in the Time of Cholera*, p. 112–116.

205 For the complex reasons behind this important paradigmatic shift see the interesting discussion by Evans, *Death in Hamburg*, pp. 502–507. The widespread criticism which Koch's theories still encountered during the epidemic is discussed on pp. 490–497.

206 Briusgin, "Epidemiia asiatskoi kholery v gorode Saratov v 1892 g.", p. 538; A.D. Pavlovskii, "Ob organisatsii i primenenii mediko-sanitarnykh mer, priniatykh protiv kholery v Povolzh'e mezhdu Nizhnim Novgorodom i Astrakhan'iu i v Kamskom krae, po rekam Kame, Viatke i Beloi, v epidemiiu 1892 goda", *Trudy s"ezda vrachei*, pp. 363–383, see p. 368.

207 Pavlovskii, "Ob organisatsii i primenenii mediko-sanitarnykh mer", pp. 363–383.

208 S.A. Lias', "Kholernye zametki i vpechatleniia", *Sbornik otchetov vrachei i studentov*, p. 82.

209 An extensive report on treatment methods in Russia during the 1892 epidemic is T.I. Bogomolov, "Ocherk sposobov lecheniia kholery, primeniavshikhcia v epidemiiu 1892 goda", *Sovremennaia klinika*, 1893, no. 6–7, pp. 353–456.

210 Hot baths had been used against cholera since the first epidemic in 1831 and were still standard treatment everywhere in Europe by the end of the nineteenth century. Evans, *Death in Hamburg*, pp. 327–346; Snowden, *Naples in the Time of Cholera*, pp. 121–138.

211 For a discussion on cholera treatment over the whole period from 1831 until 1892 see Evans, *Death in Hamburg*, pp. 327–346; with emphasis on Italy until 1884 Snowden, *Naples in the Time of Cholera*, pp. 112–138.

212 Treatment methods varied from hospital to hospital. My information is based on an account of the epidemic in the zemstvo hospital, the biggest cholera hospital in the city in 1892. The (untitled) article is written by V. Devlezerskii and published in *Vrach*, no. 40, 1892, p. 1014. It is noteworthy, that in many aspects Hamburg's physicians in 1892 were not much more advanced than Saratov's and administered the same or equally poisonous substances. By contrast, Naples' physicians in 1884 no longer experimented with purgatives, emetics, strychnin, or bloodletting. See Evans, *Death in Hamburg*, pp. 337–338 and Snowden, *Naples in the time of Cholera*, p. 128.

213 The "bismuth treatment" was the most famous cholera cure of the first pandemic, developed by Dr Leo of Warsaw. See the discussion by McGrew, *Russia and the Cholera*, pp. 140–141. For calomel and depletive therapies in general during the first pandemic including bloodletting, purgatives, and emetics, see Evans, *Death in Hamburg*, pp. 337–338 and Snowden, *Naples during the Time of Cholera*, pp. 123–125. Calomel was also the most frequently employed remedy in St Petersburg's hospitals in 1892. Other substances used in the capital included castor oil, camphor, strychnine, thymol, creolin and naphthol. There is no mentioning of these disinfectants in the sources available on Saratov. The treatment methods in St Petersburg are described by Frank Clemow, *The Cholera Epidemic of 1892*, chap. 10; also art. 1747 in *Vrach*, no. 36, 1892.

214 Of the 615 cases who entered the hospital between 15 June and 28 August, 345 died. For mortality figures in the hospital see *Vrach*, no. 40, 1892.

215 Galanin, *Meropriiatiia protiv kholery*, p. 59. For traditional forms of commemoration of death in late imperial Russia see Catherine Merridale, *Night of Stone. Death and Memory in Russia* (London, 2000).

216 Galanin, *Meropriiatiia protiv kholery*, p. 56. For burial practices during the epidemic see also Frieden, *Russian Physicians*, p. 147.
217 *Saratovskii Dnevnik*, no. 137, 1.7.1892; *Saratovskii Listok*, no. 177, 3.7.1892.
218 *Saratovskii Dnevnik* no. 138, 2.7.1892.
219 *Saratovskii Dnevnik*, no. 139, 3.7.1892.
220 The newspapers report all kinds of attempts to evade official instructions. For the given examples see *Saratovskii Dnevnik*, no. 142, 6.7.1892; *Saratovskii Dnevnik*, no. 143, 7.7.1892; also "Protokol 87-zasedaniia obshchestva Saratovskikh sanitarnykh vrachei 30 oktiabria 1892 goda", *Protokoly*, pp. 195–199; *Sbornik otchetov vrachei i studentov*.
221 *Saratovskii Listok*, no. 184, 22.6.1892.
222 *Saratovskii Dnevnik*, no. 138, 2.7.1892; *Saratovskii Listok*, no. 177, 3.7.1892.
223 My account of the course of the cholera riot is based primarily on newspaper reports in *Saratovskii Listok*, no. 182, 4.7.1892; *Russkie Vedomosti*, no. 286, 26.10.1892; *St Peterburgskie Vedomosti*, no. 179, 3.7.1892.
224 *Saratovskii Listok*, no. 137, 1.7.1892.
225 A report of the meeting in *Saratovskii Dnevnik*, no. 140, 4.7.1892.
226 *Saratovskii Listok*, no. 177, 3.7.1892.
227 See the comments on the riots in *Saratovskii Listok*, no. 142, 7.7.1892, *Saratovskii Dnevnik*, no. 137, 1.7.1892.
228 *Saratovskii Listok*, no. 177, 3.7.1892.
229 Otchet Gubernatora Saratovskoi Gubernii za 1892, RGIA, f. 1284, op. 223, d. 201, 1892.
230 Daniel R. Brower, "Labor Violence in Russia in the Late Nineteenth Century", *Slavic Review* 41 (autumn 1982), pp. 417–431.
231 Ibid., p. 427.
232 Robert E. Johnson, "Primitive Rebels? Reflections on Collective Violence in Imperial Russia", *Slavic Review*, 41 (autumn 1982), pp. 432–435; Ronald Grigor Suny, "Violence and Class Consciousness in the Russian Working Class", *Slavic Review* 41 (autumn 1982), pp. 436–442; Diane Koenker, "Collective Action and Collective Violence in the Russian Labor Movement", *Slavic Review* 41 (autumn 1982), pp. 443–448; Daniel R. Brower, "Labor Violence – a Reply", *Slavic Review* 41 (autumn 1982), pp. 449–453.
233 Theodore H. Friedgut, "Labor Violence and Regime Brutality in Tsarist Russia: The Iuzovka Cholera Riots of 1892", *Slavic Review*, 1988, pp. 245–265.
234 Ibid., p. 257.
235 Cholera riots have been extensively analysed in the international historiography on the epidemic. See in particular the recent works by Dettke, *Die Asiatische Hydra* und Catherine J. Kudlick, *Cholera in Post-Revolutionary Paris. A Cultural History* (Berkeley, 1996).
236 *Russkie Vedomosti*, no. 296, 26.10.1892. Also *Saratovskii Listok*, no. 286, 26.10.1892. With regard to the sources I have used to analyse the cholera riot in 1892 it is striking that the disturbances are not only described in full detail in the newspapers. Also, the public reports offer different and contradictory perspectives on one and the same event and thus to a considerable extent undermine whatever censorship might have controlled public reporting on the riots.
237 *Russkie Vedomosti*, no. 297, 27.10.1892; *Russkie Vedomosti*, no. 298, 28.10.1892.
238 Of the 152 people at the riot, 21 were under 20 years old, 48 were between 20 and 30, 39 were between 30 and 40, 32 were between 40 and 50, and 12 were over 50 years old. *Russkie Vedomosti*, no. 297, 27.10.1892.
239 Friedgut, "Labor Violence and Regime Brutality in Tsarist Russia", pp. 259–260.
240 Michael Melancon, "Athens or Babylon?", p. 84.
241 Rudé, *The Crowd in History*, p. 245; Snowden, *Naples in the Time of Cholera*, pp. 138–141.

242 Orlando Figes, *Peasant Russia, Civil War. The Volga Countryside in Revolution (1917–1921)* (Oxford, 1986), chap. 1; I.V. Parokh, *Ocherki istorii Saratovskogo Povolzh'ia*, 2 vols, (Saratov, 1995), vol. 1 (1855–1894), chap. 8.

243 Pamela Sears McKinsey, "Populists, Workers, and Peasants", Rex A. Wade, Scott J. Seregny (eds), *Politics and Society in Provincial Russia: Saratov, 1590–1917* (Ohio, 1989), pp. 66–67.

244 Plekhanov noted that the social composition of Saratov's worker circles differed from those in St Petersburg. In Saratov, worker circles were frequently dominated by shop owners and independent craftsmen. See McKinsey, "Populists, Workers, and Peasants", p. 66. For a direct account of these meetings in Saratov see the report by Kanatchikov, Reginald E. Zelnik (ed. and trans.), *A Radical Worker in Tsarist Russia: The Autobiography of Semen Ivanovich Kanatchikov* (Stanford, 1986).

245 The announcement was reprinted in the *Saratovskii Listok,* no. 139, 4.7.1892.

246 Pavlovskii, *Kholernye gody v Rossii*, p. 371.

247 *Vrach*, no. 29, 1892, p. 738.

248 Frieden, *Russian Physicians*, p. 145.

249 *Vrach*, no. 29, 1892, p. 738. Reports on the difficulties the physicians encountered in the districts and villages of Saratov province are abundant in the collection on the course of the epidemic in Saratov province, published by the provincial zemstvo in 1893.

250 *Vrach*, no. 29, 1892, p. 738.

251 *Vrach*, no. 29, 1892, p. 738.

252 *St Peterburgskie Vedomosti*, no. 178, 4.7.1892.

253 Reports on the meeting in *Saratovskii Dnevnik*, no. 140, 4.7.1892; *Saratovskii Dnevnik*, no. 137, 1.7.1892.

254 *Sbornik otchetov vrachei i studentov.*

255 The eight cholera cases by far do not match the reality. The fact that the 28 June was the day of the riot might account for the strikingly low figure. "Protokol 87-go zasedaniia obshchestva Saratovskikh sanitarnykh vrachei, 30.10.1892," *Protokoly*, p. 197.

256 *Saratovskii Dnevnik*, no. 141, 5.7.1892.

257 Morris, *Cholera 1832*, p. 17.

258 Evans, "Epidemics and Revolutions", p. 127.

259 Robbins, *Famine in Russia*, pp. 175–176.

260 For this view see for instance Orlando Figes, *A People's Tragedy. The Russian Revolution, 1891–1924* (London, 1996), esp. pp. 157–164; Geoffrey Hosking, *Russia. People and Empire, 1552–1917* (Cambridge, MA., 1997), pp. 398–399; Frieden, *Russian Physicians*, pp. 138–143 and 158–162.

261 Pavlovskii, "Ob organisatsii i primenenii mediko-sanitarnykh mer", p. 377.

262 The measures along the railway lines were issued by the Ministry of Ways and Communications on 27 June.

4 Sanitised politics and the politics of medicine

1 See in particular the contributions in the *Trudy s"ezda vrachei prinimavshikh neposredstvennoe uchastie v bor'be s kholernoi epidemiei 1892 g. v Rossii s 13. po 20. dekabriia 1892 goda* (St Petersburg, 1893).

2 Durey, *The Return of the Plague*, p. 1.

3 Rosenberg, *The Cholera Years 1832–1859*, p. 452.

4 See for this view the discussion by Snowden, *Naples in the Time of Cholera*, p. 177.

5 Snowden, *Naples in the Time of Cholera*, p. 177; Evans, *Death in Hamburg*, pp. 475–476.

6 Snowden, *Naples in the Time of Cholera*, p. 178.

7 Figes, *A People's Tragedy*, p. 162.

8 Frieden, *Russian Physicians*, p. 161.

9 For this evaluation see also, for instance, Alan K. Wildman, *The Making of a Workers' Revolution: Russian Social Democracy, 1891–1903* (Chicago, 1967), pp. 1–14; Leopold H. Haimson, *The Russian Marxists and the Origins of Bolshevism* (Boston, 1955), pp. 49–51; more recently, Geoffrey Hosking, *Russia. People and Empire* (Cambridge, Mass., 1997), esp. pp. 398–399.

10 Amsterdamskii, "Kholernaia Epidemiia 1892 goda v Saratove", p. 92.

11 Ibid., p. 92.

12 The epidemic had much less of an impact during the following three years. According to Vladykin, the province counted 1,417 cases and 645 deaths in 1893 and 453 cases and 251 deaths in 1894. It was cholera free in 1895. Vladykin, *Materialy k istorii kholernoi epidemii 1892–1895*, pp. 20–21.

13 Morris, *Cholera 1832*, p. 2.

14 This argument has been put forward most notably for the British and the German case. See for instance Terence Ranger, Paul Slack (eds), *Epidemics and Ideas. Essays on the Historical Perception of Pestilence* (Cambridge, 1992), p. 13; E.P. Hennock, "The Urban Sanitary Movement in England and Germany, 1838–1914: A Comparison", *Continuity and Change*, vol. 15, no. 2 (2000), pp. 269–296; Florian Tennstaedt, *Sozialgeschichte der Sozialpolitik in Deutschland. Vom 18. Jahrhundert bis zum Ersten Weltkrieg* (Göttingen, 1982), pp. 207–210.

15 Durey, *The Return of the Plague*, p. 205; also Morris, *Cholera 1832*, p. 198.

16 Rosenberg, "Cholera in Nineteenth-Century Europe", p. 455.

17 Pelling, *Cholera, Fever, and English Medicine*, p. 6.

18 Evans, *Death in Hamburg*, chap. 6.

19 Snowden, *Naples in the Time of Cholera*, chap. 5.

20 Evans, *Death in Hamburg*, pp. 513–522.

21 Snowden, *Naples in the Time of Cholera*, pp. 191–201.

22 McGrew, *Russia and the Cholera*, p. 15.

23 The Medical Department of the Ministry of Internal Affairs supported this development through the publication of two major medical journals, the *Archive of Forensic Medicine and Public Hygiene* (1865–1871) and the *Medical Topographical Collection* (1870–1876).

24 Frieden, *Russian Physicians*, pp. 113–122.

25 Erisman had first arrived in Russia in 1869 but then went back to western Europe in order to study with Max von Pettenkofer in Munich. He returned to Russia in 1875 and established his reputation with a monumental 19-volume study on the sanitary conditions in the factories of Moscow province. Between 1879 and 1896, Erisman played a key role in the development of medical preventive programmes in the Moscow zemstvo, Russia's most progressive and exemplary zemstvo in the field of public health organisation. For a short biography of Friedrich Erisman and his work in Russia see Frieden, *Russian Physicians*, pp. 99–104.

26 Hutchinson, *Politics and Public Health in Revolutionary Russia*, esp. pp. 85–107.

27 "Protokol 86 ocherednogo zasedaniia obshchestva Saratovskikh sanitarnykh vrachei, 14.10.1892", *Protokoly zasedanii obshchestva Saratovskikh sanitarnykh vrachei za 1890,91,92*, pp. 180–190. The exception among Saratov's physicians was Amsterdamskii, who conducted the special investigation into the cholera epidemic in 1892 and actually knew more about the epidemic than anybody else in the city. He held the contagionist position, scientifically proven by Robert Koch, which considered the decisive factor in the spread of cholera to be the water supply. The link of bad sanitation with disease can be traced back to Edwin Chadwick's public health reforms in Britain in the mid-nineteenth century. However, Russia's physicians were looking to Germany for reform ideas.

28 S. Gusev, A. Khovanskii, *Saratovets*, p. 81.

29 Amsterdamskii, "Kholernaia epidemiia 1892 goda v Saratove", p. 96.

30 Ibid., p. 97.

31 For examples see *Saratovskii Listok*, no. 140, 5.7.1892; no. 143, 8.7.1892; no. 130, 21.6.1892.

32 *Russkie Vedomosti*, no. 234, 25.8.1892.

33 P. Sokolov, "O sanitarnom sostoianii Saratovskikh ovragov", *SZN*, 1905, no. 4, p. 23.

34 Amsterdamskii, "Kholernaia Epidemiia 1892 goda v Saratove", pp. 96–97 and 101.

35 RGIA, f. 1287, op. 33, d. 2446, 1892.

36 For the work of the commission and the history of Saratov's sewage system in the 1890s in general see M.I. Krotkov, *O neobkhodimosti i vozmozhnoi zamene nyne proektiruemykh sposobov udaleniia iz goroda Saratova nechistot i otbrosov gorodskoi zhizni i uborki ikh na svalochnom uchastke gorodskoi zemli luchshimi sposobami ikh udaleniia i uborki* (Saratov, 1898), pp. 7–27; also V.I. Almazov, "O kanalizatsii v Saratove", *ISGD*, 1907, no. 1, pp. 115–136.

37 Krotkov, *O neobkhodimosti i vozmozhnoi zamene nyne proektiruemykh sposobov udaleniia iz goroda Saratova nechistot*, pp. 20–27.

38 Ibid., p. 20 and 25–26.

39 Ibid., p. 19.

40 N. Savel'ev, "K voprosu o prinuditel'nom ozdorovlenii russkikh gorodov", *Gorodskoe Delo*, 1908, no. 15, pp. 731–739.

41 V.I. Likhachev, *Sanitarnoe opisanie Povol'zhia* (St Petersburg, 1898), p. 5.

42 The full report of the 'commission to prevent the outbreak of plague in the empire and to fight against it' (komissiia o preduprezhdenii zaneseniia v imperiiu chumnoi zarazy i o bor'be s neiu) can be found in RGIA, f. 1298, op. 1, 1892 g., d. 2871. For the account on Saratov see ll. 202–211. Likhachev had been elected mayor of St Petersburg in 1885.

43 This was the *kommissiia dlia ozdorovleniia gorodov Astrakhani, Tsaritsyna, Saratova, i Samary*, soon known as the *ozdorovitel'naia kommissiia*. For the commission's report see G.V. Khlopin, *Materialy po ozdorovleniiu Rossii. Sanitarnoe opisanie gorodov Astrakhani, Samary, Saratova, Tsaritsyna s ukazaniem mer, neobkhodimykh dlia ikh ozdorovleniia* (St Petersburg, 1911).

44 The new municipal statute of 1892, in particular, restricted the possibilities of gaining revenue from local taxation. V.A. Nardova, *Samoderzhavie i gorodskie dumy v Rossii v kontse XIX-nachale XX veka* (St Petersburg, 1994).

45 Nardova, *Samoderzhavie i gorodskie dumy v Rossii*, p. 53. Saratov had a substantially greater budget than most Russian cities and its income ranked among one of the highest: St Petersburg (16.7 million), Moscow (13.8 million), Odessa (6 million), Riga (4 million), Kiev (2.5 million), Khar'kov (1.9 million), Rostov-na-Donu (1.5 million), Samara (1.5 million). Ibid., p. 53. As compared to western European cities, however, Russia's municipal budgets looked rather meagre. Paris, for instance, disposed of 123 million rubles at the end of the nineteenth century; London of 84,338,140 rubles; Berlin 55 million rubles whereas in Russia the income of all cities together amounted to 112 million rubles. See M. Volynskii, "Pervyi s"ezd russkikh gorodskikh deiatelei i ego blizhaishie zadachi", *Gorodskoe Delo*, no. 16, 1908, pp. 795–802, here: p. 800. Also Nardova, cited above, p. 49. The exact costs of Chizhov's canalisation were 1,580,000 rubles. See Khlopin, *Materialy po ozdorovleniiu*, p. 222.

46 *Ves' Saratov. Spravochnik-Kalendar'* (Saratov, 1916), p. 38.

47 *Doklad biudzhetnoi kommissii gorodskoi dumy* (Saratov,1909), p. 145.

48 Nardova, *Samoderzhavie i gorodskie dumy v Rossii*, pp. 62–66.

49 Frederick W. Skinner, "Odessa and the Problem of Urban Modernization", Michael F. Hamm (ed.), *The City in Late Imperial Russia* (Bloomington, 1986), pp. 209–248, here: p. 222; see also his "Trends in Planning Practices: The Building of Odessa, 1794–1917", Michael F. Hamm (ed.), *The City in Russian History* (Lexington, 1976), pp. 139–195, in particular pp. 148–152.

50 Nardova, *Samoderzhavie i gorodskie dumy v Rossii*, p. 62.

51 Ibid., p. 62. Saratov received the loan in 1902. Khlopin, *Materialy po ozdorovleniiu Rossii*, p. 223.

52 Protokol zasedaniia Saratovskoi Gorodskoi Dumy, *ISGD* 1907, no. 3, pp. 186–194.

53 Khlopin, *Materialy po ozdorovleniiu Rossii*, p. 223.

54 Ibid., pp. 223–224.

55 Ibid., p. 223.

56 This was in particular due to the new municipal statute from 1892. V.A. Nardova, *Samoderzhavie i gorodskie dumy v Rossii*, pp. 20–21. The percentage reflected the situation in most other Russian cities. See the articles on individual cities in Hamm (ed.), *The City in Late Imperial Russia*.

57 Nardova, *Samoderzhavie i gorodskie dumy v Rossii*, p. 23.

58 "Protokol 87-go zasedaniia obshchestva Saratovskikh sanitarnykh vrachei, 30.10.1892 goda", pp. 191–205.

59 "Protokol 86-go zasedaniia obshchestva Saratovskikh sanitarnykh vrachei, 14.10.1892 goda", pp. 180–189.

60 "Protokol zasedaniia Saratovskoi gorodskoi sanitarnoi kommissii, 21.8.1907", *ISGD*, 1907, no. 4, p. 284.

61 See the discussion in "Protokol zasedaniia Saratovskoi gorodskoi sanitarnoi kommissii, 7.11.1907", *ISGD*, 1907, pp. 430–412; also V.I. Almazov, "O kanalisatsii v Saratove. Doklad gorodskoi dume", *ISGD*, 1907, no. 1, pp. 114–136.

62 "Protokol zasedanii Saratovskoi gorodskoi kanalizatsionnoi kommissii, 22.5.1907", *ISGD*, 1907, no. 4, pp. 53–64, esp. pp. 56–61.

63 "Doklad gorodskoi upravy v Saratovskuiu gorodskuiu dumu", *ISGD*, 1907, no. 4, pp. 294–299.

64 I.N. Kokshaiskii, *Predvaritel'nye dannye perepisi naseleniia g. Saratova i ego prigorodov, proizvedennoi v 1916 godu* (Saratov, 1922), pp. 52–56.

65 "Protokol zasedanii Saratovskoi gorodskoi kanalizatsionnoi kommissii, 22.5.1907", pp. 60–64; Khlopin, *Materialy po ozdorovleniiu Rossii*, pp. 224–226.

66 For the details of the plan see Matveev, *Glebuchev ovrag (1871–1906 gg.)*, pp. 12–16; Khlopin, *Materialy po ozdorovleniiu Rossii*, pp. 211–212; Lutz Häfner, " 'Lebst Du nicht im Graben, fressen Dich die Raben.' Politische Partizipation und sozialpolitischer Diskurs im Spiegel städtischer Sanierung an der städtischen Peripherie von Saratov 1860 bis 1914", *JfGO*, 1996, pp. 190–209, here: pp. 193–195.

67 Khlopin, *Materialy po ozdorovleniiu Rossii*, p. 211.

68 Matveev, *Glebuchev ovrag (1871–1906 gg.)*, p. 14; Khlopin, *Materialy po ozdorovleniiu Rossii*, pp. 212–213.

69 Khlopin, *Materialy po ozdorovleniiu Rossii*, p. 212; Matveev, *Glebuchev ovrag (1871–1906 gg.)*, p. 16; Lutz Häfner, "Leben sie im Graben fressen sie die Raben", p. 194.

70 Matveev, *Glebuchev ovrag (1871–1906 gg.)*, p. 18; Khlopin, *Materialy po ozdorovleniiu Rossii*, p. 212.

71 Matveev, *Glebuchev Ovrag (1871–1906 gg.)*, pp. 22–31; Khlopin, *Materialy po ozdorovleniiu Rossii*, pp. 212–213.

72 Khlopin, *Materialy po ozdorovleniiu Rossii*, p. 215.

73 Matveev, *Glebuchev ovrag (1871–1906 gg.)*, pp. 29–30; Khlopin, *Materialy po ozdorovleniiu Rossii*, p. 212.

74 With regard to Russia's cities the link between urban renewal, urban welfare and social reform has been established by Joseph Bradley, *Muzhik and Muscovite. Urbanization in Late Imperial Russia* (Berkeley, 1985), esp. chs. 7 and 8.

75 *Saratovskii Vestnik*, no. 133, 25.6.1892.

76 *Saratovskii Vestnik*, no. 130, 21.6.1892.

77 *Saratovskii Vestnik*, no. 133, 25.6.1892.

78 *Saratovskii Vestnik*, no. 132, 24.6.1892.

79 For examples see *Saratovskii Vestnik*, no. 124, 24.6.1892; no. 133, 25.6.1892; *Saratovskii Listok*, no. 130, 21.6. 1892 and many more.

80 Already on 22 June, for instance, Princess M.A. Meshcherskaia, the governor's wife, organised a committee for the care of orphans whose parents had died of cholera. *Saratovskii Listok*, no. 133, 25.6.1892.

81 "Protokol soedinennogo zasedaniia obshchestva Saratovskikh sanitarnykh vrachei s chlenami fiziko-meditsinskogo obshchestva, 24.6.1892", *Protokoly zasedanii obshchestva Saratovskikh sanitarnykh vrachei za 1890,91,92 gg.* (Saratov, 1894), pp. 175–179. *Saratovskii Vestnik*, no. 133, 25.6.1892; *Saratovskii Listok*, no. 124, 24.6.1892.

82 V.I. Miropol'skii, *Obshchii ocherk deiatel'nosti 'Obshchestva Saratovskikh sanitarnykh vrachei', s maia 1886 g. po ianvar' 1893 goda*, pp. 46–47.

83 *Protokoly zasedanii obshchestva Saratovskikh sanitarnykh vrachei za 1890,91,92 gg.*, p. 209.

84 GASO, f. 576, op. 1., d. 3, l. 60.

85 *Saratovskii Vestnik*, no. 133, 25.6.1892.

86 Lindenmeyr, *Poverty is Not a Vice*, esp. pp. 48–72.

87 Ibid., esp. chap. 3.

88 Ibid., pp. 72–73.

89 The basic legal problem concerning public relief was similar to that in the field of public health. Two statutes, the Zemstvo Statute and the Statute on Public Assistance, established parallel jurisdictions. In contrast to public health, the Zemstvo Statute made the provision of poor relief obligatory to the *zemstva*. For municipal governments, however, public welfare was optional. Lindenmeyr, *Poverty is Not a Vice*, pp. 48–50; p. 61 and 67.

90 Ibid., p. 10. See also Hubertus Jahn, "Health Care and Poor Relief in Russia, 1700–1856", Ole Peter Grell, Andrew Cunningham, Robert Jütte (eds), *Health Care and Poor Relief in 18th and 19th Century Northern Europe* (Aldershot, 2002), pp. 157–171, esp. p. 159.

91 The secularisation of poor relief took its original beginning with Peter the Great. However, the state continued to play a limited role in the provision of public welfare. As Lindenmeyr has shown, one of the reasons for limited state assistance to the poor was the difference made between beggars, who were to be eradicated by law, and poverty, which was considered as inevitable. Adele Lindenmeyr, *Poverty is not a Vice*, chap. 2, pp. 26–47.

92 Ibid., esp. chap. 3.

93 Lindenmeyr, *Poverty is not a Vice*, pp. 82–88.

94 See in particular the studies by I.N. Matveev, "Sanitarnye ocherki. Nochlezhnye doma, artel'nye kvartiry i postoialye dvory goroda Saratova", *SZN*, 1896, no. 39, pp. 502–521; 1898, no. 9–10, pp. 79–113; 1898, no. 13–14, pp. 115–128; 1898, no. 24, pp. 125–164; also his "Bani goroda Saratova", *SZN*, 1897, no. 15, pp. 212–228. Studies and articles on Saratov's social question in the 1890s are too numerous to be cited here in full. The vast majority of them were published in the *SSO*. The most important works have provided the basis for the analysis of Saratov's vulnerability to cholera in Chapter 1. In Saratov, the social question emerged later when compared with St Petersburg and Moscow, where authorities began to confront the problem in the 1870s. See Joseph Bradley, *Muzhik and Muscovite*, pp. 273–291; also his "Once You've Eaten Khitrov Soup, You'll Never Leave!': Slum Renovation in Pre-revolutionary Moscow", *Russian History*, vol. 11 (1984), pp. 1–28.

95 The real number of charitable organisations was probably higher since it also included the institutions led by factories and other enterprises. Matveev gives the number of 49 charitable organisations in 1898, N.I. Matveev, "Saratovskie bogadel'ni. Sanitarnye ocherki", *SZN*, 1898, no. 9–10, p. 158–159.

96 Matveev, "Saratovskie bogadel'ni, esp. pp. 100–101.

97 For the principles of the Elberfeld system of poor relief see Evans, *Death in Hamburg*, pp. 99–100; Lindenmeyr, *Poverty is not a Vice*, p. 149.
98 N.I. Matveev, "Sanitarnye ocherki. Doma prizreniia", *SZN*, 1898, no. 24, pp. 148–149.
99 Matveev, "Sanitarnye ocherki berega Volgi", pp. 42–43.
100 N.I. Matveev, "Sanitarnye Ocherki", *SZN*, 1896, no. 39, pp. 502–511, esp. p. 502.
101 N.I. Matveev, "Sanitarnye ocherki berega Volgi", p. 16.
102 Ibid., p. 39.
103 Matveev, *Gorod Saratov v sanitarnom otnoshenii*, p. 89.
104 Ibid., pp. 42–63.
105 Typhus is transmitted by the human body louse. Typhoid, by contrast, is transmitted through water and foodstuffs which have been infected by the faeces of an infected individual. The connection between the two diseases and conditions of filth and dirt is clearly explained by Evans, *Death in Hamburg*, p. 189.
106 D.N. Zhbankov, "Neskol'ko zametok o kholere 1892 i 1893 gg. i o bor'be s neiu", *Vrach*, 1894, no. 51, pp. 1–26, p. 21.
107 *Vrach*, 1892, no. 29, p. 738.
108 Frieden, *Russian Physicians*, esp. chap. 5; Hutchinson, "Society, Corporation or Union? Russian Physicians and the Struggle for Professional Unity (1890–1913)", *JfGO*, vol. 30 (1982), pp. 37–53.
109 The papers and discussions of the conference are published in the already mentioned *Trudy s"ezda vrachei neposredstvenno prinimavshikh uchastie v bor'be s kholernoi epidemiei 1892 goda v Rossii* (St Petersburg, 1893); see also the report by A.V. Pogozhev, "S"ezd vrachei pri meditsinskom departamente 13–20 dekabria 1892 g.", *Meditsinskoe Obozrenie*, vol. 39, no. 2, pp. 197–207; Frieden, *Russian Physicians*, p. 155.
110 For a concise summary of the resolutions of the conference see the reprint of the resolutions in *SSO*, 1893, no. 1–2, pp. 20–28.
111 A.A. Ternovskii, "Doklad kommissii s"ezda zemskikh vrachei o meropriiatiiakh na sluchai vozobnovleniia kholery v 1893 godu", *SSO*, 1893, no. 1 and 2, pp. 1–10.
112 A.V. Pogozhev, "S"ezd vrachei pri meditsinskom departamente 13–20 dekabriia 1892 g.", esp. p. 203.
113 The resolutions of the Medical Department taken in the wake of the cholera conference are reprinted in *SSO*, 1893, no. 1–2, pp. 20–45. For the continuation of the Sanitary Executive Commissions and their tasks and rights see pp. 20–22.
114 Frieden, *Russian Physicians*, pp. 154–158.
115 This important point is accurately stressed by Nancy Frieden in her interpretation of the commissions. Frieden, *Russian Physicians*, pp. 154–158.
116 See the resolution of the Medical Department as reprinted in the *SSO*, 1893, no. 1–2, § 2, p. 21.
117 For the minutes of the meeting see "Zhurnaly zasedanii gubernskoi zemskoi sanitarno-ispolnitel'noi kommissii", *SSO*, 1893, no. 5–6, pp. 176–181.
118 *Sbornik otchetov vrachei i studentov rabotavshikh po kholernoi epidemii 1892 goda v Saratovskoi gubernii*, ed. Saratovskoe gubernskoe zemstvo (Saratov, 1893).
119 In fact, contemporaries expected a much more severe attack in 1893 since in the past the second cholera year had usually been more virulent than the first one. Frieden, *Russian Physicians*, p. 154.
120 For a thorough analysis of miasmatist theory see in particular Evans, *Death in Hamburg*, pp. 232–243; also Ackerknecht, "Anticontagionism between 1821 and 1867", esp. p. 57; with specific focus on Russia Frieden, *Russian Physicians*, esp. pp. 78–84.
121 Hutchinson, *Tsarist Russia and the Bacteriological Revolution*, pp. 420–439.
122 D.A. Zhbankov, "Kratkii istoricheskii obzor deiatel'nosti sanitarnykh biuro i obshchestvenno-sanitarnykh uchrezhdenii v zemskoi Rossii", *Vrach*, no. 51, p. 3.

123 Ackerknecht, "Anticontagionism between 1821 and 1867," pp. 562–593.

124 Frieden, *Russian Physicians*, pp. 122–127.

125 This important transformation is stressed by Frieden, *Russian Physicians*, pp. 128–131.

126 The commission was renamed the *sanitarnoe biuro* in 1906. For its history see M.I. Matveev, *Gorod Saratov v sanitarnom otnoshenii v 1906 godu. Otchet sanitarnogo vracha* (Saratov, 1908), pp. 3–25.

127 Ibid., pp. 105–128. In 1901, the sanitary commission established a fifth district at the *gory*, and in 1906 a sixth district at the banks.

128 Ibid., pp. 124–126.

129 Ibid., p. 105.

130 Ibid., p. 112.

131 Frieden, *Russian Physicians*, pp. 87–90.

132 *Vrach*, 1892, no. 29, p. 738.

133 Frieden, *Russian Physicians*, pp. 161–162.

134 For the development and tasks of the *sanitarnoe biuro* in general see D. Zhbankov, *Kratkii istoricheskii obzor deiatel'nosti sanitarnykh biuro i obshchestvenno-sanitarnykh uchrezhdenii v zemskoi Rossii* (Moscow, 1910), pp. 1–4. See also the analysis by Frieden, *Russian Physicians*, pp. 159–160. The activity of Saratov's *sanitarnoe biuro* is best reflected in the *Saratovskii Sanitarnyi Obzor*, which has been widely used as a major source of material for this study.

135 E Nikolaev, "Saratovskoe sanitarnoe obshchestvo", *SZN*, 1905, no. 6–7, pp. 59–65.

136 GASO, f. 3, op. 1, d. 4319; f. 4, op. 1, d. 2496, l. 10. For an exhaustive account of the history of the university see V.A. Solomonov, *Imperatorskii Nikolaevskii Saratovskii Universitet. Istoriia otkrytiia i stanovleniia (1909–1917)* (Saratov, 1999). Besides Saratov, competing applications came from Tsaritsyn, Samara, Minsk, Vitebsk, Smolensk, Voronezh, Iaroslavl', Nizhnii Novgorod and Astrakhan'.

137 GASO, f. 4, op. 1, d. 2796, l.1. Solomonov, *Imperatorskii Nikolaevskii Saratovskii Universitet*, p. 38.

138 The State Duma gave its go-ahead on 8 May 1909, the State Council on 10 June 1909. V.A. Solomonov, *Imperatorskii Nikolaevskii Saratovskii Universitet*, p. 11.

139 Solomonov, *Imperatorskii Nikolaevskii Saratovskii Universitet*, chap. 2.

140 Frieden, *Russian Physicians*, p. 128.

141 Ibid., p. 128.

142 Hutchinson, *Tsarist Russia and the Bacteriological Revolution*, p. 430.

143 Evans, *Death in Hamburg*, esp. pp. 167–273.

144 Ibid., pp. 270–275.

145 For the ascendancy of Russian laboratory medicine and the reforms in medical education following the Great Reforms see in particular Mirko Grmek, "The History of Medical Education in Russia", C.D. O'Malley (ed.), *The History of Medical Education*, UCLA Forum in Medical Sciences, no. 12 (Berkeley, 1970), pp. 303–327 and Alexander S. Vuchinich, *Science in Russian Culture, 1861–1917* (Stanford, 1970).

146 Hutchinson, *Tsarist Russia and the Bacteriological Revolution*, esp. pp. 424–426.

147 Khlopin, *Materialy po ozdorovleniiu Rossii*, p. 231.

5 The revival of cholera: 1904–1910

1 Apart from the lower Volga, the most affected places in 1904 were the Erivan and Baku provinces. See Z. Frenkel', *Kholera i nashi goroda* (Moscow, 1909), pp. 3–4. Snowden mentions a full-scale epidemic in Russia in 1904, which alarmed the Italian state. However, the available sources do not confirm a major epidemic throughout the empire in 1904. Snowden, *Naples in the Time of Cholera*, p. 233.

2 For reasons discussed below, the sixth pandemic did not produce as much material as the outbreak in 1892. My figures are from V.I. Binshtok, "Kholernaia epidemiia 1910 goda v Rossii", *Vrachebnaia gazeta*, 1910, no. 45, pp. 1353–1357, here: p. 1353. Binshtok's figures are based on the *Otchety o sostoianii narodnogo zdraviia*, edited by the *upravlenie glavnogo vrachebnogo inspektora*. For further statistical information on the country as a whole throughout the sixth cholera pandemic see the following works: N.S. Avdakov, *Geografichesko-Statisticheskii ocherk kholernoi epidemii v Rossii v 1910 g.* (Khar'kov, 1910); Frenkel', *Kholera i nashi goroda*; N.F. Gamaleia, "Kholera", (St Petersburg, 1910); V.I. Binshtok, S.A. Novosel'skii, "Kholera i vodosnabzhenie v gorodakh Rossii", *Vrachebnaia gazeta*, 1912, no. 8, pp. 21–23; also M.M. Gran', "Poslednie epidemii v Rossii v sviazi s sostoianiem sovremennykh epidemiologicheskikh znanii", *Zhurnal ORVP*, 1908, no. 6, pp. 627–640; N.G. Freiberg, "Kholernye epidemii 1907 i 1908 gg. v Rossii", *Vrachebnaia gazeta*, 1909, no. 35, pp. 97–103.

3 Again, figures refer to European Russia. Binshtok, "Kholernaia epidemiia", p. 1353.

4 Snowden, *Naples in the Time of Cholera*, p. 360.

5 Briggs, *Cholera and Society in the Nineteenth Century*, pp. 76–96. The role of cholera in revolutions has been probed most deeply by Evans, *Epidemics and Revolutions*, pp. 123–146.

6 Rosenberg, *Cholera in Nineteenth-Century Europe*, pp. 425–463.

7 Pelling, *Cholera, Fever and English Medicine*.

8 Snowden, *Naples in the Time of Cholera*, pp. 244–246.

9 The reduced reporting about cholera in Saratov's newspapers reflects public reporting about the disease between 1904 and 1910 in general.

10 A detailed account of the epidemic in the Far East can be found in N.V. Kirilov "Kholernaia epidemiia Dal'nego Vostoka i mery bor'by s nimi v Kitae i v nashikh predelakh", *Pirogovskii s"ezd po bor'be s kholeroi, Moskva, 21–23 marta 1905 g., Trudy s"ezda* (Moscow, 1905), pp. 1–11. For descriptions of the course of cholera throughout the sixth pandemic from 1902 onwards, see G.I. Dembo, "Dvizhenie kholery v Rossii v epidemii 1908 goda", *Vrachebnaia gazeta*, 1908, no. 51, pp. 1521–1526; Avdakov, *Geografichesko-Statisticheskii ocherk*; Frenkel', *Kholera i nashi goroda*; Binshtok, "Kholernaia epidemiia", pp. 1353–1357; Binshtok and Novosel'skii, "Kholera i vodoshabzheniie v gorodakh Rossii", pp. 21–23; Gamaleia, *Kholera*.

11 The outbreak in 1902 officially recorded 2,131 cholera cases and 1,389 deaths. My figures are taken from Dembo, "Dvizhenie kholery v Rossii v epidemii 1908 goda", p. 1521. Dembo's account is based on the report of the *upravlenie glavnogo vrachebnogo inspektora*; see also Frenkel', *Kholera i nashi goroda*, pp. 1–4.

12 The Transsiberian railway was opened in 1904. Parts of it had been opened in 1897 (west Siberian railway) and 1898 respectively (central Siberian railway). James N. Westwood, *A History of Russian Railways* (London, 1964), p. 111.

13 Kirilov "Kholernaia epidemiia Dal'nego Vostoka", pp. 1–11.

14 The following figures provide a sense of the severity of the epidemic in Persia, which worried Russian authorities: In Herat, a city of 250,000 inhabitants and thus slightly bigger than Saratov at the eve of the First World War, the epidemic in 1904 killed 35,000 people within a few months; Tauride, of approximately the same size, counted 15,000 victims. Frenkel', *Kholera i nashi goroda*, p. 3.

15 Dembo, "Dvizhenie kholery v Rossii", pp. 1521–1526; Frenkel', *Kholera i nashi goroda*, pp. 3–4. For a report on the fight against the epidemic in Baku see I.M. Leplinskii, "Deiatel'nost' prozektorskogo kabineta Bakinskoi gorodskoi Mikhailovskoi bol'nitsy vo vremia kholernoi epidemii v 1904 g. v g. Baku", *Pirogovskii s"ezd po bor'be s kholeroi*, pp. 87–89.

16 Baku province recorded 2,529 cholera cases and 2,036 deaths; Erivan 4,615 cases and 2,679 deaths. Frenkel', *Kholera i nashi goroda*, p. 4.

17 On the outbreak in 1904 see Frenkel', *Kholera i nashi goroda*, pp. 3–5; also Avdakov, *Geografichesko-Statisticheskii ocherk*, pp. 3–4.
18 Frenkel', *Kholera i nashi goroda*, p. 4.
19 The outbreak affected chiefly the Privislinskii region adjacent to Prussia, which recorded a (successfully contained) cholera epidemic in 1905. Frenkel', *Kholera i nashi goroda*, p. 10.
20 These patterns of the epidemic in Russia are elaborated for the first pandemic by McGrew, *Russia and the Cholera*, pp. 54–55 and pp. 70–71; they are confirmed for the following three pandemics by Arkhangel'skii, *Kholernye epidemii v Evropeiskoi Rossii*.
21 Freiberg, "Kholernye epidemii 1907 i 1908 gg. v Rossii", pp. 97–103.
22 For the debate about this possibility see in particular M. Kazanskii, *Oblastnoi Povolzhskii protivokholernyi s"ezd v g. Samare (20.–29.4. 1908 g.)* (Kazan', 1909), pp. 18–27.
23 The only source which points to this possibility is Freiberg, "Kholernye epidemii 1907 i 1908 gg. v Rossii", p. 99. Samara had been linked to Orenburg province (Ufa) via railway since 1888.
24 N.N. Klodnitskii, "Kharakter i znachenie epidemii kholery 1907 g. v Samare i Astrakhani", *Vrachebnaia gazeta*, 1908, no. 21, pp. 639–642; Freiberg, "Kholernye epidemii 1907 i 1908 gg. v Rossii", pp. 97–103; Frenkel', *Kholera i nashi goroda*, pp. 10–11. During the cholera epidemic Saratov's local physicians still reasoned that the germ had reached Samara nevertheless from Persia but had simply not been noticed on its way. See the comment by N.N. Klodnitskii in "Protokol zasedaniia Saratovskoi gorodskoi sanitarnoi kommissii 21.8.1907 goda", *ISGD*, 1907, no. 4, pp. 381–393, esp. p. 384.
25 For the significance of Astrakhan' during the sixth pandemic see N.G. Freiberg, "Kholernye epidemii 1907 i 1908 gg. v Rossii", pp. 97–103; N.N. Klodnitskii, "Kharakter i znachenie epidemii kholery 1907 g. v Samare i Astrakhani", pp. 639–642; P.P. Maslakovets, "Kholera v g. Astrakhani i ee predmestiiakh letom 1907 g.", *Vrachebnaia gazeta*, 1908, no. 21, pp. 642–645.
26 A.A. Desiatov, *Kholera 1907–1908–1909 i 1910 g.g. na vodnykh putiakh Kazanskogo okruga putei soobshcheniia* (St Petersburg, 1911), pp. 10–11; Frenkel', *Kholera i nashi goroda*, pp. 11–12.
27 Avdakov, *Geografichesko-Statisticheskii ocherk*, pp. 6–7.
28 Binshtok, "Kholernaia epidemiia 1910 goda v Rossii", p. 1353.
29 S.A. Novosel'skii, "Kholera v Peterburge", *Vrachebnaia gazeta*, no. 37, 1908, pp. 1061–1063, here: p. 1061.
30 Avdakov, *Geografichesko-Statisticheskii ocherk*, p. 11. Once again, real figures are probably much higher than those officially reported.
31 Ibid., p. 11.
32 Ibid., p. 11.
33 N.F. Gamaleia, *Kholera* (St Petersburg, 1910), p. 17. In St Petersburg, a city of 1,847,609 inhabitants, cholera caused more than 8,963 cases and 3,986 deaths in 1908; in 1909, the city reported 8,326 cases; and in 1910, the disease incidence was 4,863 cases and 1,365 deaths. For figures see Avdakov, *Geografichesko-Statisticheskii ocherk*, pp. 5–9; also V.I. Binshtok, S.A. Novosel'skii, "Kholera i vodosnabzhenie v gorodakh Rossii", *Vrachebnaia gazeta*, 1912, no. 8, pp. 21–23.
34 For the history of the Anti-Plague Commission see Frieden, *Russian Physicians*, esp. pp. 290–292; also Hutchinson, *Politics and Public Health in Revolutionary Russia*, pp. 6–7.
35 This point is in particular made by Hutchinson, *Politics and Public Health in Revolutionary Russia*, p. 6.
36 "Vysochaishe utverzhdennykh 11-go avgusta 1903 g. pravil o priniatii mer k prekrash-cheniiu kholery i chumy", *Vrachebno-sanitarnaia khronika Saratovskoi gubernii*, 1904, no. 7, pp. 619–625.

37 The decisive battle between Pettenkofer and Koch took place in the immediate aftermath of the cholera epidemic in Hamburg in 1892. See Evans, *Death in Hamburg*, pp. 490–507.
38 Ibid., pp. 502–507.
39 See the analysis by Hutchinson, *Tsarist Russia and the Bacteriological Revolution*, pp. 420–439; also his *Politics and Public Health in Revolutionary Russia*, pp. 35–38.
40 A thorough discussion of both the significance of the Paris Convention in 1903 and of the endless possibilities to violate the agreement even in 1910 is provided by Snowden, *Naples in the Time of Cholera*, esp. chap. 7.
41 My information on the basic agreements of the convention are derived from Snowden, *Naples in the Time of Cholera*, pp. 302–305; for the Russian interpretation of the treaty see N.G. Freiberg, "Mezhdunarodnye mery protiv kholery i chumy. Parizhskaia konventsiia 1903 goda", *VOGSPM*, 1906, pp. 122–125.
42 Freiberg, "Mezhdunarodnye mery protiv kholery i chumy", p. 123. In the course of Plehve's reform of the MVD, V.K. Anrep replaced L.F. Ragozin in 1904 as director of the Medical Department of the MVD. Ragozin was appointed president of the Medical Council.
43 Freiberg, "Mezhdunarodnye mery protiv kholery i chumy", p. 123.
44 An extensive report on the expedition in 1904 and 1905 and its activity is provided by S.I. Zlatogorov, "O deiatel'nosti vrachebno-sanitarnogo otriada, komandirovannogo v mae 1905 goda v Tavriz v ozhidanii kholery", *Vrachebnaia Gazeta*, 1908, no. 2, pp. 252–257 and *Vrachebnaia gazeta*, 1908, no. 10, pp. 295–297; see also his report about treatment methods applied in Persia: "O predokhranitel'nykh privivkakh protiv kholery", *Pigorovskii s"ezd po bor'be s kholeroi. Moskva 21.–23.3.1905, Trudy s"ezda* (Moscow, 1905), pp. 42–58.
45 S.I. Zlatogorov, "O deiatel'nosti vrachebno-sanitarnogo otriada, komandirovannogo v mae 1905 goda v Tavriz v ozhidanii kholery", pp. 252–257.
46 V.P. Krasnukha, "Bor'ba s kholeroi v Zakaspiiskoi oblasti", *Pirogovskii s"ezd po bor'be s kholeroi. Moskva 21.–23.3.1905, Trudy s"ezda* (Moscow, 1905), pp. 90–96.
47 Ibid., p. 93.
48 Among them were the links between Balashov and Khar'kov (1895); Iaroslavl' and Arkhangel (1899); the Trans-Caspian railway had been completed in 1898.
49 E.A. Vodarskii, *Volga. Vodnye puti Volzhskogo basseina v predelakh Kazanskogo okruga putei soobshcheniia. Tekhnichesko-statisticheskii ocherk* (Moscow, 1908), p. 44.
50 A.A. Desiatov, Ocherk sanitarno-ekonomicheskogo polozheniia rabochikh na parokhodakh basseina r. Volgi", *8. Sbornik otchetov i dokladov vrachei sanitarnogo nadzora na r.r. Volge i Kame i na Mariinskom sisteme za 1903 g.* (St Petersburg, 1904), pp. 119–132, here: p. 119.
51 For the regulations issued by the Anti-Plague Commission to contain cholera on rivers see *Vysochaishe utverzhdennykh 11-go avgusta 1903 g. pravil o priniatii mer k prekrashcheniiu kholery i chumy*, §§ 23–43.
52 A.A. Desiatin, *Kholera 1907–1908–1909–1910 na vodnykh putiakh Kazanskogo okruga putei soobshcheniia* (St Petersburg, 1911), pp. 23–27.
53 This measure was introduced only in 1908. In 1910, the vessels were employed in Astrakhan', Tsaritsyn, Nizhnii Novgorod and Rybinsk, the four most important migrant centres at the river. A.A. Desiatin, *Kholera 1907–1908–1909–1910*, pp. 43–44; also "Iz namechennykh meropriiatii dlia bor'by s kholeroi v 1908 g.", *Vrachebnaia gazeta*, 1908, no. 21, pp. 651–652.
54 Desiatin, *Kholera na vodnykh putiakh*, p. 44.
55 Ibid., pp. 55–64.
56 This binding decree (*obiazatel'noe postanovlenie*) was issued in 1908. Ibid., p. 42.
57 Friedgut, *Labor Violence and Regime Brutality in Tsarist Russia*, here: p. 251.
58 Frieden, *Russian Physicians*, esp. pp. 295–301.

59　*Pirogovskii s"ezd po bor'be s kholeroi, Trudy s"ezda*, esp. pp. 90–162.
60　For examples see Saratov's zemstvo edited *Kholernaia epidemiia v Saratovskoi gubernii v 1908 godu. Sbornik otchetov* (Saratov, 1909).
61　Freiberg, "Mezhdunarodnye mery protiv kholery i chumy", p. 123. Exceptionally for Europe, Greece and Serbia still continued to establish old-style quarantines, allegedly as a response to Turkey's quarantine policies against these two countries. Another exception in Europe was Italy, where military force was employed to control cholera as late as 1910. Snowden, *Naples in the Time of Cholera,* esp. pp. 237–241.
62　These provinces reported together 67,491 cholera cases in 1910 as opposed to 70,481 in 1892. The Volga provinces from Iaroslavl' to Astrakhan', to compare, counted 154,008 cholera cases in 1892 and only 34,000 in 1910. Avdakov, *Geografichesko-Statisticheskii ocherk,* p. 10.
63　Snowden, *Naples in the Time of Cholera*, pp. 237–241; see also his "Cholera in Barletta 1910".
64　It is, of course, impossible to generalise this observation for the empire as a whole. A case study on the course of the cholera epidemic in 1910 at a particular locality in Russia's south, especially Rostov on Don, which was severely ravaged in 1910, would probably be most revealing for understanding the sixth pandemic in Russia. My assessment of the significance of social upheaval during the sixth pandemic is derived from the perspective on Saratov and the lower Volga. However, the lower Volga after all had been the centre of cholera riots in 1892 from where social unrest was carried up the river. In this region, still one of the country's epicentres, the epidemic's social impact was far different from that in 1892.
65　P.P. Maslakovets, "Kholera v g. Astrakhani i ee predmestiiakh letom 1907 g.", *Vrachebnaia gazeta*, 1908, no. 21, pp. 642–645, here: p. 644.
66　M. Kazanskii, *Oblastnoi Povolozhskii protivokholernyi s"ezd v g. Samare* (Kazan', 1909), pp. 73–76.
67　Ibid., p. 75.
68　The commission included the hygienists Khlopin and Sidlovskii, the chemist Dianin and the physician Shmid (Astrakhan'). The report of the commission can be found in G.V. Khlopin, "Vlianie neftianykh produktov na rybnoe naselenie rek i na kachestvo ikh vody", *Vrach*, 1898, no. 51., pp. 217–223.
69　My information about the institution is derived from Desiatov, *Kholera 1907– 1908–1909–1910*, which analyses in detail the measures taken along the Volga River.
70　The results of these investigations, which provide the first and very valuable information about working and living conditions at the Volga River, were published in several monumental volumes. Kazanskii okrug putei soobshcheniia, *Obzor o deiatel'nosti vrachebno-sanitarnogo nadzora na rr. Volge i Kame i na Mariinskoi sisteme za 1904 g.* (St Petersburg, 1905); za 1908 (St Petersburg, 1909); za 1910 (St Petersburg, 1911).
71　The reports of these expeditions were published in major medical journals. Among them are the above-mentioned articles on Astrakhan', Saratov, Tsaritsyn and Samara by S.I. Zlatogorov, N.N. Klodnitskii, V.A. Taranukhin, and P.P. Maslakovets.
72　S.I. Zlatogorov, "O kholere 1907 g. v Saratovskoi gubernii", *Vrachebnaia gazeta*, 1908, no. 12, pp. 42–48, here: p. 47.
73　For the operation of the cholera commission in 1830 and the structural problems inherent in the attempt to centralise the nation's defence against the disease see McGrew, *Russia and the Cholera,* pp. 58–63.
74　My information on the history and personnel composition of the Anti-Plague Commission is drawn from Frieden, *Russian Physicians*, p. 291; and Hutchinson, *Politics and Public Health in Revolutionary Russia,* pp. 6–7.
75　The Medical Department was replaced by the Main Administration for Local Economic Affairs. The Medical Council was only abolished by the Bolsheviks in 1917. Likewise, the non-governmental Anti-Plague Commission, despite prodigious efforts to reform Russia's medical administration after the revolution in 1905, also survived

until the revolution. See Hutchinson, *Politics and Public Health in Revolutionary Russia*, pp. 167 and 188; also Frieden, *Russian Physicians*, pp. 288–291.

76 "Vysochaishe utverzhdennykh 11-go avgusta 1903 g. pravil o priniatii mer k prekrashcheniiu kholery i chumy", *Vrachebno-sanitarnaia khronika Saratovskoi gubernii*, 1904, no. 7 (July), pp. 619–625.

77 On the provincial level, the SECs included the vice governor, the representative of the nobility (*predvoditel' dvorianstva*), medical inspector, police chief (*politseimeister*), chief factory inspector (*starshii fabrichnyi inspector*), one representative of the local district of communications (*okrug putei soobshcheniia*), the military and the church. In the cities, they also included one representative from the provincial zemstvo uprava, the mayor of the provincial capital, one municipal physician and the municipal uprava in its full membership. *Vysochaishe utverzhdennykh 11-go avgusta 1903 g. pravil o priniatii mer k prekrashcheniiu kholery i chumy*, §§ 9–10.

78 Ibid., § 1.

79 Ibid., § 1.

80 Desiatov, *Kholera 1907–1908–1909 i 1910 g.g.*, p. 130.

81 P.P. Maslakovets, "Kholera v g. Astrakhani i ee predmestiiakh letom 1907 g.", *Vrachebnaia gazeta*, 1908, no. 21, pp. 642–645, here: p. 643.

82 The comment was made by Teziakov, A.A. Desiatov, and S.N. Igumnov at the cholera congress in Samara. M. Kazanskii, *Oblastnoi Povolzhskii protivokholernyi s"ezd v g. Samare (20.–29.4.1908)*, p. 77.

83 Desiatov, *Kholera 1907–1908–1909 i 1910 g.g.*, p. 45.

84 Complaints were loudly vocalised by local administrative and medical authorities across the country. At the lower Volga, the topic was discussed at a regional cholera congress in Samara in 1908. See RGIA, f. 1288, op. 13, d. 99, 1908; also M. Kazanskii, *Oblastnoi povolzhskii protivokholernyi s"ezd v g. Samare (20.–29.4.1908g)* (Kazan', 1909), pp. 60–64; for the discussions about the new legislation on the national level see P.P. Rozanov, "Ob obshchestvennykh merakh bor'by s kholeroi", *Pirogovskii s"ezd po bor'be s kholeroi. Moskva 21.–23.3.1905* (Moscow, 1905), pp. 116–124; see also the abundance of articles on the issue in the national medical press, for instance G.I. Rostovtsev, "V ozhidanii kholernoi epidemii", *Vrachebnyi vestnik*, 1905, no. 15, pp. 9–10; M. Katsaurov, "Pravila 11 avgusta 1903 g.", *Vrachebnyi vestnik*, 1905, no. 19, pp. 295–296; "Novyi tsirkuliar o pravilakh 11 avgusta 1903 g.", *Vrachebnaia gazeta*, 1908, no. 12, pp. 377–378.

85 Frieden, *Russian Physicians*, pp. 164–166.

86 RGIA, f. 1288, op. 13, 1908, d. 99.

87 Witte, the representative of the Anti-Plague Commission at the cholera congress in Samara, reported about this complaint. RGIA, f. 1288, op. 13, 1908 g., d. 99.

88 "Novyi tsirkuliar o pravilakh 11 avgusta 1903 g.", *Vrachebnaia gazeta*, 1908, no. 12, pp. 377–378, p. 377.

89 Ibid., p. 377.

90 Frieden, *Russian Physicians*, pp. 297–305; Hutchinson, *Tsarist Russia and the Bacteriological Revolution*, pp. 437–438.

91 Both papers and discussions from the Congress are published in *Pirogovskii s"ezd po bor'be c kholeroi*.

92 Hutchinson, *Tsarist Russia and the Bacteriological Revolution*, p. 438.

93 *Pirogovskii s"ezd po bor'be s kholeroi*, p. 210.

94 The decisive significance of the 'Cholera Congress' for driving the medical profession into radical politics has been analysed by Frieden, *Russian Physicians*, pp. 297–311 and 381–389; see also Hutchinson, *Politics and Public Health in Revolutionary Russia*, pp. 35–38 and 44–46.

95 *Pirogovskii s"ezd po bor'be c kholeroi*, p. 210; *Russkii vrach*, 1905, no. 52, p. 1605; also Hutchinson, *Politics and Public Health in Revolutionary Russia*, pp. 35–38.

96 Frieden, *Russian Physicians*, p. 307.

97 According to Nancy Frieden, the *Pirogov Journal* reported 1,324 repressed physicians by 1907. Frieden, *Russian Physicians*, p. 319. See also Hutchinson, "Politics and Medical Professionalization after 1905", Harley D. Balzer (ed.), *Russia's Missing Middle Class* (New York, 1996), pp. 89–116.

98 For Rein's experience of the cholera of 1910 in southern Russia see Hutchinson, *Politics and Public Health in Revolutionary Russia,* pp. 89–91.

99 M. Chervonenkis "Kratkii obzor epidemii kholery v Saratovskoi gubernii v 1904 g.", *Vrachebno-Sanitarnaia khronika Saratovskoi gubernii*, 1905, no. 3–4, pp. 241–253, p. 241.

100 For a description of cholera's arrival in Saratov in 1904 see the *Doklady upravy po otdeleniiu narodnogo zdraviia o kholere* (Saratov, 1904), pp. 3–44, esp. pp. 3–5; also Chervonenkis "Kratkii obzor epidemii kholery", esp. pp. 241–242.

101 The social and occupational profile of the cholera patients is provided by M. Chervonenkis "Kratkii obzor epidemii kholery", pp. 244–246.

102 The most detailed account of the anti-cholera campaign by local authorities is given in the *Doklady upravy po otdeleniiu narodnogo zdraviia o kholere* (Saratov, 1904), pp. 3–44, esp. pp. 7–40.

103 M. Chervonenkis "Kratkii obzor epidemii kholery", p. 244.

104 *Doklady upravy po otdeleniiu narodnogo zdraviia o kholere*, p. 6.

105 On agriculture in Saratov province after the turn of the century, see Timothy R. Mixter, "Peasant Collective Action in Saratov Province, 1902–1906", Rex A. Wade, Scott J. Seregny (eds), *Politics and Society in Provincial Russia: Saratov, 1590–1917* (Ohio, 1989), pp. 191–232; I.V. Porokh, *Ocherkji istorii Saratovskogo Povolzh'ia (1894–1917)*, vol. 2, pp. 20–43; also Theodore H. von Laue, "Russian Labor between Field and Factory 1892–1903", *California Slavic Studies*, 3 (1964), pp. 33–64. According to Mixter, the peasant population in the province grew from 1,476,700 in 1858 to 2,096,200 in 1897 (p. 193).

106 Timothy R. Mixter, "Peasant Collective Action in Saratov Province, 1902–1906", pp. 196–198.

107 Ibid., pp. 209–220. For a vivid description of social discontent as the revolution went under way see also the biographic account by Maria Stolypin Bock, "Stolypin in Saratov", *Russian Review*, July 1953, vol. 12, no. 3, pp. 187–193.

108 A. Ershov, *Ocherk chernorabochego dvizheniia v Saratovskom krae* (Saratov, 1909), p. 37.

109 For the following see in particular I.V. Porokh, *Ocherki istorii Saratovskogo Povolzh'ia (1894–1917)*, vol. 2, pp. 172–195; also Timothy R. Mixter "Peasant Collective Action in Saratov Province, 1902–1906"; Thomas Fallows, "Governor Stolypin and the Revolution of 1905 in Saratov", Rex A. Wade, Scott J. Seregny (eds), *Politics and Society in Provincial Russia: Saratov, 1590–1917* (Ohio, 1989), pp. 160–190, esp. pp. 162–163.

110 Figures from I.V. Porokh, *Ocherki istorii Saratovskogo Povolzh'ia*, vol. 2, p. 191.

111 GASO, f. 1283, op. 1, d.11, l. 67 ob.–68.

112 I.V. Porokh, *Ocherki istorii Saratovskogo Povolzh'ia*, vol. 2, p. 193.

113 *Doklady upravy po otdeleniiu narodnogo zdraviia*, p. 12–13. Some provincial districts remained without any medical care at all as a result of the war.

114 N.R. Ivanov, *Saratovskie uchenye-mediki. Stranitsy istorii. 1909–1979* (Saratov, 1982), pp. 129–133.

115 *Doklady upravy po otdeleniiu narodnogo zdraviia*, p. 13.

116 Evans, *Epidemics and Revolutions*, pp. 123–146.

117 See the argument ibid., p. 131.

118 Ibid., p. 144.

119 Evans, *Death in Hamburg*, esp. pp. 346–372.

120 There has yet to be an in-depth study of Paris's final cholera experience. Frank Snowden points to the city's tranquillity in *Naples in the Time of Cholera*, p. 244.

121 Ibid., chap. 7.

122 "Vysochaishe utverzhdennye 11 Avgusta 1903 g. pravila o priniatii mer k prekrash-cheniiu kholery i chumy pri poiavlenii ikh vnutri Imperii", *Vrachebno-sanitarnaia khronika Saratovskoi gubernii*, 1904, no. 7 (July), pp. 619–625, § 20.

123 Thomas Fallows, "Governor Stolypin and the 1905 Revolution", Rex A. Wade, Scott J. Seregny (eds), *Politics and Society in Provincial Russia: Saratov, 1590–1917*, pp. 160–191, here: p. 171; Frieden, *Russian Physicians*, pp. 308–311; on the increasing hostility against the medical intelligentsia in the province see Chervonkis, "Kratkii obzor epidemii kholery".

124 *Russkii Vrach*, 1905, no. 25, p. 823.

125 Chervonenkis, "Kratkii obzor epidemii kholery", p. 252.

126 Fallows, "Governor Stolypin and the 1905 Revolution", p. 170.

127 The incident is mentioned in N.I. Teziakov, *Ocherk kholernoi epidemii 1907 g. i protivokholernykh meropriiatii v Saratovskoi gubernii* (Saratov, 1908), p. 5.

128 The society was dissolved at the beginning of June 1905. E.P. Nikolaev, "Saratovskoe sanitarnoe obshchestvo (Istoricheskaia spravka)", *SZN*, 1905, no. 6–7, pp. 59–65.

129 Fallows, "Governor Stolypin and the 1905 Revolution", pp. 171–173; also Frieden, *Russian Physicians*, pp. 310–311.

130 Fallows, "Governor Stolypin and the 1905 Revolution", p. 177.

131 For this interpretation see in particular Frieden, *Russian Physicians*, pp. 308–311.

132 Binshtok, "Kholernaia epidemiia", pp. 1353–1357.

133 N.I. Teziakov, "Kholernaia epidemiia v Saratovskoi gubernii v 1910 godu, v sviazi s epidemiiami 1904–1909 gg.", *Kholernaia epidemiia v Saratovskoi Gubernii v 1910 godu. Sbornik otchetov* (Saratov, 1911), pp. 178–191, here: p. 180; see also G.I. Dembo, "K istorii bor'by s kholeroi v Rossii v 1910 godu", *Vrachebnaia gazeta*, 1910, no. 45, pp. 1368–1374, here: p. 1370.

134 As in 1892, the real figures were most likely higher than the officially recorded numbers suggest. Official and medical authorities still struggled with people's reluctance to report cholera or the early detection of cholera cases, for example, although to a lesser extent.

135 The differences in the medical infrastructure played a greater role during the sixth pandemic than in 1892. This was due to the fact that the "golden era" of zemstvo medicine actually fell in the 1890s. During the sixth pandemic, Astrakhan' suffered from the medical dependence on St Petersburg as much as did the province of Orenburg and the Ural region. The delegates at the Cholera Congress in Samara in 1908 therefore demanded the establishment of provincial zemstvo organisations in all three provinces. See M. Kazanskii, *Oblastnoi Povolzhskii protivokholernyi s"ezd v g. Samare (20.–29.4.1908)* (Kazan', 1909), pp. 72–73.

136 P.P. Maslakovets, "Kholera v g. Astrakhani i ee predmestiiakh letom 1907 g.", *Vrachebnaia gazeta*, 1908, no. 21, pp. 642–645, here p. 643.

137 Maslakovets, "Kholera v g. Astrakhani", p. 644; also N.N. Klodnitskii, "Kharakter i znachenie epidemii kholery 1907 g. v Samare i Astrakhani", *Vrachebnaia gazeta*, 1908, no. 21, pp. 639–642.

138 N.N. Rodionov, "Kratkii ocherk kholernoi epidemii 1908 goda v g. Tsaritsyne", *Kholernaia epidemiia v Saratovskoi gubernii v 1908 godu. Sbornik otchetov* (Saratov, 1909), pp. 42–59, p. 57.

139 Parokh, *Ocherki istorii Saratovskogo Povolzh'ia*, p. 19.

140 For the increasing commercial significance of Tsaritsyn see "Torgovlia Saratova v 1892 godu", *Vestnik finansov, promyshlennosti i torgovli*, 10.10.1893, no. 41, pp. 55–58; according to the journal, Tsaritsyn received 39.9 million pud of naphta, 4.0 million pud of fish and 2.5 million pud of salt. Saratov received 23.7 million pud of naphta, 0.6 million pud of fish and 1.7 million pud of salt.

141 N. Ponomarev, "O peredvizhenii sel'skokhoziaistvennykh rabochikh, napravliaiush-chikhcia v iugovostochnye mestnosti Rossii", *Sel'skoe khoziaistvo i lesovodstvo*, 1896, no. 2, p. 299.

142 At the beginning of the twentieth century, Tsaritsyn in fact ranked among the three main shipping centres at the middle and lower Volga alongside Astrakhan' and Nizhnii-Novgorod. Desiatov, *Kholera 1907–08–09 i 1910 g.g.*, p. 17.

143 S.I. Zlatogorov, "O kholere 1907 v Saratovskoi gubernii", *Vrachebnaia gazeta*, 1908, no. 12, pp. 363–368 and no. 13, pp. 409–412. Also N.N. Rodionov, "Kratkii ocherk kholernoi epidemii 1908 goda v g. Tsaritsyne", *Kholernaia epidemiia v Saratovskoi gubernii*, pp. 42–59.

144 In the 1890s, the zemstvo allocated 3,000 rubles for sanitary services as compared to 24,000 assigned in Saratov. D.I. Zhbankov, *Kratkii istoricheskii obzor deiatelnosti sanitarnykh biuro i obshestvenno-sanitarnykh uchrezhdenii v zemskoi Rossii* (Moscow, 1910), pp. 68–69.

145 Zhbankov, *Kratkii istoricheskii obzor deiatelnosti sanitarnykh biuro*, p. 42; for a description of the sanitary infrastructure of Samara province see also M.M. Gran', "Prishlye sel'skokhoziaistvennye rabochie Samarskoi gubernii v sanitarnom otnoshenii", *SSO*, 1901, no. 42–45, pp. 32–51; and the same author's "Zaboty Samarskogo gubernskogo zemstva o prishlykh sel'skokhoziaistvennykh rabochikh", *SSO*, 1901, no. 1–16, pp. 16–28.

146 Zhbankov, *Kratkii istoricheskii obzor deiatelnosti sanitarnykh biuro*, p. 30.

147 For the following see ibid., p. 6.

148 Desiatov, *Kholera 1907–1908–1909 i 1910 g.g.*, pp. 133–139.

149 For examples see Desiatov, *Kholera 1907–1908–1909 i 1910 g.g.*, pp. 133–139; N.N. Klodnitskii, "Kharakter i znachenie epidemii kholery", pp. 639–642; see also the reports given by V.A. Taranukhin and M.M. Gran' at the regional cholera congress in Samara in 1908, reproduced in M. Kazanskii, *Oblastnoi Povolzhskii protivokholernyi s"ezd v g. Samare (20.–29.4.1908 g.)*, pp. 15–18 and 33. At the congress, N.I. Teziakov, sanitary physician in Saratov province, pointed out that Samara's zemstvo spent 100,000 rubles on the anti-cholera campaign in 1907 as compared with 23,000 rubles assigned by Saratov's zemstvo. This was precisely because medical-sanitary organisation in Saratov province had been placed on a better footing over the last two decades. M. Kazanskii, *Oblastnoi Povolzhskii protivokholernyi s"ezd v g. Samare (20.–29.4.1908 g.)*, p. 65.

150 N.I. Teziakov, *Ocherk kholernoi epidemii 1907 g. i protivokholernykh meropriiatii v Saratovskoi gubernii* (Saratov, 1908), p. 15.

151 *Saratovskie Gubernskie Vedomosti*, 28.7.1907; also *Izvestiia Gorodskoi Dumy*, 1907, no. 3, pp. 135–136.

152 "Doklad gorodskoi upravy v Saratovskuiu gorodskuiu dumu, 22.8.1907 g.", reprinted in *ISGD*, 1907, no. 3, p. 334.

153 For the functions of the Sanitary Executive Commission and the Sanitary Commission see "Obzor deiatel'nosti gorodskoi dumy", p. 281. The institution was established in Saratov in 1904. As Teziakov pointed out, Sanitary Executive Commissions had little influence in Saratov. Frequently, they relied on already existing institutions meeting under another name. The provincial SECs, with few exceptions, usually followed the suggestions of the provincial uprava. Teziakov, *Ocherk kholernoi epidemii"*, pp. 18–22. See also the conclusion by G. Dembo in his review on Teziakov's report, *Vrachebnaia gazeta*, 1908, no. 12, pp. 378–379.

154 For the anti-cholera measures elaborated by the municipal Sanitary Executive Commission see "Doklad gorodskoi upravy v Saratovskuiu gorodskuiu dumu, 22.8.1907 g.", reprinted in *ISGD*, 1907, no. 3, pp. 332–334.

155 S.L. Raskovich "Pasterovskaia stantsiia", *SSO*, 1903, no. 3, pp. 29–41; S.L. Rashkovich "Otchet o deiatel'nosti Pasterovskoi stantsii Saratovskogo gubernskogo zemstva za pervuiu polovinu 1903 goda", *Vrachebno-Sanitarnaia khronika Saratovskoi gubernii*, 1903, no. 7, pp. 269–278.

156 S.I. Zlatogorov, "O kholere 1907 g. v Saratovskoi gubernii", *Vrachebnaia gazeta*, 1908, no. 12, p. 368. A laboratory approaching modern technical standards was only established in the city in 1912.

157 "Doklad gorodskoi upravy v Saratovskuiu Gorodskuiu Dumu", *ISGD*, 1907, no. 4, pp. 332–380.

158 'Measures of all-provincial significance' were, for instance, the organisation of medical-sanitary observation at particularly popular places or measures for the improvement of their sanitary conditions. They also included the establishment of medical observation points at the rivers or the organisation of soup kitchens and tearooms. All these measures, however, only involved the activity of the provincial zemstvo, which was supposed to support and strengthen the measures taken by municipal and district authorities. See Teziakov, *Ocherk kholernoi epidemii 1907 g.*, chap. 3, pp. 41–46.

159 The earliest beginnings of *sanitary guardianships* in Saratov city actually reach back to the year 1898. They were only put into operation for the first time because of the outbreak of cholera in 1904. After the revolution the guardianships were prohibited by the provincial zemstvo and only re-established in 1908, as temporary institutions in times of cholera. Saratov city established permanent sanitary guardianships only in 1912. For their history see Matveev, *Gorod Saratov v sanitarnom otnoshenii*, pp. 165–189; also "Doklad gorodskoi sanitarnoi komissii ob uchrezhdenii sanitarnykh popechitel'stv v gorode Saratove", *Svedeniia o deiatel'nosti vrachebno-sanitarnoi organisatsii v bol'nitse g. Saratova za fevrale 1912 g.*, 1912, no. 2, pp. 25–32.

160 "Protokol' zasedaniia Saratovskoi gubernskoi sanitarno-ispolnitel'noi kommissii 20 iuliia 1910 g.", *Vrachebno-sanitarnaia khronika Saratovskoi Gubernii*, 1910, no. 8, pp. 757–780, here: p. 761.

161 Ibid., p. 761.

162 See the reports in the zemstvo edited *Kholernaia epidemiia v Saratovskoi gubernii v 1908 godu. Sbornik otchetov* (Saratov, 1909); *v 1909 godu* (Saratov, 1910); *v 1910 godu* (Saratov, 1911).

163 S.I. Zlatogorov, "O kholere 1907 g. v Saratovskoi gubernii", pp. 367–368.

164 Ibid., p. 367.

165 Ibid., p. 366.

166 For the minutes of the first duma meeting concerning the cholera epidemic on 22.8.1907 see *ISGD*, 1907, no. 3, pp. 239–253.

167 For the measures taken by the municipal duma see "Dannye o razvitii i dvizhenii epidemii kholery v g. Saratove so dnia ee vozniknoveniia po oktiabr", *ISGD*, 1907, no. 5, pp. 616–641, esp. p. 626–630; also *ISGD*, 1907, no. 3, pp. 239–240; *Obzor deiatel'nosti Saratovskogo gorodskogo obshchestvennogo napravleniia za 1905–08 godu* (Saratov, 1909), pp. 295–301.

168 Zlatogorov, "O kholere 1907 g. v Saratovskoi gubernii", p. 365.

169 "Protokol zasedaniia Saratovskoi Gorodskoi Sanitarno-Ispolnitel'noi Kommissii 10.9.1907 goda," *Izvestiia Saratovskoi Gorodskoi Dumy*, 1907, pp. 415–453, esp. pp. 424–425; see also the report by Zlatogorov, "O kholere 1907 g. v Saratovskoi gubernii", *Vrachebnaia gazeta*, p. 365.

170 "Protokol zasedaniia Saratovskoi Gorodskoi Sanitarno-Ispolnitel'noi Kommissii 10.9.1907 goda", pp. 415–453, p. 426.

171 Ibid., pp. 415–453. The decree was issued on 10 September 1907.

172 Zlatogorov, "O kholere 1907 g. v Saratovskoi gubernii", p. 366.

173 Ibid., p. 368.

Conclusion: Saratov, cholera and the empire

1 *St Peterburgskie Vedomosti*, no. 177, 3.7.1892.

Bibliography

Primary sources

Archival material

Russkii Gosudarstvennyi Istoricheskii Arkhiv (RGIA), St Petersburg
f. 1282 Kantseliariia vnutrennikh del
f. 1284 Departament obshchikh del MVD
f. 1287 Khoziaistvennyi departament MVD
f. 1288 Glavnoe upravlenie po delam mestnogo khoziaistva MVD
f. 101 Parokhodnoe obshchestvo "Kavkaz i Merkurii"
f. 573 Departament okladnykh sborov

Selection of official documents

Freiberg, N.B. *Vrachebno-sanitarnoe zakonodatel'stvo v Rossii* (St Petersburg, 1908)
Galanin, M.I. *Meropriiatiia protiv kholery russkogo i inostrannykh pravitel'stv i ikh nauchnye osnovy dlia vrachei i administratorov* (St Petersburg, 1892)
Polnoe sobranie zakonov Rossiiskoi imperii, 2nd series
Ragozin, L.F., ed. *Svod uzakonenii i raporiazhenii pravitel'stva po vrachebnoi i sanitarnoi chasti v imperii*. 3 vols (St Petersburg, 1895–1898)
Svod Zakonov Rossiiskoi Imperii, vol. 13, *Ustav vrachebnyi*. St Petersburg, 1892, 1905, vol. 15 *Svod ugolovnyi* (St Petersburg, 1885)
Ministerstvo vnutrennikh del. Meditsinskii departament. *Otchet o sostoianii narodnogo zdraviia i organisatsii vrachebnoi pomoshchi naseleniiu v Rossii* (St Petersburg, 1899)
——, *Rossiiskii meditsinskii spisok* (St Petersburg, 1857–1912)
——, *Sanitarnoe sostoianie gorodov Rossiiskoi Imperii v 1895 godu* (St Petersburg, 1899)
——, *Spravochnaia kniga dlia vrachei*, 2 vols. (St Petersburg, 1857–1912)
——, Tsentral'nyi statisticheskii komitet. *Obshchii svod po imperii rezul'tatov razrabotki dannykh pervoi vseobshchei perepisi naseleniia, proizvedennoi 28 ianvaria 1897 goda.* Edited by N.A. Troinitskii. 2 vols. (St Petersburg, 1905)

Contemporary newspapers and journals

Gigiena i sanitariia
Gorodskoe delo
Meditsinskaia beseda

Meditsinskoe obozrenie
Mezhdunarodnaia klinika
Morskoi sbornik
Nabliudatel'
Nedelia
Obshchestvennyi vrach
Prakticheskaia meditsina
Pravitel'stvennyi vestnik
Saratovskii dnevnik
Saratovskii listok
Saratovskie gubernskie vedomosti
Saratovskii sanitarnyi obzor
Saratovskaia zemskaia nedelia
Sovremennaia klinika
Sankt Peterburgskie vedomosti
Russkaia starina
Russkie vedomosti
Russkii arkhiv
Russkii vrach
Sel'skoe khoziaistvo i lesovodstvo
Vestnik Evropy
Vestnik obshchestvennoi gigieny, sudebnoi i prakticheskoi meditsiny
Vestnik sudebnoi meditsiny i obshchestvennoi gigieny
Voenno-meditsinskii zhurnal
Vrach
Vrachebno-sanitarnaia khronika Saratovskoi gubernii
Vrachebnaia gazeta
Zhurnal mikrobiologii, epidemiologii i immunobiologii
Zhurnal ministerstva vnutrennikh del
Zhurnal obshchestva russkikh vrachei v pamiat' N.I.Pirogova
Zhurnal russkogo obshchestva okhraneniia narodnogo zdraviia

Contemporary unofficial documents

Alianchikov, P.N., "Otchet o deiatel'nosti vo vremia prikomandirovaniia k Bakinskomu karantinu", *Trudy s"ezda vrachei, prinimavshikh neposredstvennoe uchastie v bor'be s kholeroiu v Rossii v 1892 godu* (St Petersburg, 1893), pp. 320–336

Almazov, V.I., "K voprosu ob uporiadochenii Glebucheva ovraga", *ISGD*, 1907, no. 4, pp. 487–496

——, "O kanalizatsii v Saratove. Doklad gorodskoi dume", *ISGD*, 1907, no. 1, pp. 114–136

Amsterdamskii, A.V., "Kholernaia epidemiia 1892 goda v Saratove i ee sviaz' s sanitarnymi usloviiami goroda", *SSO*, 1895, no. 1–4, pp. 89–120; no. 5, pp. 180–189; no. 6, pp. 219–235

Arkhangel'skii, G.I. *Kholernye epidemii Evropeiskoi Rossii v 50-ti letnii period 1823–1872 gg.* (St Petersburg, 1847)

Avdakov, N.S., *Geografichesko-Statisticheskii ocherk kholernoi epidemii v Rossii v 1910 g.* (Khar'kov, 1910)

Binshtok, V.I., "Kholernaia epidemiia 1910 goda v Rossii", *Vrachebnaia gazeta*, no. 45, 7.11.1910, pp. 1353–1357

Blosfel'd, G.I., "Zamechaniia o vostochnoi kholere, svirepstvovavshei v gorode Kazani v 1847 godu, sobrannye is nabliudenii professorov meditsinskago fakul'teta Imperatorskago Kazanskago Universiteta", *Uchenye zapiski*, izdavaemye Imperatorskim Kazanskim Universitetom 1848, kn. 1 (Kazan', 1848), pp. 1–102

Bogomolov, T.I., "Ocherk sposobov lecheniia kholery, primeniavshikhcia v epidemii 1892 goda", *Sovremennaia Klinika*, 1893, no. 5, pp. 353–456

Briusgin, A. "Epidemiia aziatskoi kholery v g. Saratove v 1892 g.", *Zhurnal russkogo obshchestva okhraneniia narodnogo zdraviia*, 1896, no. 6–7, pp. 537–549

Bukhovtsev, I.N., Shteinberg, S.I., *Kholera i mery preduprezhdeniia ee razvitiia* (Saratov, 1885)

Chervonenkis, M., "Kratkii obzor epidemii kholery v Saratovskoi gubernii v 1904 g.", *Vrachebno-sanitarnaia khronika Saratovskoi gubernii*, 1905, no. 3–4, pp. 241–253

Clemow, Frank; Edin, M.D., *The Cholera Epidemic of 1892 in the Russian Empire* (London, New York, 1893)

Danilov, N., "Obzor epidemii aziatskoi kholery v Messopotamii i Persii v 1889 g.; mery, priniatye protiv zanosa ee v predely Rossii", *Meditsinskaia beseda*, 1890, vol. 4 (April), pp. 145–147

Dembo, G.I., "K istorii bor'by s kholeroi v Rossii v 1910 godu", *Vrachebnaia gazeta*, 1910, no. 45, pp. 1368–1374

Derbek, F.A., *Istoriia chumnykh epidemii v Rossii s osnovaniia gosudarstva do nastoiashchego vremeni* (St Petersburg, 1905)

Desiatov, A.A., "Iz namechennykh meropriiatii dlia bor'by s kholeroi v 1908 g.", *Vrachebnaia gazeta*, 1908, no. 21, pp. 651–652

——, *Kholera 1907–1908–1909 i 1910 g.g. na vodnykh putiakh Kazanskogo okruga putei soobshcheniia* (St Petersburg, 1905)

——, "Ocherk sanitarno-ekonomicheskogo polozheniia rabochikh na parokhodakh basseina reki Volga", *Materialy dlia izucheniia sanitarnogo sostoianiia vnutrennykh vodnykh putei. VIII sbornik otchetov i dokladov vrachei sanitarnogo nadzora na r.r. Volge i Kame i na Mariinskoi sisteme za 1903 g.* (St Petersburg, 1904) pp. 119–135

Diubiuk, Evgenii, "Usloviia naima na sel'sko-choziaistvennye raboty i tseny na rabochie ruki v 1905", *Sbornik svedenii po Saratovskoi Gubernii za 1905* (Saratov, 1906)

Doklady upravy po otdeleniiu narodnogo zdraviia o kholere (Saratov, 1904)

Dukhovnikov, F.V., "Pamiati M.I. Semevskogo: referat', chitannyi v Saratovskoi uchenoi arkhivnoi komissii", *Russkaia Starina*, 1892, December, pp. 685–689

Ekk, N.V., "O chrezmernoi smertnosti v Rossii i neobkhodimosti ozdorovleniia", *Mezhdunarodnaia klinika*, no. 5, 1888, pp. 685–689

Engel'gardt, A.P., *Chernozemnaia Rossiia. Ocherk ekonomicheskogo polozheniia kraia* (Saratov, 1902)

Erisman, F.F., Khlopin, G.V., "Meditsina i narodnoe zdravie v Rossii", *Brokgauz-Eifron*, 1899, vol. 27, pp. 214–227

Erisman, F.F., *Kholera: Epidemiologiia i profilaktika* (Moscow, 1893)

Ershov, A. I., *Ocherk chernorabochego dvizheniia v Saratovskom krae* (Saratov, 1909)

Ershov, C.M., "Epidemiia aziatskoi kholery v 1889 godu i mery bor'by s neiu", *Mezhdunarodnaia klinika*, 1890, no. 3 (March), pp. 1–20

Freiberg, N.G., "Kholernye epidemii 1907 i 1908 gg. v Rossii", *Vrachebnaia gazeta*, 1908, no. 35, pp. 97–103

——, "Mezhdunarodnye mery protiv kholery i chumy. Parizhskaia konventsiia 1903 goda", *VOGSPM*, 1906, pp. 122–125

Frenkel', Z., *Kholera i nashi goroda* (Moscow, 1909)

Galanin, M.I., *Meropriiatiia protiv kholery russkogo i inostrannykh pravitel'stv i ikh nauchnye osnovy dlia vrachei i administratorov* (St Petersburg, 1892)

Gamal'ia, N.F., *Kholera* (St. Petersburg, 1910)

Gets fon', P.P., "Dnevnik pastora Ioanna Gubera: kholera f Saratove, v iune I iule 1830 g.", *Russkaia starina* (August 1878), pp. 581–590

Glavatskii, P.A., "Meropriiatiia po bor'be s kholeroiu na Kavkaze", *Trudy s"ezda vrachei, prinimavshikh neposredstvennoe uchastie v bor'be s kholernoi epidemiei 1892 goda v Rossii* (St Petersburg, 1893), pp. 31–35

Gran', M.M., "Poslednie epidemii v Rossii v sviazi s sostoianiem sovremennykh epidemiologicheskikh znanii", *Zhurnal ORVP*, 1908, no. 5, pp. 627–640

——, "Zaboty Samarskogo gubernskogo zemstva o prishlykh sel'skokhoziaistvennykh rabochikh", *SSO*, 1901, no. 1–16, pp. 16–28

——, "Prishlye sel'skokhoziaistvennye rabochie Samarskoi gubernii v sanitarnom otnoshenii", *SSO*, 1901, no. 42–45, pp. 32–51

Grebenshchikov, V.I., Sokolov, D.A. *Smertnost' v Rossii i bor'ba s neiu* (St Petersburg, 1901)

Grigor'ev, N.I., "Kholera v Astrakhani v 1892 godu", *Zhurnal russkogo obshchestva okhraneniia narodnogo zdraviia*, 1893, no. 5, pp. 348–413

Gusev, S.; Khovanskii, A., *Saratovets. Ukazatel' i putevoditel' po Saratovu.* (Saratov, 1881)

Haurowiz, H., *Topographisch-medicinische Beobachtungen über den südlichen Theil des Saratowschen Gouvernements* (St Petersburg, 1836)

Kanel', V.Ia. "Obshchestvennaia meditsina v sviazi s usloviiami zhizni naroda", *Istoriia Rossii v xix veke*, 9 vols (St Petersburg, 1909–1911), vol. 8, pp. 156–262

Karchagin, L.G., "Po povodu kholernoi epidemii v Rossii v 1892", *Vrach*, 1892, no. 32, pp. 79–81

Katsaurov, M., "Pravila 11 avgusta 1903 g.", *Vrachebnyi vestnik*, 1905, no. 19, pp. 295–296

Kazanskii, M., *Oblastnoi Povolzhskii protivokholernyi s"ezd v g. Samare (20–29.4.1908)* (Kazan', 1909)

Kazanskii okrug putei soobshcheniia. Obzor o deiatel'nosti vrachebno-sanitarnogo nadzora na rr. Volge i Kame i na Mariinskoi sisteme za 1904 g. (St Petersburg, 1905); za 1908 (St Petersburg, 1909), za 1910 (St Petersburg, 1911)

Kedrov, S., "Kratkii obzor istorii Saratovskogo kraia", *Saratovskii krai. Istoricheski ocherk, vospominaniia, materialy* (Saratov, 1893), pp. 3–18

Kharitonov, L.A., "Kholernaia epidemiia v Rossii v 1892–1895 godakh", *VOGSPM*, 1902, Apr., pp. 1–16; Nov. pp. 16–23

Khlopin, G.V., *Materialy po ozdorovleniiu Rossii. Sanitarnoe opisanie g.g. Astrakhani, Samary, Saratova i Tsaritsyna s ukazaniem mer, neobkhodimykh dlia ikh ozdorovleniia* (St Petersburg, 1911)

Khlopin, G.V., "Vlianie neftianykh produktov na rybnoe naselenie rek i na kachestvo ikh vody", *Vrach*, 1898, no. 51, pp. 217–223

Kholernaia Epidemiia v Saratovskoi Gubernii v 1910 godu. Sbornik otchetov, izdanie Saratovskogo gubernskogo zemstvo (Saratov, 1911)

Kirilov, N.V., "Kholernaia epidemiia Dal'nego Vostoka i mery bor'by s nimi v Kitae i v nashikh predelakh", *Pirogovskii s"ezd po bor'be s kholeroi, Mskova, 21–23 marta 1905 g., Trudy s"ezda* (Moscow, 1905), pp. 1–11

Klodnitskii, N.N., "Kharakter i znachenie epidemii kholery 1907 g. v Samare i Astrakhani", *Vrachebnaia gazeta*, 1908, no. 21, pp. 639–642

Kokshaiskii, I.N., *Gorod Saratov v zhilishchnom otnoshenii: Predvaritel'nye dannye perepisi naseleniia goroda Saratova i ego prigorodov, proizvedennoi v 1916 godu* (Saratov, 1922)

Kolpenskii, V., "Kholernyi bunt v 1892 godu", *Arkhiv istorii truda v Rossii*, 1922, no. 3, p. 104–113

Krotkov, M.I., *Doklad o neobkhodimoi i vozmozhnoi zamene nyne praktikuemykh sposobov udaleniia iz goroda Saratova nechistot i otbrosov gorodskoi zhizni i uborki ikh na svalochnom uchastke gorodskoi zemli luchshimi sposobami ikh udaleniia i uborki* (Saratov, 1899)

Kuz'min, S.I.; Ershov, A.I., *Kratkii ocherk sostoianiia Saratovskoi Aleksandrovskoi gubernskoi zemskoi bol'nitsy v 1906,1907 i otchasti v 1905 godu. Doklad IX gubernskomu s'ezdu vrachei i predsedatelei zemskikh uprav Saratovskoi gubernii* (Saratov, 1908)

Lias, S.A., "Kholernye zametki i vpechatleniia", *Sbornik otchetov vrachei i studentov rabotavshikh po kholernoi epidemii 1892 goda v Saratovskoi gubernii*, ed. Saratovskoe gubernskoe zemstvo. Saratov 1893, pp. 82–83

Lichtenstädt, Jeremias, *Die asiatische Cholera in Russland in den Jahren 1829 und 1830* (Berlin, 1831)

——, "Fragmente aus einer ausführlichen zur Fortsetzung meiner Schriften über die asiatische Cholera in Russland bestimmten Abhandlung von Prof. Dr. Lichtenstädt", *Mittheilungen über die Cholera-Epidemie zu St. Petersburg im Sommer 1831, von praktischen Aerzten daselbst*, unter Redaktion der Herren Doktoren Lichtenstädt und Seidlitz, 2 vols (St Petersburg, 1831)

Likhachev, V.I., *Sanitarnoe opisanie povolzh'ia* (St Petersburg, 1898)

Lipskii, A.A., "Mery bor'by s kholeroiu, proektirovannye v Rossii v 1883–1885 godakh", *VOGSPM*, vol. 9, (January–March 1890), pp. 36–46

Loris-Melikov, I.Z., "Iz otcheta o poezdke v Persiiu", *VOGSPM*, vol. 27, no. 7 (January 1895), pp. 1–38

Lunkevich, A., "Obshchii otchet po komandirovkam v Zakaspiiskuiu oblast', po sluchaiu poiavleniia asiatskoi kholery, i v Persiiu, po povodu rassledovaniia slukhov o liudskoi chume", *Voenno-meditsinskii zhurnal*, vol. 176, no. 1 (Jan. 1893), pp. 49–72

Mark, C.A., "Kholera v selenii Kaakhka Zakaspiiskoi oblasti", *Voenno-meditsinskii zhurnal*, vol. 179, no. 1 (January 1894), pp. 1–47

Markus, F.C.M., *Rapport sur le choléra-morbus de Moscow* (Moscow, 1832)

Maslakovets, P.P., "Kholera v g. Astrakhani i ee predmestiiakh letom 1907 g.", *Vrachebnaia gazeta*, 1908, no. 21, pp. 642–645

Matveev, I.V., *Glebuchev ovrag, 1871 – 1906 gg.* (Saratov, 1907)

——, "Bani goroda Saratova", *SZN*, 1897, no. 5, pp. 212–228

——, *Gorod Saratov v sanitarnom otnoshchenii v 1906 godu. Otchet sanitarnogo vracha*, (Saratov, 1906)

——, "Kholera v Saratove", *Saratovskii Dnevnik*, no. 127, 17.6.1892

——, "Nochlezhie doma, artel'nye kvartiry i postoialye dvory goroda Saratova", *SZN*, 1896, no. 9–10, pp. 79–113; no. 39, pp. 502–511; 1898, no. 13–14, pp. 115–128; no. 24, pp. 125–164

——, "Sanitarnye ocherki berega Volgi u Saratova", *VOGSPM*, Nov. 1906, pp. 1–53

——, "Sanitarnye ocherki. Doma prizreniia", *SZN*, 1898, no. 24, pp. 148–149

——, "Saratovskie bogadel'ni. Sanitarnye ocherki", *SZN*, 1898, no. 9–10, pp. 79–113

Miropol'skii, V.I., *Obshhchii ocherk deiatel'nosti 'Obshchestva Saratovskikh sanitarnykh vrachei', s maia 1886 g. po ianvar' 1893 goda* (Saratov, 1893)

Molleson, I.I., "Organisatsiia dela bor'by s kholeroiu v Saratovskoi gubernii", *Trudy s"ezda vrachei, prinimavshikh neposredstvennoe uchastie v bor'be s kholeroiu v Rossii v 1892 godu* (St Petersburg, 1893), pp. 27–30

Molleson, I.I., "V ozhidanie kholery", *SZN*, 1892, no. 2, pp. 425–434

Nikolaev, E., "Saratovskoe sanitarnoe obshchestvo", *SZN*, 1905, no. 6–7, pp. 59–65

Novosel'skii, S.A., "Kholera i vodosnabzhenie v gorodakh Rossii", *Vrachebnaia gazeta*, 1912, no. 8, pp. 21–23

Obshchestvo russkikh vrachei v pamiat' N.I. Pirogova, *Trudy s"ezda vrachei prinimavshikh neposredstvennoe uchastie v bor'be s kholernoi epidemiei 1892 g. v Rossii s 13. po 20. dekabriia 1892* (St Petersburg, 1893)

Obshchestvo Saratovskikh sanitarnykh vrachei, *Protokoly zasedanii obshchestva za 1890, 91, 92 gg.* (Saratov, 1893)

Pagozhev, A.V., "S"ezd vrachei pri meditsinskom departamente 13–20 dekabria 1892 g.", *Meditsinskoe obzrenie*, vol. 39, no. 2 (1893), pp. 197–207

Pavlovskii, A.D., "Ob organisatsii i primenenii mediko-sanitarnykh mer, priniatykh protiv kholery v Povolzh'e, mezhdu Nizhnim Novgorodom i Astrakhan'iu i v Kamskom krae, po rekam Kame, Viatke i Beloi, v epidemiiu 1892 goda", *Trudy s"ezda vrachei prinimavshikh neposredstvenno uchastie v bor'be s kholernoi epidemiei 1892 goda v Rossii* (St Petersburg, 1893), pp. 368–382

Pirogovskii s"ezd po bor'be s kholeroi. Moskva 21.–23.3.1905. Trudy s"ezda (Moskow, 1905)

Poliakov, P.A., "Kholernaia epidemiia 1892 goda v g. Askhabade", *Voenno-meditsinskii zhurnal*, vol. 177, no. 5 (May 1893), pp. 43–102

Ponomarev, N., "O peredvizhenii sel'sko-khoziastvennykh rabochikh, napravliaiush-chikhsia v iugo-vostochny mestnosti Rossii", *Sel'skoe khoziaistvo i lesovodstvo*, 1896, no. 2, pp. 270–312

Popov, R.V., "Kratkii obzor meropriiatii, vypolnennykh zemstvami Moskovskoi gubernii v vidu ugrozhaiushchei kholery", *Trudy s"ezda vrachei prinimavshikh neposredstvenno uchastie v bor'be s kholernoi epidemiei 1892 goda v Rossii* (St Petersburg, 1893), pp. 35–43

Raskovich, S.L., "Otchet o deiatel'nosti Pasterovskoi stantsii Saratovskogo gubernskogo zemstva za pervuiu polovinu 1903 goda", *Vrachebno-sanitarnaia khronika Saratovskoi gubernii*, 1903, no. 7, pp. 269–278

——, "Pasterovskaia Stantsiia", *SSO*, 1903, no. 3, pp. 29–41

Reman, Dr. J., "Poiavlenie vostochnoi kholery na sredizemnom i Kaspiiskom More", *Voenno-meditsinskii zhurnal*, vol. 3, no. 1 (1824), pp. 3–14; vol. 3, no. 2 (1824), pp. 159–195

Rodionov, N.N., "Kratkii ocherk kholernoi epidemii 1908 goda v g. Tsaritsyne", *Kholernaia epidemiia v Saratovskoi gubernii v 1908 godu. Sbornik otchetov* (Saratov, 1909), pp. 42–59

Rostovtsev, G.I., "V ozhidanii kholernoi epidemii", *Vrachebnyi vestnik*, 1905, no. 15, pp. 9–10

Rozanov, P.P., "Ob obshchestvennykh merakh bor'by s kholeroi", *Pirogovskii s"ezd po bor'be s kholeroi. Moskva 21.–23.3.1905* (Moscow, 1905), pp. 116–124

Saar, G., *Saratovskaia promyshlennost' v nachale 90-kh gg.* (Saratov, 1928)

Schiemann, Theodor, *Geschichte Russlands unter Kaiser Nikolaus I.*, Bd. 3: *Kaiser Nikolaus im Kampf mit Polen und im Gegensatz zu England und Frankreich. 1830–1840* (Berlin, 1913)

Semenov T'ian Shanskii, V.P. (ed.) *Rossiia. Polnoe geograficheskoe opisanie nashego otechestva*. 9 vols (St Petersburg, 1901), vol. 6

Sokolov, P.N., "O sanitarnom sostoianii ovragov Beloglinskogo i Glebucheva", *SZN*, 1905, no. 3, pp. 29–46; 1905, no. 4, pp. 13–34

——, "Sanitarnyi ocherk g. Saratova", *SZN*, 1904, no. 5, pp. 51–69 and 1904, no. 6–7, pp. 116–123

Ternovskii, A.A., "Doklad kommissii s"ezda zemskikh vrachei o meropriiatiiakh na sluchai vozobnovleniia kholery v 1893 godu", *Saratovskii sanitarnyi obzor*, 1893, no. 1, pp. 1–10

Teziakov, N.I., *Materialy po izucheniiu detskoi smertnosti v Saratovskoi gubernii s 1899 po 1901 g.* (Saratov, 1904)

——, "Kholernaia epidemiia v Saratovskoi gubernii v 1910 godu, v sviazi s epidemiiami 1904–1909 gg.", *Kholernaia epidemiia v Saratovskoi gubernii v 1910 godu. Sbornik otchetov*, ed. Saratovskoe gubernskoe zemstvo (Saratov, 1911), pp. 178–191

——, "Kratkii ocherk kholernoi epidemii 1908 g. v Saratovskoi gubernii", *Kholernaia epidemiia v Saratovskoi gubernii v 1908 godu. Sbornik otchetov*, ed. Saratovskoe gubernskoe zemstvo (Saratov, 1909), pp. 132–139

——, "*Materialy dlia kharakteristiki Saratovskoi Aleksandrovskoi gubernskoi zemskoi bol'nitsy, kak obshche-gubernskogo lechebnogo uchrezhdeniia. Doklad VIII gubernskomu s"ezdu vrachei i predsedatelei zemskikh uprav Saratovskoi gubernii* (Saratov, 1907)

——, *Ocherk kholernoi epidemii 1907 g. i protivokholernye meropriiatiia v Saratovskoi gubernii* (Saratov, 1908)

——, "Otkhozhie promysly i rynki naima sel'sko-khozaistvennykh rabochikh v Saratovskoi gubernii", *SZN*, 1903, no. 1, pp. 1–39

——, "Kholernaia epidemiia v Saratovskoi gubernii v 1910 godu, v sviazi s epidemiiami 1904–1909 gg.", *Kholernaia epidemiia v Saratovskoi gubernii v 1910 godu. Sbornik otchetov*, ed. Saratovskoe gubernskoe zemstvo (Saratov, 1911), pp. 178–191

Ukke, "Epidemii i nashi meditsinskie poriadki", *Vestnik Evropy*, 1882, vol. 5, pp. 827–852

Ves' Saratov. Spravochnik-Kalendar' (Saratov, 1916)

Vladykin, B.V., *Materialy k istorii kholernoi epidemii 1892–1895 v predelakh evropeiskoi Rossii* (St Petersburg, 1899)

Vodarskii, E.A., *Volga. Vodnye puti Volzhskogo basseina v predelakh Kazanskogo okruga putei soobshcheniia. Tekhnicheskii-statisticheskii ocherk* (Moskva, 1908)

Vorob'ev, V.V., "O nekotorykh faktorakh, sposobstvovavshikh vozniknoveniiu kholernykh besporiadkov v epidemiiu 1892 goda", *Trudy s"ezda vrachei, prinimavshikh neposredstvennoe uchastie v bor'be s kholeroiu v Rossii v 1892 godu* (St Petersburg, 1893), pp. 137–144

Zhbankov, D.I., *Kratkii istoricheskii obzor deiatel'nosti sanitarnykh biuro i obshchestvenno-sanitarnykh uchrezhdenii v zemskoi Rossii* (Moscow, 1910)

——, "Neskol'ko zametok o kholere 1892 i 1893 gg. i o bor'be s neiu", *Vrach*, 1894, no. 51, pp. 1–26

Zlatogorov, S.I., "O deiatel'nosti vrachebno-sanitarnogo otriada, komandirovannogo v mae 1905 goda v Tavriz v ozhidanii kholery", *Vrachebnaia gazeta*, 1908, no. 2, pp. 252–257; no. 10, pp. 285–297

——, "O kholere 1907 v Saratovskoi gubernii", *Vrachebnaia gazeta*, 1908, no. 12, pp. 363–368; no. 13, pp. 409–412

——, "O predokhranitel'nykh privivkakh protiv kholery", *Pirogovskii s"ezd po bor'be s kholeroi, Moskva 21.–23.3.1905, Trudy s"ezda* (Moskva, 1905), pp. 42–58

General reference materials

Bol'shaia meditsinskaia entsiklopediia. Edited by A.N. Semashko. 35 vols (Moscow, 1928–1936); edited by A.N. Bakulev. 36 vols, 2nd ed. (Moscow, 1956–65)

Chernova, E.N. (ed.), *Sistematicheskii katalog otechestvennykh periodicheskikh i prodolzhaiushchikhsia izdanii po meditsine*, 1792–1960 (Leningrad, 1965)

Entsiklopedicheskii slovar' Brokgauz i Efrona, 86 vols (St Petersburg, 1890–1907)

Entsiklopedicheskii slovar' voennoi meditsiny, 6 vols (Moscow, 1946–1948)

Fadeev, T.D.; Ramazaev, E.F.; Efimov, T.P. *Kholera. Bibliografiia otechestvennoi literatury 1823–1962* (Saratov, 1966)

Kaufman, I.M., *Russkie biograficheskie i biobibliograficheskie slovari* (Moscow, 1956)

Khovanskii, N.F., *Ocherki po istorii goroda Saratova i Saratovskoi gubernii* (Saratov, 1884), vol. 1, chap. 4, Nashi pisateli, uchenye, voiny i gosudarstvennye liudi, pp. 37–184

Levit, M.M., *Meditsinskaia periodicheskaia pechat' Rossii i SSSR* (1792–1962) (Moscow, 1963)

Lotova, E.I., *Bibliografiia i obzor osnovnykh rabot po istorii gigeny i sanitarii (1917–1957gg.)* (Moscow, 1959)

Petrov, B.D. and Matskina, R. Iu. (eds), *Istoriia razvitiia meditsiny i zdravookhraneniia v Rossii: Obzor dokumental'nykh materialov* (Moscow, 1958)

Rossiiskii, D.M., *Istoriia vseobshchei i otechestvennoi meditsiny i zdravookhraneniia: Bibliografiia (996–1954 gg.)*, edited by B.D. Petrov (Moscow, 1956)

Rossiiskii, D.M., *Bibliograficheskii ukazatel' russkoi literatury po istorii meditsiny s 1789 g. po 1928 g.* (Moscow, 1928)

Russkii biograficheskii slovar', 25 vols (St Petersburg, 1896–1918)

Sokolov, S.L., "Saratovtsy-pisateli i uchenye (Materialy dlia biobibliograficheskogo slovaria)", *Trudy Saratovskoi uchenoi arkhivnoi komissii*, vol. xxx, xxxii, xxxiii (Saratov, 1913–1916)

Valk, S.N. and Bedin, V.V., *Tsentral'nyi gosudarstvennyi istoricheskii arkhiv SSSR v Leningrade: Putevoditel'* (Leningrad, 1956)

Zhbankov, D.N., *Bibliograficheskii ukazatel' po obshchestvennoi meditsinskoi literature za 1890–1905 gg.* (Moscow, 1907)

Secondary literature

Ackerknecht, Erwin H., "Anticontagionism between 1821 and 1867", *Bulletin of the History of Medicine*, XX (1948), pp. 562–593

Alexander, John T., *Bubonic Plague in Early Modern Russia: Public Health and Urban Disaster* (Baltimore, London: Johns Hopkins University Press, 1980)

—— , "Catherine II, Bubonic Plague, and the Problem of Industry in Moscow", *American Historical Review* 79 (June 1974), pp. 637–671

—— , "Communicable Disease, Anti-epidemic Policies, and the Role of Medical Professionals in Russia, 1752–62", *Canadian-American Slavic Studies* 12 (spring 1978), pp. 154–169

—— "Medical Developments in Petrine Russia", *Canadian-American Slavic Studies* 7 (summer 1974), pp. 198–221

—— "Medical Professionals and Public Health in 'Doldrums' Russia, 1725–1762", *Canadian-American Slavic Studies* 12 (spring 1978), pp. 116–135

Alpern-Engel, Barbara, *Between the Fields and the City. Women, Work, and Family in Russia, 1861–1914* (Cambridge: Cambridge University Press, 1995)

—— , "Russian Peasant View of City Life: 1861–1914", *Slavic Review*, vol. 52, no. 3 (1993), pp. 446–459

Altstadt-Mirhadi, Audrey. "Baku. Transformation of a Muslim Town", Michael F. Hamm (ed.), *The City in Late Imperial Russia* (Bloomington: Indiana University Press, 1986), pp. 238–318

Anderson, Barbara, *Internal Migration during Modernization in Late Nineteenth Century Russia* (Princeton: Princeton University Press, 1980)

Arnold, David, *Colonizing the Body. State Medicine and Epidemic Disease in Nineteenth-Century India* (Berkeley: University of California Press, 1993)

——, "Cholera and Colonialism in British India", *Past and Present*, vol. 113 (1986), pp. 118–151

—— (ed.), *Warm Climates and Western Medicine: The Emergence of Tropical Medicine, 1500–1900* (Amsterdam: Rodopi, 1996)

Ascher, A. *The Revolution of 1905. Russia in Disarray*, 2 vols (Stanford, Calif.: Stanford University Press, 1988)

——, *P.A. Stolypin: The Search for Stability in Late Imperial Russia* (Stanford, Calif.: Stanford University Press, 2001)

Balzer, Harley D. (ed.), *Russia's Missing Middle-Class: The Professions in Russian History* (Armonk, N.Y.: M.E. Sharpe, 1996)

Bater, James M., *St Petersburg: Industrialization and Change* (Montreal: McGill-Queen's University Press, 1976)

——, "Some Dimensions of Urbanization and the Response of Municipal Government: Moscow and St Petersburg", *Russian History*, vol. 5, no. 1 (1978), pp. 46–63

——, "St Petersburg and Moscow on the Eve of Revolution", Kaiser, D.H. (ed.), *The Workers' Revolution in Russia, 1917. The View from Below* (Cambridge: Cambridge University Press, 1987), pp. 20–58

—— "Transcience, Residential Persistence, and Mobility in Moscow and St Petersburg, 1900–1914", *Slavic Review*, 39, no. 2 (June 1980), pp. 239–254

Berman, Marshall, *All that is Solid Melts into Air: The Experience of Modernity* (New York: Simon & Schuster, 1982)

Bilson, Geoffrey, *A Darkened House: Cholera in Nineteenth-Century Canada* (Toronto, 1980)

Black, Cyril E., *The Dynamics of Modernization. A Study in Comparative History* (New York: Harper & Row, 1966)

Blackwell, William L., *The Beginnings of Russian Industrialization 1800–1860* (Princeton: Princeton University Press, 1968)

——, "Modernization and Urbanization in Russia", Michael Hamm (ed.), *The City in Russian History* (Lexington: University Press of Kentucky, 1976)

Bonnell, Victoria E., *Roots of Rebellion: Workers' Politics and Organizations in St Petersburg and Moscow, 1900–1914* (Berkeley: University of California Press, 1983)

——, *The Russian Worker: Life and Labor under the Tsarist Regime* (Berkeley: University of California Press, 1983)

——, "Urban Working Class Life in Early Twentieth-Century Russia: Some Problems and Patterns", *Russian History*, vol. 8, no. 3 (1981), pp. 360–378

Bradley, Joseph, *Muzhik and Muscovite: Urbanization in Late Imperial Russia* (Berkeley: University of California Press, 1985)

——, "'Once You've Eaten Khitrov Soup You'll Never Leave!': Slum Renovation in Late Imperial Russia", *Russian History*, vol. 11 (1984), pp. 1–28

——, "The Moscow Workhouse and Urban Welfare Reform in Russia", *Russian Review* 41, no. 4 (1892), pp. 427–444

——, "Voluntary Associations, Civic Culture, and Obshchestvennost' in Moscow", Clowes, Edith W., Kassow, Samuel D., West, James L. (eds), *Between Tsar and People. Educated Society and the Quest for Public Identity in Late Imperial Russia* (Princeton: Princeton University Press, 1991), pp. 131–148

Briese, Olaf, *Angst in den Zeiten der Cholera; vol. 1, Über kulturelle Ursprünge des Bakteriums; vol. 2, Panik-Kurve. Berlins Cholerajahr 1831–32; vol. 3, Auf Leben und Tod. Briefwelt als Gegenwelt; vol. 4, Das schlechte Gedicht. Strategien literarischer Immunisierung* (Berlin: Akademie Verlag, 2003)

Briggs, Asa, "Cholera and Society in the Nineteenth Century", *Past and Present*, 19 (Apr. 1961), pp. 76–96

——, "The Human Aggregate", in Dyos, H.J. and Wolff, Michael (eds), *The Victorian City. Images and Realities*, 2 vols, (London, New York: Routledge, 1973), vol. 1, pp. 83–104

Brower, Daniel, *The Russian City between Tradition and Modernity, 1850–1900* (Berkeley, Oxford: University of California Press, 1990)

Brower, Daniel, "Labor Violence in Russia in the Late Nineteenth Century", *Slavic Review* vol. 41, no. 3 (Fall 1992), pp. 417–431

Brower, Daniel R.; Lazzerini, Edward J. (eds), *Russia's Orient: Imperial Borderlands and Peoples, 1700–1917* (Bloomington: Indiana University Press, 1997)

Burbank, Jane; Ransel, David L. (eds), *Imperial Russia: New Histories for the Empire* (Bloomington: Indiana University Press, 1998)

Champion, Justin A.I. (ed.), *Epidemic Disease in London* (London: Centre for Metropolitan History, working papers 1, 1993)

Chevalier, Louis, *Laboring Classes and Dangerous Classes in Paris During the First Half of the Nineteenth Century*, translated by Frank Jellinek (New York: H. Fertig, 1973)

——, (ed.), *Le choléra: la première épidémie du XIX siècle* (La Roche-sur-Yon: Impr. Centrale de l'Ouest, 1958)

Clowes, Edith W., Samuel D. Kassow, and James L. West (eds), *Between Tsar and People: Educated Society and the Quest for Public Identity in Late Imperial Russia* (Princeton: Princeton University Press, 1991)

Curtin, Philip D., *Death by Migration: Europe's Encounter with the Tropical World in the Nineteenth Century* (Cambridge: Cambridge University Press, 1989)

Defoe, Daniel, *A Journal of the Plague Year* (Oxford: Oxford University Press, 1990)

Delaporte, François, *Disease and Civilization: The Cholera in Paris, 1832*, translated by Arthur Goldhammer (Cambridge, Mass.: MIT Press, 1986)

Dettke, Barbara, *Die Asiatische Hydra. Die Cholera 1830/31 in Berlin und den preußischen Provinzen Posen, Preußen und Schlesien* (Berlin: de Gruyter, 1995)

Dinges, Martin, "Kann man medizinische Aufklärung importieren? Kulturelle Probleme im Umfeld deutscher Ärzte in Rußland in der zweiten Hälfte des 18. Jahrhunderts" Beer Mathias, Dahlmann Dittmar (eds.), Migration nach Ost- und Südosteuropa vom 18. bis zum Beginn des 19. Jahrhunderts. Ursachen – Formen – Verlauf – Ergebnis (Stuttgart: Jan Thorbecke Verlag, 1999), pp. 209–234

Douglas, Mary, *Purity and Danger: An Analysis of Concepts of Pollution and Taboo* (London: Routledge, 1966)

Durey, Michael, *The Return of the Plague: British Society and the Cholera, 1831–32* (Dublin: Gill and Macmillan, 1979)

Dyos, H.J. and Wolff, Michael, *The Victorian City. Images and Realities*, 2 vols (London and New York: Routledge, 1973)

Economakis, E.G., *From Peasant to Petersburger* (Basingstoke, London: Macmillan, 1998)

Eklof, Ben; Bushnel, John; Zakharova, Larissa (eds), *Russia's Great Reforms, 1855–1881* (Bloomington: Indiana University Press, 1994)

Eklof, Ben, *Russian Peasant Schools: Officialdom, Village Culture, and Popular Pedagogy* (Berkeley: University of California Press, 1986)

Ely, Christopher, "The Origins of Russian Scenery: Volga River Tourism and Russian Landscape Aesthetics", *Slavic Review*, vol. 62, no. 4 (2003), pp. 666–682

Emmons, Terence and Wayne S. Vucinich (eds), *The Zemstvo in Russia: An Experiment in Local Self-Government* (Cambridge: Cambridge University Press, 1983)

Engelstein, Laura, *The Keys to Happiness. Sex and the Search for Modernity in Fin-de-Siècle Russia* (Ithaca: Cornell University Press, 1992)

——, *Moscow 1905: Working-Class Organization and Political Conflict* (Stanford, Calif.: Stanford University Press, 1982)

Evans, Richard J., *Death in Hamburg. Society and Politics in the Cholera Years 1830–1910* (Oxford: Oxford University Press, 1987)

——, "Epidemics and Revolutions: Cholera in Nineteenth-Century Europe", *Past and Present*, vol. 120 (August 1988), pp. 123–146

——, "Review of Peter Baldwin's *Contagion and the State in Europe, 1830–1930*", *European History Quarterly*, vol. 31 (2000), pp. 447–454

Fedor, Thomas S, *Patterns of Urban Growth in the Russian Empire during the Nineteenth Century* (Chicago: University of Chicago Press, 1975)

Field, Daniel, *Rebels in the Name of the Tsar* (Boston: Houghton Mifflin, 1976)

Field, Mark G, "Medical Organization and the Medical Profession", Black, Cyril E. (ed.), *The Transformation of Russian Society: Aspects of Social Change since 1861* (Cambridge, Mass: Harvard University Press, 1960)

Figes, Orlando, *A People's Tragedy. The Russian Revolution 1891–1924* (London: Pimlico, 1996)

——, *Peasant Russia, Civil War. The Volga Countryside in Revolution (1917–1921)* (Oxford: Clarendon Press, 1989)

Freeze, Gregory L. "The *Soslovie* (Estate) Paradigm and Russian Social History." *American Historical Review,* vol. 91, no. 1 (1986), pp. 11–36

Frieden, Nancy A., *Russian Physicians in an Era of Reform and Revolution, 1856–1905* (Princeton: Princeton University Press, 1981)

——, "The Russian Cholera Epidemic, 1892–93, and Medical Professionalization", *Journal of Social History*, vol. 10 (1977), pp. 538–559

——, "Physicians in Pre-Revolutionary Russia: Professionals or Servants of the State", *Bulletin of the History of Medicine*, vol. 49 (1975), pp. 20–29

Friedgut, Theodore H., "Labor Violence and Regime Brutality in Tsarist Russia: The Iuzovka Cholera Riots of 1892", *Slavic Review*, vol. 46, no. 2 (1988), pp. 245–265

Gleason, William, "Public Health, Politics, and Cities in Late Imperial Russia", *Journal of Urban History*, vol. 16, no. 4 (August 1990), pp. 341–365

Gradmann, Christoph, "Indivisible Enemies. Bacteriology and the Language of Politics in Imperial Germany", *Science in Context*, vol. 13 (2000), pp. 9–30

Graham, Loren R, *Science in Russia and the Soviet Union* (Cambridge: Cambridge University Press, 1993)

Grmek, Mirko, "The History of Medical Education in Russia", C.D. O'Malley (ed.), *The History of Medical Education*, UCLA Forum in Medical Sciences, no. 12 (Berkeley: University of California Press, 1970), pp. 303–327

Gross Solomon, Susan; Hutchinson, John F. (eds), *Health and Society in Revolutionary Russia* (Bloomington: Indiana University Press, 1990)

Hachten, Elizabeth A., "In the Service to Science and Society", *Osiris*, vol. 17 (2002), pp. 171–209

Häffner, Lutz, "Stadtdumawahlen und soziale Eliten in Kazan' 1870 bis 1913: Zur rechtlichen Lage und politischen Praxis der lokalen Selbstverwaltung", *JfGO*, vol. 44, no. 2 (1996), pp. 217–252

——, "Politische Partizipation und sozialpolitischer Diskurs im Spiegel städtischer Sanierung an der städtischen Peripherie von Saratov, 1860–1914", *JfGO*, vol. 48 (2000), pp. 190–209

Haimson, Leopold, "The Problem of Social Stability in Urban Russia, 1905–1917", *Slavic Review*, vol. 23, no. 4 (December 1964), pp. 629–642; 1965, pp. 1–22

Halliday, Stephen, *The Great Stink of London. Sir Joseph Bazalgette and the Cleansing of the Victorian Metropolis* (Gloucestershire: Sutton Publishing, 1999)

Hamm, Michael F., *Kiev. A Portrait, 1800–1917* (Princeton, NJ: Princeton University Presss, 1993)

——, "Khar'kov's Progressive Duma, 1910–1914: A Study in Russian Municipal Reform", *Slavic Review*, vol. 40 (1981), pp. 17–36

——, "The Modern Russian City. A Historiographical Analysis", *Journal of Urban History*, vol. 4, no. 1 (Nov. 1977), pp. 39–75

—— (ed.), *The City in Late Imperial Russia* (Bloomington: Indiana University Press, 1986)

—— (ed.), *The City in Russian History* (Lexington: University of Kentucky Press, 1976)

Hardy, Anne, *The Epidemic Streets: Infectious Disease and the Rise of Preventive Medicine, 1856–1900* (Oxford: Clarendon Press, 1993)

Harrison, Mark, "A Question of Locality: The Identity of Cholera in British India, 1860–1890", David Arnold (ed.), *Warm Climates and Western Medicine: The Emergence of Tropical Medicine 1500–1890* (Amsterdam: Rodopi, 1996), pp. 133–159

Hausmann, Guido, "Die russische Stadt in der Geschichte", *JfGO*, vol. 27 (1979), pp. 481–497

——, *Universität und städtische Gesellschaft in Odessa, 1865–1917: Soziale und nationale Selbstorganisation an der Peripherie des Zarenreiches* (Stuttgart: Frank Steiner Verlag, 1998)

Haywood, Richard Mowbray, *Russia Enters the Railway Age, 1842–1855* (Boulder: East European Monographs, 1988)

Heilbronner, Hans, "The Russian Plague of 1878–79", *Slavic Review*, vol. 21 (March 1962), pp. 89–112

Herlihy, Patricia, *Odessa: A History, 1794–1914* (Cambridge, Mass: Harvard University Press, 1981)

——, "Death in Odessa: A Case Study of Population Movements in a Nineteenth-Century City", *Journal of Urban History*, vol. IV, no. 4 (August 1978), pp. 417–442

Heyningen, William E. and Seal, John R., *Cholera: The American Scientific Experience, 1947–1980* (Boulder, Col.: Westview Press, 1983)

Hildermeyer, Manfred, *Bürgertum und Stadt in Rußland 1760–1860. Rechtliche Lage und soziale Struktur* (Köln-Wien: Böhlau Verlag, 1986)

——, "Sozialer Wandel im städtischen Rußland in der zweiten Hälfte des 19. Jahrhunderts", *JfGO*, vol. 25 (1977), pp. 525–566

Hittle, Michael, *The Service City: State and Townsmen in Russia, 1600–1800* (Cambridge, Mass: Harvard University Press, 1979)

Hoffmann, David L.; Kotsonis, Yanni (eds), *Russian Modernity. Politics, Knowledge, Practices* (London: Macmillan Press, 2000)

Hosking, Geoffrey, *Russia. People and Empire* (Cambridge, Mass.: Harvard University Press, 1997)

Howard-Jones, Norman, "Cholera Therapy in the Nineteenth Century", *Journal of the History of Medicine*, vol. 17 (1972), pp. 373–395

Huber, Valeska, "Unification of the Globe by Disease? The International Sanitary Conferences on Cholera, 1851–1894", *Historical Journal*, vol. 49, no. 2 (2006), pp. 453–467

Hutchinson, John F., *Politics and Public Health in Revolutionary Russia, 1890–1918* (Baltimore, London: Johns Hopkins University Press, 1990)

——, "Politics and Medical Professionalization after 1905", Balzer, Harley D. (ed.), *Russia's Missing Middle Class* (New York, London: M.E. Sharpe, 1996), pp. 89–116

——, "Society, Corporation or Union? Russian Physicians and the Struggle for Professional Unity (1890–1913)", *JfGO*, vol. 30 (1982), pp. 37–53

——, "Tsarist Russia and the Bacteriological Revolution" *Journal of the History of Medicine and Allied Sciences*, vol. 40 (1985), pp. 420–439

——, " 'Who Killed Cock Robin?' An Inquiry into the Death of Zemstvo Medicine", Gross Solomon, Susan and Hutchinson, John F. (eds), *Health and Society in Revolutionary Russia* (Bloomington: Indiana University Press, 1990), pp. 3–26

Ivanov, N.R., *Saratovskie uchenye-mediki. Stranitsy istorii. 1909–1979* (Saratov: Izdatel'stvo Saratovskogo Universiteta: 1982)

Jahn, Hubertus, "Health Care and Poor Relief in Russia, 1700–1856", Ole Peter Grell, Andrew Cunningham, Robert Jütte (eds), *Health Care and Poor Relief in 18th and 19th Century Northern Europe* (Aldershot: Ashgate, 2002), pp. 157–171

——, "Der St. Petersburger Heumarkt im 19. Jahrhundert. Metamorphosen eines Stadtviertels", *JfGO*, vol. 44 (1996), pp. 162–177

Johnson, Robert E., *Peasant and Proletarian: The Working Class of Moscow in the Late Nineteenth Century* (New Brunswick, N.J.: Rutgers University Press, 1979)

——, "Primitive Rebels? Reflections on Collective Violence in Imperial Russia", *Slavic Review*, vol. 41, no. 3 (fall 1982), pp. 432–435

——, "Peasant Migration and the Russian Working Class. Moscow at the End of the Nineteenth Century", *Slavic Review*, vol. 35, no. 4 (Dec. 1976), pp. 652–664

Kahan, Arcadius, "Social Aspects of the Plague Epidemics in 18th-Century Russia", *Economic Development and Cultural Change*, vol. 27 (1979), pp. 255–266

Kizevetter, A.A., *Na rubezh'e dvukh stoletii: Vospominaniia, 1881–1914* (Prague: Orbis, 1929)

Koenker, Diane, *Moscow Workers and the 1917 Revolution* (Princeton: Princeton University Press, 1981)

——, "Collective Action and Collective Violence in the Russian Labor Movement", *Slavic Review*, vol. 41, no. 3 (fall 1982), pp. 443–448

Korolenko, V.G., "V kholernyi god", *Polnoe sobranie sochinenii* 9 vols (St Petersburg, 1914), vol. 3, pp. 369–421

Krug, Peter F., "The debate over the delivery of Health Care in Rural Russia: The Moscow Zemstvo, 1864–1878", *Bulletin of the History of Medicine*, vol. 50 (1976), pp. 226–241

Kudlick, Catherine J., *Cholera in Post-Revolutionary Paris. A Cultural History* (Berkeley, CA.: University of California Press, 1996)

Labisch, A., "Gesundheitskonzept und Medizin im Prozeß der Zivilisation", Spree R. (ed.), *Medizinische Deutungsmacht im sozialen Wandel des 19. und frühen 20. Jahrhunderts* (Bonn: Psychiatrie Verlag, 1989)

Lampard, Eric E., "The Urbanizing World", in Dyos, H.J. and Wolff, Michael (eds), *The Victorian City. Images and Realities*, 2 vols (London and New York: Routledge, 1973), vol. 1, pp. 3–57

Laue, Theodore von, "Russian Labor Between Field and Factory, 1892–1903", *California Slavic Studies*, vol. 3 (1964), pp. 33–64

——, "Russian Peasants in the Factory, 1892–1904" *Journal of European History*, vol. 21 (March 1961), pp. 61–80

Levit, M.M., *Stanovlenie obshchestvennoi meditsiny v Rossii* (Moskva, 1974)

Lincoln, W. Bruce, *Nicholas I. Emperor and Autocrat of All the Russians* (Bloomington: Indiana University Press, 1978)

——, "The Russian State and its Cities: A Search for Effective Municipal Government, 1786–1842", *JfGO*, vol. 17, no. 4 (1969), pp. 531–541

Lincoln Fitzpatrick, Anne, *The Great Russian Fair: Nizhnii Novgorod, 1840–1890* (Basingstoke: Macmillan, 1990)

Lindenmeyr, A., *Poverty is not a Vice. Charity, Society, and the State in Imperial Russia* (Princeton: Princeton University Press, 1996)

——, "A Russian Experiment in Voluntarism. The Municipal Guardianships of the Poor, 1894–1914", *JfGO*, vol. 30, no. 3 (1982), pp. 429–451

Longmate, Norman, *King Cholera: The Biography of a Disease* (London: H. Hamilton, 1966)

Luckin, Bill, "States and Epidemic Threats", *Bulletin of the Society for the Social History of Medicine*, vol. 34 (June, 1984), pp. 25–27

Mann, Thomas, *Der Tod in Venedig* (Frankfurt, 14th ed. 2001)

Manning, Roberta Thompson, *The Crisis of the Old Order in Russia: Gentry and Government.* (Princeton: Princeton University Press, 1990)

Manzoni, Alessandro, *The Betrothed* (London: Penguin, 1972)

Markel, Howard, *Quarantine! East European Jewish Immigrants and the New York City Epidemics of 1892* (Baltimore, MD, 1997)

——, " 'Knocking out the Cholera': Cholera, Class, and Quarantine in New York City, 1892", *Bulletin of the History of Medicine*, vol. 69 (1995), pp. 420–457

Marquez, Gabriel Garcia, *Love in the Time of Cholera*, trans. Edith Grossman (London, 1989)

Matiko, Ogawa, "Uneasy Bedfellows: Science and Politics in the Refutation of Koch's Bacterial Theory of Cholera", *Bulletin of the History of Medicine*, vol. 74 (2000), pp. 761–707

McGrew, Roderick E., *Russia and the Cholera, 1823–1832* (Madison: University of Wisconsin Press, 1965)

——, "The First Cholera Epidemic and Social History", *Bulletin of the History of Medicine*, vol. 24 (1960), pp. 61–73

McNeill, William H., *Plagues and Peoples* (Oxford: Blackwell, 1977)

McReynolds, Louise, *The News under Russia's Old Regime: The Development of a Mass-Circulation Press* (Princeton: Princeton University Press, 1991)

——, "Urbanism as a Way of Russian Life", *Journal of Urban History*, vol. 20, no. 2 (February 1994), pp. 240–251

Merridale, Catherine, *Night of Stones. Death and Memory in Russia* (London: Granta Books, 2000)

Mespoulait, Martine, "Statisticiens des *Zemstva*. Formation d'une nouvelle profession intellectuelle en Russie dans la période prérévolutionnaire (1880–1817). Le cas de Saratov", *Cahiers du Monde Russe*, vol. 40, no. 4 (Oct. – Dec. 1999), pp. 573–623

Metchnikoff, Olga, *Life of Elie Metchnikoff 1845–1916* (London: Constable and Company, 1921)

Michaels, Paula, *Curative Powers: Medicine and Empire in Stalin's Central Asia* (London: Eurospan, 2003)

Mironov, B.N., "Buereaucratic- or Self-Government: The Early Nineteenth Century Russian City", *Slavic Review*, vol. 52, no. 2 (1993), pp. 233–255

———, *Russkii Gorod v 1740–1860 gody: demograficheskoe, sotsial'noe i ekonomicheskoe razvitie* (Leningrad: Nauka, 1990)

———, *Sotsial'naia istoriia Rossii perioda imperii*, 2 vols (St Petersburg: Bulanin, 1999)

Mitchell, B.R., *European Historical Statistics 1750–1970* (London: Macmillan, 1975)

Mixter, Timothy, "Of Grandfather-Beaters and Fat-Heeled Pacifists: Perceptions of Agricultural Labor and Hiring Market Disturbances in Saratov, 1872–1905", *Russian History*, vol. 7, no. 1–2 (1980), pp. 139–168

———, "The Hiring Market as Workers' Turf: Migrant Agricultural Laborers and the Mobilization of Collective Action in the Steppe Grainbelt of European Russia, 1853–1913", Esther Kingston Mann and Timothy Mixter (eds), *Peasant Economy, Culture, and the Politics of European Russia, 1800–1921* (Princeton: Princeton University Press, 1991), pp. 294–340

Moon, David, *The Abolition of Serfdom in Russia, 1762–1907* (Harlow: Longman, 2001)

———, "Peasant Migration, the Abolition of Serfdom and the Internal Passport System in the Russian Empire, c. 1800–1914", Eltis, D. (ed.), *Free and Coerced Migration: Global Perspectives* (Stanford, CA: Stanford University Press, 2002)

Morris, R.J., *Cholera, 1832: The Social Response to an Epidemic* (London: Croom Helm, 1976)

Morrissey, Susan K., *Suicide and the Body Politic in Imperial Russia* (Cambridge: Cambridge University Press, 2006)

———, "Suicide and Civilization in Late Imperial Russia", *JfGO*, vol. 43 (1995), pp. 201–217

Nardova, V.A., *Gorodskoe samoupravlenii v Rossii v 60-kh-nachale 90-kh godov XIX v.* (Leningrad: Nauka, 1984)

———, *Samoderzhavie i gorodskie dumy v Rossii v kontse XXIX-nachale XX veka* (St Petersburg: Nauka, 1994)

Netchkina, M.V.; Sivkov, K.V.; Sidorov, A.L., "La Russie", in Louis Chevalier (ed.), *Le choléra. La première épidémie du XIXe siècle* (La Roche-sur-Yon 1958), pp. 143–155

Neuberger, Joan, *Hooliganism: Crime, Culture, and Power in St. Petersburg, 1900–1914* (Berkeley: University of California Press, 1993)

Olzscha, Reiner, "Die Epidemiologie und Epidemiographie der Cholera in Russland. Ein Beitrag zur Geomedizin", *Zeitschrift für Hygiene und Infektionskrankheiten*, vol. 121, no. 1 (Berlin, 1939), pp. 1–26

Panzac, Daniel, *Quarantaines et Lazarets. L'Europe et la Peste d'Orient (xvii-xx siècles)* (Edisud, 1987)

Parokha, I.V. (ed.), *Ocherki istorii Saratovskogo povolzh'ia* (Saratov: Izdatel'stvo Saratovskogo Universiteta, 1999)

Patterson, David K., "Cholera Diffusion in Russia, 1823–1923", *Social Science and Medicine*, vol. 38, no. 9 (1994), pp. 1171–1191

Pearson, Thomas F., *Russian Officialdom in Crisis: Autocracy and Local Self-Government, 1861–1900* (Cambridge: Cambridge University Press, 1981)

Pelling, Margaret, *Cholera, Fever and English Medicine, 1825–1865* (Oxford: Oxford University Press, 1978)

Petrov, B.D, *Ocherki istorii otechestvennoi meditsiny* (Moscow,1962)

Pettenkofer, Max von, *Untersuchung und Beobachtung über Verbreitung der Cholera, nebst Betrachtungen über Massregeln derselben Einhalt zu thun* (Munich, 1855)

Phoofuto, Pule, "Epidemics and Revolutions: The Rinderpest Epidemic in Late Nineteenth Century Southern Africa", *Past and Present*, no. 138 (February 1993), pp. 112–143

Pollitzer, R., *Cholera* (Geneva, 1959)

Prshad, Bijay, "Native Dirt/Imperial Ordure. The cholera of 1832 and the morbid resolutions of modernity", *Journal of Historical Sociology*, vol. 7 (1994), pp. 243–260

Raeff, Marc, *Understanding Imperial Russia: State and Society in the Old Regime* (New York: Columbia University Press, 1984)

——, *The Well-Ordered Police State: Social and Institutional Change Through Law in the Germanies and Russia, 1600–1800* (New Haven: Yale University Press, 1983)

Raleigh, Donald J., *Experiencing Russia's Civil War: Politics, Society and Revolutionary Culture in Saratov, 1917–1922* (Princeton: Princeton University Press, 2002)

——, (ed.), *A Russian Civil War Diary. Alexis Babine in Saratov, 1917–1922* (Durham and London: Duke University Press, 1988)

——, "Co-optation *Amid* Repression. The Revolutionary Communists in Saratov Province 1918–1920", *Cahiers du Monde Russe*, vol. 40, no. 4 (1999), pp. 625–656

——, "A Provincial Kronstadt. Popular Unrest in Saratov at the End of the Civil War", idem (ed.), *Provincial Landscapes. Local Dimensions of Soviet Power, 1917–1953* (Pittsburgh: University of Pittsburgh Press, 2001)

——, "Revolutionary Politics in Provincial Russia: The Tsaritsyn 'Republic' in 1917", *Slavic Review*, vol. 40, no. 2 (summer 1981), pp. 194–209

Ramer, Samuel C., "Who was the Russian Feldsher?" *Bulletin of the History of Medicine*, vol. 50 (1976), pp. 213–225

——, "Professionalism and Politics: The Russian Feldsher Movement", Harley D. Balzer (ed.), *Russia's Missing Middle Class* (New York: M.E. Sharpe, 1996), pp. 117–142

Ransel, David L., *Mothers of Misery: Child Abandonment in Russia.* (Princeton: Princeton University Press, 1988)

Rashin, A.G., *Naselenie Rossii za 100 let, 1811–1913* (Moscow, 1956)

Reid, Donald, *Paris Sewers and Sewermen. Realities and Representations* (Cambridge, MA and London: Harvard University Press, 1991)

Rieber, Alexander J., *Merchants and Entrepreneurs in Imperial Russia* (Chapel Hill: University of North Carolina Press, 1982)

Robbins, Richard G., *Famine in Russia, 1891–1892. The Imperial Government Responds to a Crisis* (New York: Columbia University Press, 1975)

——, *The Tsar's Viceroys: Russian Provincial Governors in the Last Years of the Empire* (Ithaca, NY: Cornell University Press, 1987)

Rogger, H. *Russia in the Age of Modernisation and Revolution 1881–1917* (London, New York: Longman, 1983)

Rosenberg, Charles, *The Cholera Years: The United States in 1832, 1849 and 1866* (Chicago: University of Chicago Press, 1962)

——, "Cholera in Nineteenth-Century Europe: A Tool for Social and Economic Analysis", *Comparative Studies in Society and History*, vol. 8 (1965–66), pp. 452–483

Rozman, Gilbert, *Urban Networks in Russia, 1750–1800 and Premodern Periodization* (Princeton: Princeton University Press, 1976)

Rudé George, *The Crowd in History: A Study of Popular Disturbances in France and England, 1730–1848*, 2nd ed. (London: Lawrence and Wishart, 1981)

——, *The Crowd in the French Revolution* (Oxford: Clarendon Press, 1959)

Sanders, Jonathan, "Lessons from the Periphery: Saratov, January 1905", *Slavic Review*, vol. 46, no. 2 (1987), pp. 229–244

Saunders, David, "A Pyrrhic Victory: The Russian Empire in 1848", Evans, R.J.W., Strandmann, Hartmut Pogge von (eds), *The Revolutions in Europe 1848–1849* (Oxford: Oxford University Press, 2000), pp. 135–154

Schaeffer Conroy, Mary, *In Health and in Sickness. Pharmacy, Pharmacists, and the Pharmaceutical Industry in Late Imperial, Early Soviet Russia* (New York: Columbia University Press, 1994)

Schaeffer Conroy, Mary, "Malaria in Late Tsarist Russia", *Bulletin for the History of Medicine*, vol. 56, no. 1 (1982), pp. 41–55

Schlögel, Karl, *Jenseits des Großen Oktober. Das Laboratorium der Moderne. Petersburg 1909–1921* (Berlin: Siedler Verlag, 1988)

Semenov, V.N., Semenov, N.N., *Saratov Kupecheskii* (Saratov, 1995)

——, *V Starinu Saratovskuiu* (Saratov, 1994)

Slack, Paul, *The Impact of Plague in Tudor and Stuart England* (London: Clarendon Press, 1985)

Snowden, Frank, *Naples in the Time of Cholera, 1884–1911* (Cambridge: Cambridge University Press, 1995)

——, "Cholera in Barletta 1910", *Past and Present*, vol. 132 (August 1991), pp. 67–103

Sparr, Frank, *Die Ausbreitung der Cholera in der britischen Flotte im Schwarzen Meer während des Krimkrieges im August 1854. Eine Auswertung von Schiffsjournalen der Royal Navy* (Frankfurt am Main, 1989)

Starr, Frederick S., *Decentralization and Self-Government in Russia, 1830–1870* (Princeton: Princeton University Press, 1972)

Steel, David, "Plague Writing: From Boccaccio to Camus", *Journal of European Studies*, XI (1981), pp. 88–110

Stevenson, Lloyd G., "Science Down the Drain. On the Hostility of Certain Sanitarians to Animal Experimentation, Bacteriology and Immunology", *Bulletin of the History of Medicine*, vol. 39, no. 1 (1955), pp. 1–26

Stolberg, Michael, "Die Cholera im 19. Jahrhundert – zum Umgang mit einer neuen Krankheit", Heinz Schott (ed.), *Medizin, Romantik und Naturforschung. Bonn im Spiegel des 19. Jahrhunderts* (Bonn, 1993), pp. 87–109

——, "Gottesstrafe oder Diätsünde. Zur Mentalitätsgeschichte der Cholera", *Medizin, Gesellschaft und Geschichte. Jahrbuch des Instituts für Geschichte der Medizin der Robert Bosch Stiftung*, vol. 8 (Stuttgart, 1989), pp. 9–25

——, "Public Health and Popular Resistance. Cholera in the Grand Duchy of Tuscany", *Bulletin of the History of Medicine*, vol. 68 (1994), pp. 254–277

Stolypin Bock, Maria, "Stolypin in Saratov", *Russian Review*, vol. 12, no. 3 (July 1953), pp. 187–193

Suny, Ronald Grigor, "Violence and Class Consciousness in the Russian Working Class", *Slavic Review* 41 (fall 1982), pp. 436–442

Szreter, S., Mooney, G., "Urbanisation, mortality and the standard of living debate: new estimates of the expectation of life at birth in nineteenth-century cities", *Ec.HR*, 2nd series, 51 (1998), pp. 84–112

Taylor, Kim, *Chinese Medicine in Early Communist China, 1945–1963. A Medicine of Revolution* (London, New York: Routledge Curzon, 2005)

Thurston, Robert W., *Liberal City, Conservative State: Moscow and Russia's Urban Crisis, 1906–1914* (New York, Oxford: Oxford University Press, 1987)

Wade, Rex A., Seregny, Scott J. (eds), *Politics and Society in Provincial Russia: Saratov, 1590–1917* (Ohio: Ohio State University Press, 1989)

Walkowitz, Judith, *Cities of Dreadful Delight. Narratives of Sexual Danger in Late-Victorian London* (Chicago: University of Chicago Press, 1992)

Weinberg, Robert, *The Revolution of 1905 in Odessa: Blood on the Steps* (Bloomington: Indiana University Press, 1993)

Weindling, Paul Julian, *Epidemics and Genocide in Eastern Europe 1890–1945* (Oxford, 2000)

Weissmann, Neil, *Reform in Tsarist Russia. The State Bureaucracy and Local Government, 1900–1914* (New Brunswick: Rutgers University Press, 1981)

Westwood, James N., *A History of Russian Railways* (London: George Allen & Unwin, 1964)

Wheatcroft, Steven G., "Famine and Epidemic Crises in Russia, 1918–1922: The Case of Saratov", *Annales de démographie historique*, 1983, pp. 329–352

Wohl, Anthony S., *Endangered Lives. Public Health in Victorian Britain* (London: Methuen, 1983)

——, *The Eternal Slum. Housing and Social Policy in Victorian London* (London: Edward Arnold, 1977)

Yaney, George L., *The Systematization of Russian Government: Social Evolution in Domestic Administration of Imperial Russia, 1711–1905* (Urbana: University of Illinois Press, 1973)

Zabludovskii, P.E. *Istoriia otechestvennoi meditsiny* (Moscow, 1960)

Zaionchkovskii, P.A., *Rossiiskoe samoderzhavie v kontse XIX stoletiia* (Moscow, 1970)

Zakharova, L.G., Ben Eklov, and J. Bushnell (eds.), *Velikie reformy v Rossii, 1856–1874* (Moscow: Izdatel'stvo Moskovskogo Universiteta, 1992)

Zelnik, Reginald E., "The Peasant and the Factory", Vucinich, Wayne S. (ed.), *The Peasant in Nineteenth Century Russia* (Stanford: Stanford University Press, 1968)

Zelnik, Reginald E., (ed. and trans.), *A Radical Worker in Tsarist Russia: The Autobiography of Semen Ivanovich Kanatchikov* (Stanford, Calif.: Stanford University Press, 1986)

——, *Law and Disorder on the Narova River: The Kreenholm Strike of 1872* (Berkeley, London: University of California Press, 1995)

——, *Labor and Society in Tsarist Russia: The Factory Workers of St. Petersburg, 1855–1870* (Stanford, Calif: Stanford University Press, 1971)

Index

apothecaries: raise prices on disinfection means 74; pillaged in Saratov in 1892 88

Anti-Plague Commission: set up in 1899 127; composition and function 135; lacking medical expertise 135; criticised by local authorities 136; charged with anti-cholera combat in 1903 127, 134; directs policy along Persian–Russian border in 1904 128; regulates quarantine on waterways 129

Astrakhan': 22, 25, 27, 29, 40, 57, 59, 60, 61, 67, 70, 78, 81, 131, 144; cholera's classic entry to Europe 11, 12; and cholera in 1823 12; and cholera in 1830 14, 17, 18; establishes military regime (1892) 62–3; unprepared for cholera (1892) 62–3; anti-cholera campaign (1892) 62–3; riots (1892) 63, 80; governor encourages flight (1892) 82; and cholera in 1907 1910; and cholera in 1910 123, 125

bacteriology (*see also* diagnosis) rejected by majority of Russian physicians in 1890s 71–2, 114–15; advocated in St Petersburg 115; triumphs in Russia 119; explains cholera

Baku 12, 19, 27, 29, 39, 40, 44, 57, 59, 60, 61, 70, 126; and cholera in 1830 17; unprepared for cholera (1892) 61–2; in state of sanitary neglect 61; ravaged by cholera in 1892 61–2; and cholera in 1904 125

Balashov 143

Baltic Sea 29

banks (at Volga River): closure of shops 73, 83, 84; cholera spreads from (1892) 77; temporary cholera accomodation at 74; as Saratov's sewer 34–5, 37; spread

diseases 35; centre of cholera infection (1892) 77

barracks, cholera 25; construction of (1892); built up in Saratov 73

Black Sea 29

Botkin, Sergei chair of bacteriology at Military-Medical Academy 54; studied with Robert Koch 54

Botkin, Sergei head of Botkin Commission 32

Briggs, Asa 2–3, 7, 52,76, 80, 97

Britain: cholera in 1831 16, 20, 58

Bulletin of Finances, Industry, and Commerce (Vestnik finansov, promyshlennosti i torgovli) 29

Caucasus 29, 38, 40, 57, 61, 126; major epicentre in 1830 17; invaded by cholera in 1846 19; particularly vulnerable to epidemics 49; course of cholera in 1892 62; epicentre in 1910 126

caravans: carry cholera from Central Asia to Russia 13

Caspian Sea 23, 29, 38, 81; and cholera in 1830 14; and maritime quarantine (1892) 55, 57–61; and cholera in 1904 124, 125

Catherine II: influenced by German cameralism 45; medical reform 45

Central Cholera Council for the Russian Empire established in 1823 12; re-established in 1830 in Saratov 27

Central Medical Council 13

charity: provides medical services 107; activities in 1892 epidemic 107, 109; flourishes after 1892 109; as moral reform and social control 109–10; and social inequality 111

Chernigov: province 17, 18, 19, 20, 62; city 27